# PERSONALIZED NUTRITION

## Principles and Applications

Edited by
Frans Kok
Laura Bouwman
Frank Desiere

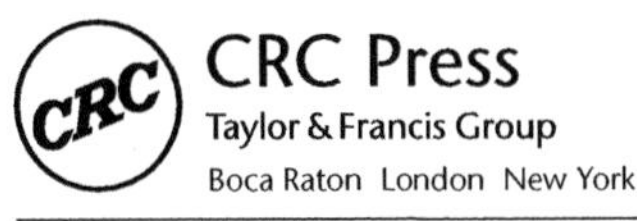


CRC Press is an imprint of the
Taylor & Francis Group, an **informa** business

CRC Press
Taylor & Francis Group
6000 Broken Sound Parkway NW, Suite 300
Boca Raton, FL 33487-2742

First issued in paperback 2019



ISBN-13: 978-0-8493-9281-8 (hbk)
ISBN-13: 978-0-367-38871-3 (pbk)



**Library of Congress Cataloging-in-Publication Data**

Personalized nutrition : principles and applications / editors, Frans Kok, Laura Bouwman, and Frank Desiere.
p. cm.
Includes bibliographical references and index.
ISBN 978-0-8493-9281-8 (alk. paper)
1. Nutrition--Genetic aspects. 2. Genomics. I. Kok, Frans. II. Bouwman, Laura, 1971- III. Desiere, Frank. IV. Title.

QP144.G45P47 2007
612.3--dc22 2007012503

**Visit the Taylor & Francis Web site at**
**http://www.taylorandfrancis.com**

**and the CRC Press Web site at**
**http://www.crcpress.com**

# Table of Contents

# Foreword

## PERSONALIZED NUTRITION: HISTORY AND PROMISES?

Personalized nutrition is an emerging but controversial new discipline among nutrition scientists. Due to its possible genetic component, it has become an attractive topic for the media. So far, the "science fiction" stories of a lady doing food shopping, guided by a PDA containing her genome information are not taken very seriously. Of course, in the developed world, personalized food choice is taken for granted. Did you realize that while ordering Italian three-taste gelato, you can choose from over a million combinations and variations, if you consider tastes, sizes, toppings, and packaging? The same is true for coffee or take-away pizzas.

In the context of this book, personalized nutrition is related to a differentiated health effect, with the key questions targeted at the possible scientific basis for this phenomenon. In order to put this in the right perspective, let us have a look at the historical development of the diet and health relationship. Until the early twentieth century, nutritional sciences dealt with hygiene and processing. This was followed by the incorporation of biochemistry and (molecular) physiology: the vitamins were described, energy metabolism was understood, etc. During the second half of the twentieth century, knowledge of cellular and molecular biological processes allowed for further optimizing of our diet toward a balanced macro- and micronutrient composition. This contributed to a prolongation of life span and produced a commercial wave of supplements.

Gradually, nutrition scientists indicated the involvement of diet in a large number of diseases and disorders (e.g., colon cancer, cardiovascular disorders, type 2 diabetes mellitus, a number of inflammation-related health problems, and many more. During the 1990s, this development triggered the introduction of functional foods, dietary components with "added health value." So far, these functional foods, apart from the aforementioned supplements (vitamins, cofactors, minerals, and so forth, which I do not consider to be real functional foods), have resulted in only a limited number of successful products (cholesterol-lowering stanols, probiotics, a number of specific fatty acids). Except for the cholesterol-lowering products, where an established biomarker (the relationship between CVD and HDL/LDL cholesterol) was established by the biomedical research community, it was very difficult to obtain scientific proof of efficacy for most other functional foods. In many cases, the advertisement and PR efforts by far outreached the scientific efforts accompanying the market introduction.

Why does nutrition science have such a hard job in providing evidence for health claims related to a dietary component? In pharmacological and biomedical research, bioactive compounds are developed to treat a well-characterized disease. In contrast, nutrition deals with prevention of disease and optimizing health. Here, biomarkers quantifying the health status are essentially missing, and much of the nutrition research (the large observational and intervention cohorts) rely on disease endpoints instead of health endpoints. Also in the "gold standard" of diet and health research, the (cross-over) dietary intervention trial, the quantification of the effect is a major issue. Usually, the observed effects are small, and great efforts have to be made to unravel the intervention effect from potential confounding variables. In other words, the confounding parameters have a larger impact than the intervention effects. The recent omics-related observations in human intervention studies, using very accurate biomarkers, confirm that intraindividual variation is much smaller than interindividual variation. Differences between study subjects may be much larger than differences affected by the dietary treatment.

The keys for personalized nutrition actually are these "confounders" that make the life of nutrition scientists so difficult. Age, gender, lifestyle (e.g., exercise), phenotype (e.g., body mass index), genetic makeup, and epi-genomic imprinting — all possibly determine our nutritional needs, the way we respond to nutrition, and thus our "personal diet-and-health relationship." Infant nutrition clearly differs from a sports diet. Now, a triad of questions arise:

1. To what extent is this personal diet-and-health relationship practically valid?
2. How can nutrition science demonstrate this?
3. What is the proposition of stakeholders in society, including the consumer?

This book at least attempts to answer these questions. My personal opinion is that indeed this relationship exists to a much greater extent than assumed until now, and that nutrition science will need to do a much better job in accurately identifying and quantifying the subtle differences in health status related to dietary treatment. A complete merger of nutrition with a number of fundamental scientific disciplines (molecular biology, biochemistry, bioinformatics, statistics, etc.) will be essential to reach the goal.

Now, what about this specific and overemphasized part of personalized nutrition, the impact of genetic differences? Of course, we know the examples of cholesterol and folate, where genetic predisposition partly determines plasma concentration and related health effects. In the case of cholesterol, a phenotypic assessment of LDL and HDL provides a solid phenotypic biomarker, which makes genetic testing (at least partly) unnecessary. In fact, this phenotypic readout is the gross result of at least 20 genetic different makeups. The HDL/LDL relationship partly determines biomedical intervention and the consumer's food choice. In the case of folate, the occurrence of a genetic polymorphism in one of the enzymes involved in folate biotransformation results in a relatively low plasma folate concentration. In extreme cases, this leads to embryonic deformation (spina bifida) due to impaired DNA synthesis. Folate is essential for DNA synthesis as it provides the methyl group for nucleotide synthesis. Folate is cheap, and some countries have turned to folate supplementation to the general population (e.g., by fortification of bread). In other words, a genetically based differential dietary advice is overruled by mass treatment.

Possible negative consequences in persons efficiently dealing with folate (high folate levels have been shown to overmethylate DNA and are thus potentially mutagenic and carcinogenic) were considered nonrelevant. Time will tell whether a personalized approach would be better.

A number of disorders related to nutrition are packed with genetic variation, but the effect of nutritional modulation of the phenotypic outcome of these variations is difficult to assess as yet. Nutrition is the worst-case scenario for this approach in science as multiple minor genetic differences can occur, possibly modulated by multiple food bioactives, usually with low receptor affinity, and resulting in multiple minor changes in gene expression and resulting phenotypic expression.

Eventually, nutrition science may very likely determine a large number of personalized nutrition and health relationships. However, this is only a small part of the equation. Food consumption nowadays is only partially driven by health concerns. It is still much more driven by convenience and price. "Food is pleasure" rightfully is a universally held credo, and science will have a hard job in promoting healthy diet if this aspect is compromised. Therefore, a personalized diet needs to be both optimized toward personal health and also for personal convenience, pleasure, and affordability. What a challenge!

**Ben van Ommen**
*Senior Research Fellow, Nutritional Systems Biology*
*Director, European Nutrigenomics Organisation (NuGO)/TNO Quality of Life*
*Zeist, The Netherlands*

# Preface

The primary role of diet is to provide an individual with optimal levels of nutrients to meet metabolic requirements, and to give the consumer a feeling of satisfaction and well being through the pleasure of eating. In addition, particular diets, foods and food components can provide additional physiological, cognitive and psychological benefits, and result in biological activities beyond their widely accepted nutritional effects. Moreover, diet not only helps to achieve and maintain optimal health and development but can also play an important role in reducing the risk of specific diseases and disorders.

However, a diet that serves the health of one individual does not necessarily work for all individuals due to differences in (genetic) predisposition, and environmental and lifestyle factors. Hence, diagnostic tools that reflect both the overall health status and (genetic) predisposition of a particular person at a given time need to be developed. The knowledge obtained thereby will facilitate appropriate nutritional advice to individuals according to their immediate and long-term health needs and, ultimately, we can foresee the time when nutritional products will be tailored for individual consumers.

The success of the introduction of personalized nutrition in society depends on many factors. The scientific background for this must be established, the regulatory system must be in place, ethical issues need to be addressed, services and products with clear health benefits must be available, and the accompanying communication must be clear.

This textbook has the aim of defining the area of personalized nutrition both from a biomedical and social science perspective. A selected group of leading scientists in the field will comprehensively address the molecular, physiological, epidemiologic, and public health aspects of personalized nutrition, highlighted with examples from major diseases. Another group of well-known social scientists will discuss the behavioral, ethical, and consumer perspectives that will influence a legitimate successful introduction of personalized nutrition.

We expect our book will be useful for the education of students in several disciplines, for example, nutrition, behavioral and communication science. Moreover, stakeholders involved in personalized nutrition in government, health care, and business may use the book as a reference guide.

Our book is divided in three sections: (1) Scientific Principles of Personalized Nutrition, (2) Personalized Nutrition: Consumer and Society, and (3) Future Perspectives on Personalized Nutrition.

In the first section, Scientific Principles of Personalized Nutrition, the state of the art of nutrigenomics technologies, including transcriptomics, proteomics, and metabolomics, are discussed. Subsequently, the use of genomics technology for a better understanding of the molecular mechanisms involved in major diet-related chronic disorders — i.e., chronic inflammation, cardiovascular disease, type 2 diabetes, cancer, and obesity — is addressed.

Next, the consequences of metabolic programming during pregnancy and the potential of new molecular biomarkers, as well as the gatekeeper role of taste in personalized nutrition, are covered. In the last chapter in this section, the epidemiologic aspects of genomic testing and the health benefits for the individual vs. the population are described.

Besides providing the most recent knowledge, all authors discuss opportunities and pitfalls of nutrigenomics in the development of personalized nutrition.

The second section, Personalized Nutrition: Consumer and Society, starts with a stakeholder analysis in which five interest groups (scientists, food companies, consumers, competitive athletes, and health-care providers) are compared regarding their practices and opinions of personalized nutrition. Based on behavioral change strategies, the next chapter is focusing on whether and how personalized nutrition will contribute to a healthier dietary pattern.

Two chapters specifically target the consumer perspective. The first reviews the marketing potential of personalized nutrition; in the second, consumer attitudes are discussed. The section is completed with a contribution on ethical issues related to personalized advice on diet and health and the customization of food products.

In the final section, Future Perspectives on Personalized Nutrition, the challenges of nutrigenomics research and its applications are presented in two chapters. One chapter focuses on the need to address the humanitarian issues related to developing countries and issues a call for international efforts to develop best practices, fostering international collaborations and sharing data sets. The final chapter provides an outlook of personalized nutrition in the context of ongoing innovations in food technology, nutrigenomics, and food delivery systems.

We sincerely hope that you enjoy reading this guide to a scientific underpinning of personalized nutrition.

**Frans J. Kok**
**Laura Bouwman**
**Frank Desiere**

# The Editors

**Frans J. Kok PhD**, is full professor of nutrition and health and head of the Division of Human Nutrition at Wageningen University, The Netherlands. Moreover, as dean of Wageningen Graduate Schools, he is responsible for securing the quality of academic research and training at the university.

Dr. Kok was trained in human nutrition at Wageningen University and in epidemiology at Harvard University, Cambridge, Massachusetts. His scientific expertise covers topics such as energy balance and body composition, diet in disease prevention, and sensory science. He has authored more than 250 original scientific publications and is a member of the Dutch Health Council and the Academic Board of Wageningen University. As a faculty member, he has lectured in many courses on nutrition and health, including the European Nutrition Leadership Program, as well as in courses in the U.S., Africa, and Asia.

**Laura Bouwman** is a PhD researcher in the department of communication science at Wageningen University. Her research is focused on whether and how innovations in personalized nutrition can be used for the development of more effective nutrition interventions. Two topics are central: 1) how stakeholders in science, healthcare, health education, government, and industry perceive their roles and responsibilities in the innovation process, and 2) the representation of personal factors in food choice, with emphasis on the representation of genetic background. Laura is involved in the development of communication activities for diverse stakeholder-groups regarding personalized nutrition in the European Nutrigenomics Organisation. Before her current PhD research, Laura worked for six years at a communication bureau for the oils and fats industry.

**Frank Desiere, PhD, MBA,** started his scientific career in the earlier days of biotechnology doing research in fermentation technology, microbiology, and biological conversion of xenobiotics, and later joined the Nestlé Research Center in Lausanne, Switzerland, to work on the ecology and evolution of bacteriophages in milk fermentation. Later, he initiated a bioinformatics effort at Nestlé and worked on microbial genomics, transcriptomics, and proteomics. Dr. Desiere also initiated Peptideatlas (www.peptideatlas.org) for the integration of proteomics data with human and other genomes. He was then responsible for a project involving personalized nutrition at Nestlé that initiated consumer and patient applications of personalized nutrition concepts in the marketplace. As a result of this initiative, his interests evolved into the commercial application of scientific concepts in science and nutrition, management of innovation and new business ideas. After having completed an MBA at IMD Lausanne, Dr. Desiere now works as business development manager at Roche Diagnostics in Basel, Switzerland. His scientific activities have resulted in more than 30 peer-reviewed publications and numerous presentations at international scientific conferences.

# Contributors

**Lydia A. Afman**
Nutrition, Metabolism, and Genomics
Division of Human Nutrition
Wageningen University
Wageningen
The Netherlands

**Elizabeth Baily**
International Food Information Council
Washington, D.C.

**Laura I. Bouwman**
Wageningen University
Sub-Department of Communication
Science, Communication
Management Group
Wageningen
The Netherlands

**Lorraine Brennan**
UCD School of Biomolecular
and Biomedical Science
UCD Conway Institute
University College
Dublin
Ireland

**Josh Conway**
Cogent Research, LLC
Cambridge, Massachusetts

**Dolores Corella**
Department of Preventive Medicine
University of Valencia
Genetic and Molecular Epidemiology
Unit
Valencia
Spain

**Hannelore Daniel**
Molecular Nutrition Unit
Center of Life and Food Sciences
Technical University of Munich
Freising-Weihenstephan
Germany

**Aldona Dembinska-Kieć**
Department of Clinical Biochemistry
Jagiellonian University
Medical College
Krakow
Poland

**Lynnette R. Ferguson**
Discipline of Nutrition
University of Auckland
Grafton, Auckland
New Zealand

**Edith J.M. Feskens**
Division of Human Nutrition
Wageningen University
Wageningen
The Netherlands

**J. Bruce German**
University of California–Davis
Davis, California

**Michael J. Gibney**
UCD Agriculture and Food Science
Centre
University College
Dublin
Ireland

**Gerrit J. Hiddink**
Wageningen University
Sub-Department of Communication Science, Communication Management Group
Wageningen
The Netherlands

**Hans-Georg Joost**
German Institute of Human Nutrition Potsdam-Rehbruecke
Nuthetal
Germany

**Ellen Kampman**
Division of Human Nutrition
Wageningen University
Wageningen
The Netherlands

**Wendy Reinhardt Kapsak**
International Food Information Council
Washington, D.C.

**Jim Kaput**
Laboratory of Nutrigenomic Medicine
Department of Surgery
University of Illinois Chicago
Chicago, Illinois

**Maria A. Koelen**
Wageningen University
Sub-Department of Communication Science, Communication and Innovation Group
Wageningen
The Netherlands

**Michiel Korthals**
Applied Philosophy
Social Sciences
Wageningen University
Wageningen
The Netherlands

**Simon C. Langley-Evans**
University of Nottingham
School of Biosciences
Sutton Bonington, Loughborough
United Kingdom

**John C. Mathers**
Human Nutrition Research Centre, School of Clinical Medical Sciences
University of Newcastle
Newcastle-on-Tyne
United Kingdom

**Michael Müller**
Nutrition, Metabolism, and Genomics Division of Human Nutrition
Wageningen University
Wageningen
The Netherlands

**Jose M. Ordovas**
Nutrition and Genomics Laboratory
Jean Meyer USDA Human Nutrition Research Center on Aging
Tufts University
Boston, Massachusetts

**Martin Philpott**
Discipline of Nutrition
University of Auckland
Grafton, Auckland
New Zealand

**Danielle R. Reed**
Monell Chemical Senses Center
Philadelphia, Pennsylvania

**Manuela Rist**
Molecular Nutrition Unit
Technical University of Munich
Freising-Weihenstephan
Germany

**Amber Ronteltap**
Marketing and Consumer Behavior Group
Wageningen University
Wageningen
The Netherlands

**David B. Schmidt**
International Food Information Council
Washington, D.C.

**Toshiko Tanaka**
Nutrition and Genomics Laboratory
Jean Mayer USDA Human Nutrition Research Center on Aging
Tufts University
Boston, Massachusetts

**Hans C.M. van Trijp**
Marketing and Consumer Behavior Group
Wageningen University
Wageningen
The Netherlands

**Pieter van't Veer**
Division of Human Nutrition
Wageningen University
Wageningen
The Netherlands

**Marianne Walsh**
UCD Agriculture and Food Science Centre
University College
Dublin
Ireland

**Heribert J. Watzke**
Nestlé Research Centre
Lausanne
Switzerland

**Christy White**
Cogent Research, LLC
Cambridge, Massachusetts

**J. T. Winkler**
London Metropolitan University
London
United Kingdom

# *Section I*

## *Scientific Principles of Personalized Nutrition*

# 1 Nutrigenomics and Transcriptomics: Applications of Microarray Analyses in Nutrition Research

*Lydia A. Afman and Michael Müller*

## CONTENTS



## 1.1 INTRODUCTION

This chapter describes how nutrients can influence gene expression and describes how this knowledge can be applied in nutritional research by utilization of transcriptional profiling. Two research approaches are discussed: a mechanistic approach and a biomarker profiling approach. The mechanistic approach is a commonly applied method in transcriptomics research and has been extremely useful in the identification of the molecular pathways and signaling routes involving nutrients. The biomarker profiling approach is under development but will have significant impact, especially in human research. For both methods, nutrition-specific pitfalls are discussed, in addition to an outline of potential applications of gene expression profiling in humans and animal models, with examples of nutrition-related transcriptomics studies published so far. Furthermore, transcriptional profiling is discussed in relation to its current and future applications in personalized nutrition.

A major drawback in the investigation of molecular mechanism of nutrients in human studies is the accessibility of organ and tissues material in healthy volunteers, hampering the investigation of organ-specific functions of nutrients. In case tissue material is available, factors such as genetic diversity present among even quite isolated populations, in addition to environmental and lifestyle factors, such as physical activity, dietary behavior, and stress, provoke such great variability in nutrient-induced responses that large, expensive study populations are required. Therefore, evidence-based nutritional research generally exploits model systems such as animal models. One of the major advantages of the use of animal models in dietary research is that dietary intake and environmental factors can be precisely controlled. In order to minimize the variability caused by genetic background, genetically identical inbred strains can be used. Moreover, transgenic and knockout models are only available in animal models and are of great benefit in identification of functional effects of nutrients. For example, mice with an overexpression or knockout of genes encoding nutrient-activated transcription factors can be used for functional genomics studies to characterize nutrient-specific induced changes in gene expression and the specific involvement of the particular transcription factor (Kersten, Seydoux et al. 1999). Another advantage of animal models is the possibility of studying molecular mechanisms of nutrients in specific organs or tissues. The enormous amount of data derived from transcriptomics studies can be used to identify nutrient-specific changes in pathways, networks, and signaling routes. Ultimately, this type of study will facilitate the unraveling of the underlying molecular mechanism of a wide variety of nutrients, with the goal of improving dietary advice via evidence-based nutrition. Another advantage of such a large data set is the identification of nutrient-induced changes in organ-specific potentially secreted proteins. These proteins are excreted by the organ in body fluids such as plasma and urine, making them promising biomarker candidates that can easily be verified in human intervention studies and consequently be used as markers for organ-specific function and health.

Another application of transcriptomics, which is not feasible yet, is the identification of predisease biomarkers of nutritional-related chronic diseases such as cardiovascular diseases, type 2 diabetes, and cancer. In order to identify those markers, monitoring of transcriptional changes during the development of diet-induced chronic diseases is required, enabling the identification of early biomarker profiles (Afman and Müller 2006). As the development of chronic diseases require long-term dietary exposure, this approach requires time- and cost-consuming long-term nutritional intervention studies that will not result in identification of early biomarkers in the near future.

## 1.2 NUTRIENTS AND TRANSCRIPTION

### 1.2.1 NUTRIENT-ACTIVATED TRANSCRIPTION FACTORS

It is widely recognized that nutrients (macro- and micronutrients) can have profound effects on gene regulation and gene transcription. These important modulatory effects of dietary components can be monitored on a genomewide scale by using state-of-the-art oligonucleotide microarrays. The exact mechanisms of how nutrients influence gene transcription is not completely known yet; however, knowledge regarding this is emerging (Müller and Kersten 2003; Desvergne, Michalik et al. 2006). Nutrients and their metabolites, such as fatty acids and certain eicosanoids, cholesterol metabolites (bile salts, oxysterols), or vitamin A metabolites (retinoic acid), serve as ligands for certain ligand-activated transcription factors such as PPARs, FXRs, LXRs, or RARs and RXRs, all members of the large superfamily of nuclear receptors (Zhang and Mangelsdorf 2002; Müller and Kersten 2003). During ligand binding, nuclear receptors undergo a conformational change that results in the coordinated dissociation of corepressors and the recruitment of coactivator proteins to enable transcriptional activation. These nutrient-sensing receptors (PPARs, FXRs, LXRS) form heterodimers with RXR and bind to specific nucleotide sequences (response elements) in the promoter regions of a large number of genes. The response elements are specific for the nuclear receptor, and each nutrient will induce a characteristic set of genes, also depending on the recruited coactivators (Figure 1.1). Through these transcription factors, nutrients are able to influence a wide variety of cellular functions.

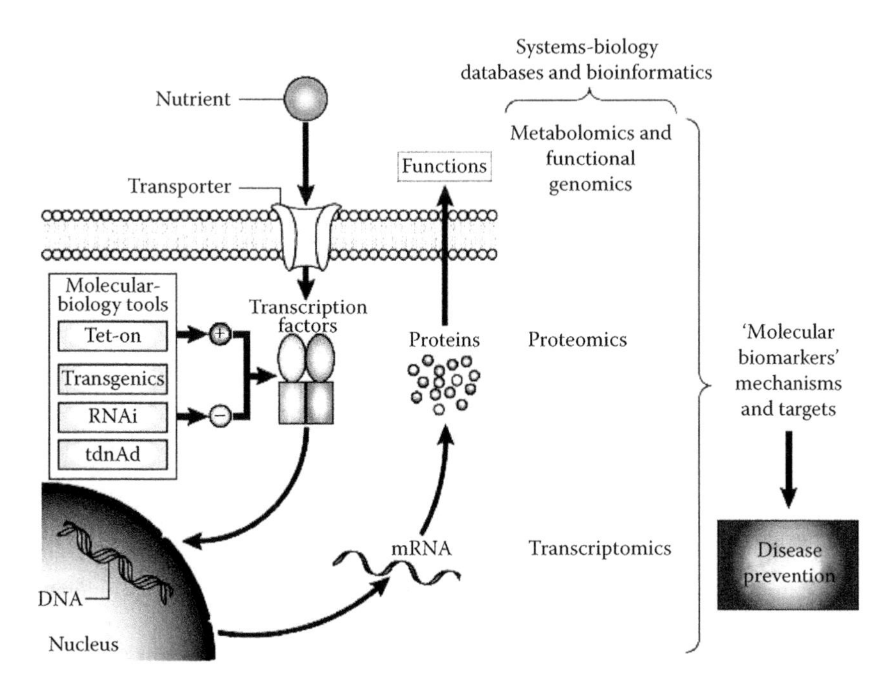


**FIGURE 1.1** The "smart" combination of molecular nutrition and nutrigenomics.

### 1.2.2 Role of the Transcription Factor PPARα

Unsaturated fatty acids, for example, can activate gene transcription by activating the fatty acid sensor PPARα, which is expressed in liver, heart, muscle, and small intestine and other organs. In the liver PPARα controls the transcription of up to 3000 genes involved in numerous metabolic and regulatory processes, including fatty acid oxidation, ketogenesis, gluconeogenesis, amino acid metabolism, cellular proliferation, and the acute-phase response (Kersten, Seydoux et al. 1999). Hepatic PPARα has an important role during fasting, when increased levels of free fatty acids are released from adipose tissue and enter the liver. These fatty acids bind to PPARα and control as a consequence several important processes, including their degradation, TG synthesis, lipid transport, or, on the other hand, gluconeogenesis. In particular, the last process that in part uses glycerol also released from the adipose tissue (Patsouris, Mandard et al. 2004) as a precursor for glucose synthesis is of crucial importance for glucose homeostasis (Kersten, Seydoux et al. 1999).

The role of hepatic PPARα for dietary fats and in obesity is less clear but most likely relevant to our understanding of the obesity-linked pathophysiology of type 2 diabetes (Patsouris, Müller et al. 2004). Visceral obesity is linked to increased free fatty acid levels (Moller and Kaufman 2005), and these molecules may be recognized by the liver as being “in need of glucose” signals, resulting in increased gluconeogenesis, which may contribute to a more pathophysiological phenotype, particularly under conditions of hepatic insulin resistance.

## 1.3 TRANSCRIPTOMICS

### 1.3.1 Technology

Transcriptomics is both a sensitive and well-validated technique, which employs high-density oligonucleotide microarray analysis to study the number of mRNA copies per gene for virtually all actively transcribed genes. This technique enables determination of expression levels of genes of the whole genome, meaning hundreds to thousands of genes at the same time and within one study. As nutrients influence transcription of genes, this technique can be applied to measure diet-induced changes in every tissue of interest. A challenge in nutritional research is the relatively small effect of dietary interventions on physiological parameters. Similarly, the effects of nutrition on gene expression patterns are also rather small and not easy to detect. Consequently, the development of a highly sensitive and validated microarray analysis platform is required along with a robust research hypothesis that is adequately addressed by the experimental design to avoid so-called fishing expeditions.

### 1.3.2 Transcriptomics and Study Design

In order to draw causal relations between nutrients and transcriptional changes, dietary adjustments should be limited when two or more diets are compared within the experiment. In addition, circadian rhythms are prevalent in several organs and tissues and potentially influence biological pathways; therefore, collection of tissue material is of crucial importance in increasing the signal-to-noise ratio

(Ptitsyn, Zvonic et al. 2006; Zvonic, Ptitsyn et al. 2006). Another undesirable factor is pooling of samples, but increasing the number of biological replicates will enhance accuracy by decreasing the false-positive rate and result in reliable data (Kendziorski, Irizarry et al. 2005). Once a transcriptomics study is performed, RNA quality and quantity should be verified and subsequent labeling and hybridization of RNA should preferably be conducted by the same technician to keep variation between arrays low. Preprocessing of data requires specific attention, as the small gene expression changes in dietary studies require a highly reliable algorithm (Irizarry, Warren et al. 2005). The most challenging part of the process occurs after the array data are obtained, when the data have to be analyzed in terms of their biological meaning. Several commercial and noncommercial tools have been developed that assist with the extraction of significantly changed genes and the visualization of changed pathways or related networks (Curtis, Oresic et al. 2005).

## 1.4 APPLICATION OF TRANCRIPTOMICS IN HUMAN STUDIES

### 1.4.1 Requirements for Human Transcriptomics Studies

The execution of a transcriptomics study requires the accurate collection of organ or tissue material for the extraction of RNA, which is a bottleneck in human studies. Biopsies can be obtained from both unhealthy as well as surrounding healthy tissue of patients who have to undergo surgical procedures. The disadvantage of this approach is that the pathological state of diseased tissue is often reflected in the surrounding nondiseased tissue as well. A major drawback in studies with healthy volunteers, which is quite common in nutrition research, is the very limited accessibility of tissues and organ material. The only way to obtain material from healthy volunteers is via biopsies from tissues such as muscle and subcutaneous adipose tissue. Although other metabolically relevant organs such as small intestine and liver are not accessible with this approach, transcriptional profiling of muscle and adipose tissue biopsies are extremely useful as these organs fulfill important physiological functions, have a central role in energy metabolism, and play crucial roles in certain diet-related diseases. A disadvantage of the collection of muscle and adipose tissue biopsies is the invasiveness of this method and the low yield of tissue and, consequently, low RNA quantity. A less invasive alternative is the use of blood cells for transcriptional profiling. These cells travel through the whole body and react on internal threats to body homeostasis, and may therefore serve as functional markers for whole-body health. Moreover, disease-specific gene expression patterns have been identified in blood cells (Martin, Graner et al. 2001; Valk, Verhaak et al. 2004), and although interindividual variety in gene expression is high, the much smaller within-person variation makes them suitable for use in dietary intervention studies (Whitney, Diehn et al. 2003; Radich, Mao et al. 2004; Cobb, Mindrinos et al. 2005). An additional difficulty in human studies is the diverse genetic background, requiring a powerful study design to obtain relevant and consistent data. One of the features of such a design is sampling within a person before and after intervention, with preferably a cross-over design. The invasiveness of tissue biopsy collection makes this method less suitable for application in short or time-course intervention studies. Another characteristic of an appropriate nutrigenomics design is a high number of replicates; the accompanying high costs, however, are often the limiting factor in this respect. A third aspect of a sound study design is the magnification of the signal-to-noise ratio, leading to an increased change on selecting the correct but rather small diet-induced effects. Such an effect could be achieved by magnifying the response through a nutritional challenge of the body.

The number of human studies that describe nutrition-related transcriptome profiling is limited. Most of the papers describe differential gene expression in muscle and adipose tissue biopsies in nutrition-related chronic diseases.

### 1.4.2 Application of Adipose Tissue Transcriptomics

In a transcriptomics study on adipose tissue, gene expression profiles were analyzed of subcutaneous white adipose tissue from obese individuals before and after a very low caloric diet intervention of 28 d (Clement, Viguerie et al. 2004). Microarray analyses were performed before and after 2 and 28 d of caloric restriction. Two days of diet intervention did not result in any considerable changes; 28 d of caloric restriction, however, induced significant gene expression changes that were mostly related to inflammatory processes. Genes related to this process could be classified into upregulation of anti-inflammatory genes and downregulation of proinflammatory genes. Other changed genes were involved in cell–cell and cell–matrix adhesion or in cell proliferation, growth, and differentiation; the latter two were mostly downregulated on caloric restriction. This study also managed to locate the genes to specific adipose tissue fractions; i.e., most genes were expressed in the stromavascular fraction of adipose tissue. Microarray analysis of adipose tissue may explain why caloric restriction delays onset of conditions frequently associated with an increase in basal inflammation, such as type 2 diabetes and cardiovascular disease, or with conditions in which cell proliferation is of pivotal importance, such as cancer.

Another often-used approach is to search for gene expression changes in animal models followed by subsequent confirmation of changes in genes of interest in human volunteers. As an example, microarray analyses of white adipose tissue of diet-induced obese mice revealed changes in several markers of inflammation that were also differently expressed in adipose tissue of obese and lean subjects. (Weisberg, McCann et al. 2003; Xu, Barnes et al. 2003). This transcriptomics study revealed that adipose tissue is not only of importance as a storage source of energy but that it might also play an essential role in the development of inflammatory conditions associated with obesity, such as metabolic syndrome and type 2 diabetes. Further studies are required to elucidate how dietary interventions, besides caloric restriction, can reduce, or preferably prevent, the inflammation in adipose tissue.

### 1.4.3 Application of Muscle Transcriptomics

Microarray profiling studies with human muscle tissue are often associated with insulin resistance and type 2 diabetes. A study on gene expression profiles in muscle tissue demonstrated a reduced expression of genes involved in oxidative phosphorylation and mitochondrial function in diabetic and insulin-resistant subjects

(Mootha, Lindgren et al. 2003; Patti, Butte et al. 2003). Moreover, they showed that these changes have most likely been mediated by the peroxisome proliferator-activated receptor γ coactivator-1 (PGC1), which was found to be downregulated in these subjects as well. Similarly, microarray analyses performed on muscle biopsies before and after 3 d of high-fat feeding showed a downregulation in expression of genes involved in oxidative phosphorylation or mitochondrial function. This high-fat feeding intervention also resulted in the downregulation of PGC1α and PGC1β, similar to the findings in diabetic muscle tissue (Sparks, Xie et al. 2005). To confirm this, a comparable intervention study was performed with C57Bl/6 mice fed a high-fat diet for 3 weeks. The gene expression changes due to high-fat feeding in the mouse study were of a greater magnitude than those observed in the human study, but were all related to a decrease in the expression of genes involved in oxidative phosphorylation and mitochondrial biosynthesis and its master regulator, PGC1. The authors suggest that high-fat diet may explain the reduction in oxidative phosphorylation previously observed in muscle of type 2 diabetes patients and prediabetic individuals (Kelley, He et al. 2002). In conclusion, this is a good example of a nutrigenomics study demonstrating that diet-induced changes in inbred mice that are genetically identical animals are of a greater magnitude than comparable interventions performed in humans with different genotypes.

With the use of transcriptomics techniques, the aforementioned studies were able to identify pathways involved in different stages of the development of type 2 diabetes. In addition, these studies were able to demonstrate that these pathways were changed in the same direction after intervention with a high-fat diet, implying that this pathway can be influenced by diet, which points toward a mechanism in diet-induced type 2 diabetes. The question still remains whether transcriptional analyses of this pathway can be used as a diagnostic tool for the early predisease state and whether and which dietary adjustments can lead to upregulation in oxidative phosphorylation, mitochondrial biosynthesis and PGC1, and ultimately result in the prevention of type 2 diabetes.

### 1.4.4 Application of Blood Cell Transcriptomics

Although transcriptomics studies with muscle and adipose tissue have proved to be of great value in identification of nutrition-related pathways, a major drawback of these tissues is the difficult accessibility in healthy human volunteers. In the last few years, several studies have shown disease-characteristic gene expression patterns, or signatures, in human blood cells (Martin, Graner et al. 2001; Valk, Verhaak et al. 2004). In addition, injection of bacterial endotoxin in healthy human volunteers displayed time-dependent changes in blood cell gene expression (Calvano, Xiao et al. 2005). Although proved to be useful as potential diagnostic tool under these conditions, the question still remains whether blood cells can be used for the identification of nutrition-specific gene expression patterns. So far, nutrigenomics-related studies have not yet employed circulating blood cells. The advantage of blood cell profiling in comparison to tissue biopsies profiling in nutritional studies is the less invasive way of collecting blood, enabling application in time-course experiments or challenge studies.

### 1.4.5 Biomarker Profiling

The ultimate opportunity for blood cell profiling in nutrigenomics research is the identification and subsequent application of gene expression patterns as early biomarkers for a predisease state. Commonly used biomarkers are often indicative of the onset or presence of diseases, and once the disease is diagnosed, drug treatment is unavoidable. The identification of early biomarkers that are indicative for a phenotype of an out-of-balance system would be very valuable in the development of nutritional strategies to regain normal healthy homeostasis. The latter is of specific relevance in the assessment of nutritional effects on disease outcome, as this requires long-term and expensive human intervention studies. The ultimate goal of the characterization of early biomarkers is the identification of subjects in the predisease state with the long-run prevention of disease outcome, achieved by adequate dietary interventions.

In summary, to our knowledge only a few nutrition-related human intervention studies have been carried out, pointing to the infant state of nutrigenomics research, in particular in humans. The aforementioned microarray studies performed in muscle and adipose tissue, especially the ones that applied the smart combinations between animal and human studies, provide the first evidence for the feasibility of nutrigenomics-related research in human intervention studies.

## 1.5 HOW CAN TRANSCRIPTOMICS BE USED IN PERSONALIZED NUTRITION?

Although the term *personalized nutrition* implies tailor-made nutritional advice, currently this is not a reality and may not even be possible in the near future. More promising results, however, can be expected from exploring the influences of specific nutrients on cellular function and their ultimate effects on health and disease. With such information, better knowledge-based dietary advice can be given to specific groups in the population, including elderly people, pregnant women, athletes, children, etc. In addition, this knowledge can lead to the development of subpopulation-specific functional foods. A following step is the identification of biomarkers that are specific for either the healthy or predisease state. One of the characteristics of the predisease state is that the body homeostasis is out of balance. A way to identify an out-of-balance system is by studying the flexibility or resilience of the body, i.e., the capability of the body to cope with challenges. For example, in subjects in the predisease state the impact of a challenge may be higher and the recovery time longer than in healthy individuals. The use of transcriptional profiling during such a challenge will assess the flexibility of the body by determination of both the magnitude of the gene expression changes and the time required for regaining the basal gene expression profile. Similarly, transcriptional profiles from diseased individuals may differ from predisease subjects through a more pronounced or an even completely different profile, in addition to a longer recovery time than predisease people. The response identified with transcriptomics can serve as a phenotype specific for an out-of-balance system representing a predisease state. For a more comprehensive phenotyping, metabolomics and proteomic parameters should be combined with transcriptomics data, preferable before and after a nutritional challenge.

## 1.6 FUTURE PERSPECTIVES FOR PERSONALIZED NUTRITION

The identification of early biomarkers of the predisease state requires time-consuming and expensive long-term nutritional intervention studies that will not result in identification of early biomarkers in the near future. Therefore, results in the near future concerning biomarker profiling will mainly be expected via animal studies, with subsequent translation of these animal biomarkers to the human situation. Promising results are, however, also expected from the previously described challenges studies, in which the flexibility of the human body is tested by measuring the adaptation and recovery of the body after intervening with dietary stressors. The latter has still to be proved useful and demonstrates that the biomarker profiling approach is currently under development. Nevertheless, the identification of early biomarkers will have high future impact, especially in human research.

Although early biomarkers will be essential for the identification of subjects in a predisease state, additional knowledge is required about the underlying molecular mechanisms of nutrients for an adequate nutritional intervention with the ultimate goal of regaining normal homeostasis. Undoubtedly, the combination of evidence-based nutrition and early biomarker-based diagnostics will be mandatory to enable accurate, tailor-made nutritional advice in the future.

## KEY READINGS

Afman, L. and Müller, M. (2006). Nutrigenomics: from molecular nutrition to prevention of disease. *J Am Diet Assoc* 106(4): 569–76.

Desvergne, B., Michalik, L. et al. (2006). Transcriptional regulation of metabolism. *Physiol Rev* 86(2): 465–514.

Müller, M. and Kersten, S. (2003). Nutrigenomics: goals and strategies. *Nat Rev Genet* 4(4): 315–22.

Mutch, D.M., Wahli, W., and Williamson, G. Nutrigenomics and nutrigenetics: the emerging faces of nutrition. *FASEB J* 19(12): 1602–16, October 2005.

## REFERENCES

Afman, L. and Müller, M. (2006). Nutrigenomics: from molecular nutrition to prevention of disease. *J Am Diet Assoc* 106(4): 569–76.

Calvano, S.E., Xiao, W. et al. (2005). A network-based analysis of systemic inflammation in humans. *Nature* 437(7061): 1032–7.

Clement, K., Viguerie, N. et al. (2004). Weight loss regulates inflammation-related genes in white adipose tissue of obese subjects. *FASEB J* 18(14): 1657–69.

Cobb, J.P., Mindrinos, M.N. et al. (2005). Application of genome-wide expression analysis to human health and disease. *Proc Natl Acad Sci USA* 102(13): 4801–6.

Curtis, R.K., Oresic, M. et al. (2005). Pathways to the analysis of microarray data. *Trends Biotechnol* 23(8): 429–35.

Desvergne, B., Michalik, L. et al. (2006). Transcriptional regulation of metabolism. *Physiol Rev* 86(2): 465–514.

Irizarry, R.A., Warren, D. et al. (2005). Multiple-laboratory comparison of microarray platforms. *Nat Methods* 2(5): 345–50.
Kelley, D.E., He, J. et al. (2002). Dysfunction of mitochondria in human skeletal muscle in type 2 diabetes. *Diabetes* 51(10): 2944–50.
Kendziorski, C., Irizarry, R.A. et al. (2005). On the utility of pooling biological samples in microarray experiments. *Proc Natl Acad Sci USA* 102(12): 4252–7.
Kersten, S., Seydoux, J. et al. (1999). Peroxisome proliferator-activated receptor alpha mediates the adaptive response to fasting. *J Clin Invest* 103(11): 1489–98.
Martin, K.J., Graner, E. et al. (2001). High-sensitivity array analysis of gene expression for the early detection of disseminated breast tumor cells in peripheral blood. *Proc Natl Acad Sci USA* 98(5): 2646–51.
Moller, D.E. and Kaufman, K.D. (2005). Metabolic syndrome: a clinical and molecular perspective. *Annu Rev Med* 56: 45–62.
Mootha, V.K., Lindgren, C.M. et al. (2003). PGC-1alpha-responsive genes involved in oxidative phosphorylation are coordinately downregulated in human diabetes. *Nat Genet* 34(3): 267–73.
Müller, M. and Kersten, S. (2003). Nutrigenomics: goals and strategies. *Nat Rev Genet* 4(4): 315–22.
Patsouris, D., Mandard, S. et al. (2004). PPARalpha governs glycerol metabolism. *J Clin Invest* 114(1): 94–103.
Patsouris, D., Müller, S. et al. (2004). Peroxisome proliferator activated receptor ligands for the treatment of insulin resistance. *Curr Opin Invest Drugs* 5(10): 1045–50.
Patti, M.E., Butte, A.J. et al. (2003). Coordinated reduction of genes of oxidative metabolism in humans with insulin resistance and diabetes: potential role of PGC1 and NRF1. *Proc Natl Acad Sci USA* 100(14): 8466–71.
Ptitsyn, A.A., Zvonic, S. et al. (2006). Circadian clocks are resounding in peripheral tissues. *PLoS Comput Biol* 2(3): e16.
Radich, J.P., Mao, M. et al. (2004). Individual-specific variation of gene expression in peripheral blood leukocytes. *Genomics* 83(6): 980–8.
Sparks, L.M., Xie, H. et al. (2005). A high-fat diet coordinately downregulates genes required for mitochondrial oxidative phosphorylation in skeletal muscle. *Diabetes* 54(7): 1926–33.
Valk, P.J., Verhaak, R.G. et al. (2004). Prognostically useful gene-expression profiles in acute myeloid leukemia. *N Engl J Med* 350(16): 1617–28.
Weisberg, S.P., McCann, D. et al. (2003). Obesity is associated with macrophage accumulation in adipose tissue. *J Clin Invest* 112(12): 1796–808.
Whitney, A.R., Diehn, M. et al. (2003). Individuality and variation in gene expression patterns in human blood. *Proc Natl Acad Sci USA* 100(4): 1896–901.
Xu, H., Barnes, G.T. et al. (2003). Chronic inflammation in fat plays a crucial role in the development of obesity-related insulin resistance. *J Clin Invest* 112(12): 1821–30.
Zhang, Y. and Mangelsdorf, D.J. (2002). LuXuRies of lipid homeostasis: the unity of nuclear hormone receptors, transcription regulation, and cholesterol sensing. *Mol Interv* 2(2): 78–87.
Zvonic, S., Ptitsyn, A.A. et al. (2006). Characterization of peripheral circadian clocks in adipose tissues. *Diabetes* 55(4): 962–70.

# 2 Exploring the Proteome for Markers of Health

*Manuela Rist and Hannelore Daniel*

## CONTENTS



## 2.1 INTRODUCTION

Proteome analysis of a particular cell or organ, or of body fluids such as plasma, urine, and others, makes it possible to identify biomarkers that respond to alterations in diet or any other treatment, and that may have a predictive value for the assessment of a human's health status. To date, proteomics has not been applied on a large scale in human studies related to nutrition, yet it has obvious advantages over transcriptome profiling techniques in that it directly assesses the molecular entities that carry out the biological functions. This chapter summarizes the different approaches in proteomics research and provides some examples that demonstrate the state of the art of biomarker discovery based on proteome analysis and their implications for the development of personalized nutrition approaches.

Human metabolism can be described as the orchestrated interplay of a huge number of proteins that perform different functions as receptors, enzymes, signaling molecules, and transporters or structural components, and that are expressed at the level of the cell, the organ, or whole organism. Proteins are the transmitters of metabolic functions, and therefore changes in the level of an individual protein or sets of proteins may indicate an altered metabolic condition. Protein synthesis and protein degradation, and thereby metabolic functions, can be affected by the overall composition of the diet, the levels of specific nutrients and nonnutrient components of foods and, indeed, many other aspects of lifestyle, in the most complex ways. Analysis of the proteome as the whole protein complement of the genome expressed in a particular cell, an organ, or body fluid — also called *proteomics* — allows changes in protein expression patterns, and the identity of the proteins themselves to be determined simultaneously. Moreover, for individual proteins, posttranslational modifications that may be crucial for protein function, or even amino acid substitutions (polymorphisms), can be detected. The potential value of proteomics for assessing markers of health has been recognized for some years [1], but only very few studies so far have employed proteome analysis as a tool for research in human nutrition and health [2].

## 2.2 TECHNIQUES EMPLOYED IN PROTEOMICS

Proteome analysis is beginning to emerge as a second high-throughput tool for nutrition research. The revival of the two-dimensional gel electrophoresis (2D-PAGE) with improved resolution, the advanced instrumentation, elegant software tools, databases, and the enormous advancements in mass spectrometry have made proteomics applications a practical alternative screening method that complements transcript profiling approaches. There are three different principal strategies for proteome analysis: (1) classical 2D-PAGE that separates proteins in a gel prior to analysis of individual proteins by peptide mass fingerprinting using mass spectrometry, (2) the so-called shotgun approaches, in which all proteins contained in a sample are first digested by proteases, followed by chromatographic separation of the obtained peptide fragments, which then are analyzed by mass spectrometry, and (3) a solid-phase-based enrichment of proteins depending on their different physico-chemical characteristics — mainly done on chips — followed by mass analysis that usually does not identify the proteins but provides mass patterns (Figure 2.1). The latter technique is predominantly used in clinical diagnostics.

The 2D-PAGE technique separates proteins according to charge (isoelectric point: pI) by isoelectric focusing (IEF) in the first dimension and according to size (molecular mass) in the second dimension. Therefore, it has a unique capacity to resolve complex mixtures of proteins, permitting the simultaneous analysis of hundreds or even thousands of gene products [3]. However, not all proteins are resolved and separated equally well by 2D-PAGE. Very alkaline, hydrophobic, and integral membrane proteins as well as high-molecular-weight proteins are still a problem. In some cases, a prefractionation according to cellular compartments (membranes/microsomes, cytosol, mitochondria) or according to protein solubility by classical means may be necessary [4]. In addition, proteins of low cellular abundance, which may be particularly important in view of their cellular functions, for example, in signaling pathways, are still very difficult to be resolved in the presence of large quantities of housekeeping proteins [5]. However, new techniques are constantly being developed that employ, for example, tagging techniques [6] or the enrichment of the minor proteins prior to separation in two-dimensional gels. The most common procedure for the identification of a protein spot in a gel is currently the peptide mapping or "fingerprint" analysis method, but other techniques and approaches can also be applied. For peptide mapping, protein containing spots are excised from the gel before the gel is altered chemically to make the protein accessible for hydrolysis by a protease such as trypsin [7]. Based on this site-specific enzymatic hydrolysis, a distinct and characteristic pattern of peptide fragments of a given protein is

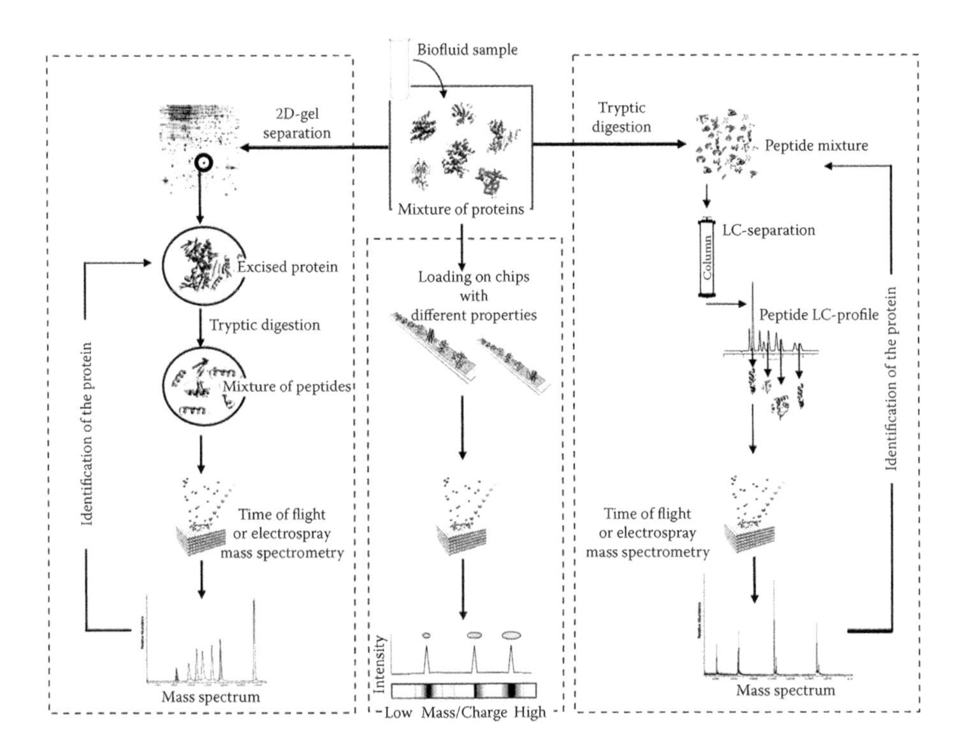


**FIGURE 2.1** The different approaches to proteome analysis.

generated. The mixture of peptides isolated from the gel spot after digestion with the protease is usually submitted to matrix-assisted laser desorption/ionization time-of-flight mass spectrometry (MALDI-TOF-MS) analysis to determine the corresponding peptide masses that are characteristic for a given protein and serve as the peptide mass fingerprint. The obtained mass spectrum is evaluated with computer programs that apply various algorithms for interpretation of the peptide pattern and predict the protein identity based on a comparison with masses predicted by "virtual digestion" of identified open-reading frames in a given genome [8].

In contrast to gel-based proteomics analysis, shotgun proteomics is a gel-free approach that uses different liquid chromatography techniques for separation of complex peptide mixtures coupled with mass spectrometry identification [9]. It starts with the isolation of the protein-containing sample, which may also be prefractionated by chromatographic or electrophoretic techniques followed by a digestion step to generate a complex mixture of peptides. Multidimensional chromatographic techniques are subsequently used to separate and further fractionate the obtained peptide mixtures, which are then submitted for analysis by electrospray ionization (ESI) or MALDI-based mass analysis. Sophisticated mathematical algorithms are used to compare the peptide sequence data derived from mass spectra with sequence information in protein databases to identify the proteins.

Major technological advancements in protein chemistry have led to chip-based protein sample arrays with different chromatographic surfaces to selectively bind proteins with specific chemical properties. One of the evolved technologies is the surface-enhanced laser desorption ionization time-of-flight (SELDI-TOF) platform for high-throughput analysis of proteins in complex biological specimens [10]. It uses a protein chip array system with different chromatographic properties, including hydrophobic, hydrophilic, anion exchange, cation exchange, or immobilized-metal affinity surfaces. After addition of an energy-absorbing matrix to the chip, the proteins are analyzed by MALDI-TOF mass analysis. The output from the proteome analysis based on chips via SELDI-TOF is a trace of relative intensity vs. $m/z$ (mass-to-charge ratio) of the detected proteins, providing a pattern that can be compared from different samples or that can be used for cluster analyses for significant protein abundance differences between samples. The future of more simple proteome analysis tools may be the use of antibody libraries that contain specific antibodies raised against an expressed open-reading frame and making proteome analysis similar to high-throughput microplate assays that allow essentially every protein to be identified and quantified easily [11].

## 2.3 BIOFLUIDS AS A SOURCE OF MARKER DISCOVERY

The analysis of the effects of nutrition on human health requires easily accessible biological samples that provide information on the metabolic status. Plasma or serum represents the fluid compartment that carries metabolites and signaling molecules from and to cells in the various body organs and therefore serves as a distribution and messenger system in interorgan metabolism (Figure 2.2). Blood is readily available in sufficient quantities, and its molecular composition appears to reflect

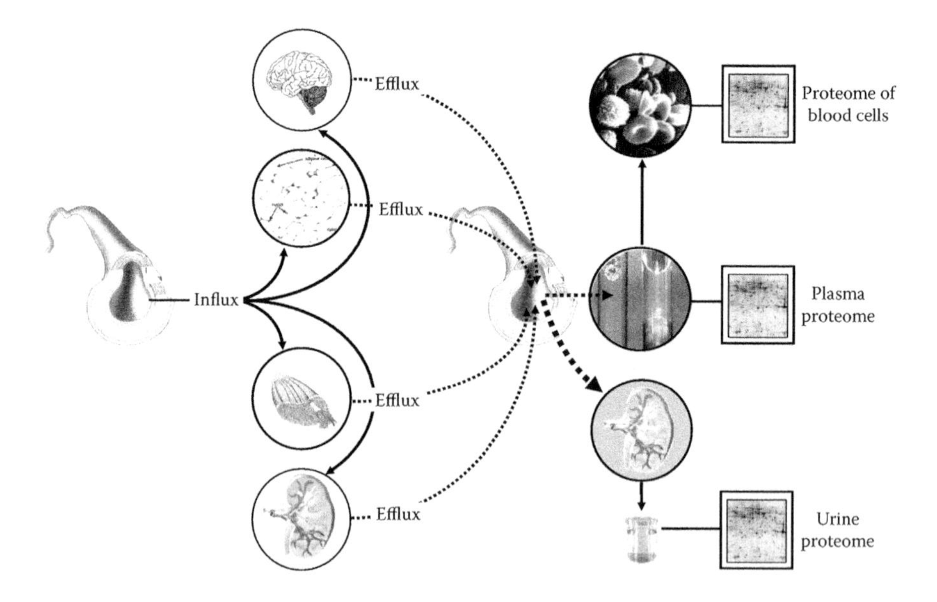


**FIGURE 2.2** The importance of human blood as a source of biological information with the possibilities of analyzing plasma, blood cell proteomes, and urine as easily obtainable samples.

the condition of individual organs and the physiological processes associated with it. Moreover, proteins in the blood are actively participating in many life-sustaining body functions such as the transport of nutrients and metabolites, inflammation, hormone signaling, and many more. The blood proteome therefore promises to be an ideal biological entity for assessing markers of health or disease.

Analysis of blood proteins, however, depends on many variables, most importantly, on the methods of sampling, sample processing, and storage. A particular problem is that plasma/serum contains around 22 abundant proteins that represent 99% of the protein mass. The most prominent protein is albumin, with around 45,000 μg/ml, whereas the concentration of other proteins, such as the alpha-fetoprotein, may be as low as 0.005 μg/ml [12]. This huge concentration difference makes analysis of the plasma proteome very difficult and requires the removal of the most abundant proteins from the sample to allow a reliable analysis of the minor components. During the course of the Human Proteome Project (HPP), a group of 38 expert labs has focused on the human plasma proteome. The Human Plasma Proteome Project (HPPP) has worked out standard operational procedures and has made recommendations for sample analysis and processing [13]. A wealth of biological information is already available from the HPPP and is in the public domain (http://www.plasmaproteomedatabase.org/). A total of 2446 unique gene products and more than 4900 protein entities were identified when specific isoforms were taken into account. *In silico* methods were employed to determine the origin and nature of the various plasma proteins (see Figure 2.3). This analysis delivered a surprisingly high number of "unexpected" protein classes, including a large number

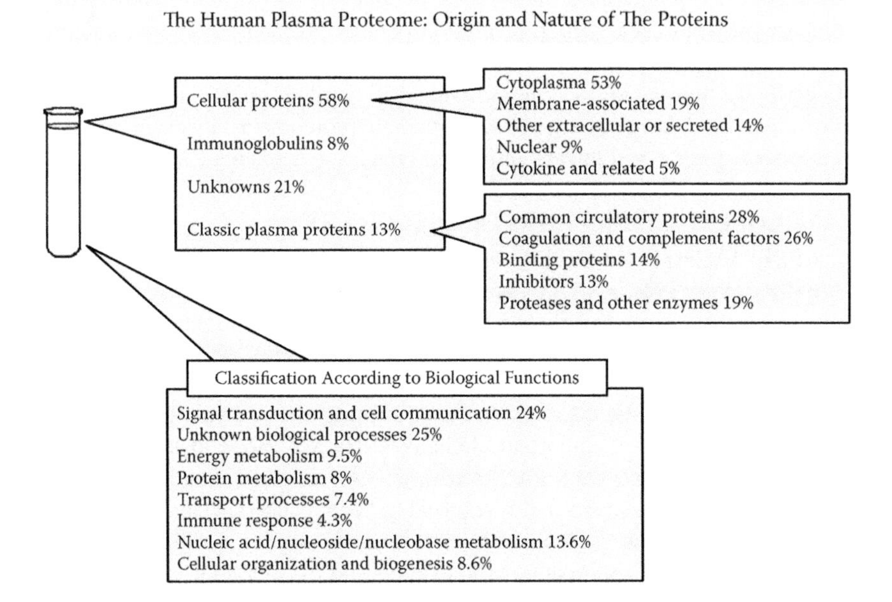


**FIGURE 2.3** The origins and nature of the proteins identified in human plasma by the HPPP.

of intracellular proteins, and even proteins of nuclear origin. Whether they are indicators of normal tissue renewal processes or a measure of tissue (organ-specific) damage is currently under investigation. In this context, the isoform-specific proteins (in case of selected enzymes, these are well-established clinical markers) in plasma are interesting for further exploration. The nutritional status is known to affect the levels of distinct plasma proteins, and organ-specific processes appear also to be detectable in plasma as some of the proteins found in plasma are derived from individual organs. In the HPPP, 362 of the plasma proteins were of hepatic origin and 345 proteins were "cardiovascular related," and about 110 proteins could be related to inflammation such as cytokines, adhesion molecules, and chemokines [14].

Plasma peptides are usually too small in molecular mass for standard proteome analysis. However, they are of particular interest because of their specific functions in biological processes in which they act as hormones, growth factors, adipokines, etc. The plasma peptidome — defined as the fraction with peptides of < 10,000 or 15,000 Da — therefore requires special techniques for separation and analysis. Usually, a prefractionation of plasma based on ultrafiltration techniques with membranes of different cutoff values is used and then further chromatographic separation steps combined with mass analysis are employed to characterize the low-molecular-weight peptides in the sample. The plasma peptidome is considered to represent up to 5000 different peptides [15].

Proteome analysis may also be applied to circulating blood cells. The fraction of mononuclear cells can easily be collected from blood samples by commercial separation kits, and these cells may serve as "reporter cells" as they are in circulation for extended time periods and reach different body compartments. Proteome analysis of human peripheral mononuclear cells has not been performed in the context of biomarker discovery or clinical diagnostics. In contrast, several studies have targeted the platelet proteome, and a high-resolution platelet proteome map that comprises more than 2000 different protein features has been generated [16,17].

Other body fluids such as urine, saliva, tears, seminal fluid, synovial fluid, and cerebrospinal fluid have also been submitted to proteome analysis in search for biomarkers of disease and toward improved clinical diagnostics [18].

## 2.4 EXAMPLES OF BIOMARKER DISCOVERY APPROACHES IN BODY FLUIDS BY PROTEOME ANALYSIS

Proteome analysis techniques are used to search for changes in the relative abundance of individual proteins or protein clusters that may be indicative of a certain disease state. Despite the fantastic accomplishments in proteome analysis in recent years, there remain a number of important challenges that will need to be addressed to pave the way for the acceptance of proteomics as a relevant diagnostic tool. The most advanced state of analysis in this respect has been reached in cancer diagnostics. Numerous studies have screened biosamples in cancer patients, including serum/plasma for identification of specific markers and for validation of the diagnostic power of the proteome approaches as compared to established clinical diagnosis strategies [19]. The ultimate goal here is to develop biomarkers that are able to reliably and accurately predict outcomes during cancer development, management, and treatment, and it is envisioned that there might in the future be a serum or urine test available for every phase of cancer that may guide clinical decision making and which may replace the invasive techniques used today [20].

Beyond cancer proteomics, there are not too many studies that have taken proteome analysis into the clinical or diagnostic environment. However, a recent study has assessed candidate protein biomarkers of rheumatoid arthritis in synovial fluid, which is found in small amounts in joints, bursas, and tendon sheaths. A total of 33 candidate biomarkers for rheumatoid arthritis were identified from a total of 418 detected proteins. Among the proteins that were elevated in the synovial fluid of patients were C-reactive protein (CRP) and six members of the S100 protein family of calcium-binding proteins [21]. Cerebrospinal fluid has also been used as a sample, and it has been hypothesized that alterations in the protein composition of CSF may reflect abnormalities in protein expression associated with trauma, neurodegenerative disorders, or multiple sclerosis. A number of proteomic approaches have recently been used to find differentially expressed proteins in patients with Alzheimer's disease [22] or multiple sclerosis [18]. Although none of the putative protein markers have been validated for these diseases, yet the efforts seem very promising.

Urine proteome analysis has the advantage that obtaining the sample does not need any invasive approaches such as drawing blood. Because it is anticipated that altered urine protein patterns or protein concentrations may reflect mainly impaired kidney functions, urine proteome analysis is currently predominantly used to characterize acute and chronic renal toxicity of compounds or for diagnostics of diseases that are known to affect kidney function. The power of urine proteomics as a diagnostic tool was recently demonstrated by identification of a large number of polypeptides in spot urine samples of type 1 diabetes patients with different stages of nephropathy [23]. Specific clusters of 54 polypeptides were only found in type 1 diabetes patients. A major challenge of urinary proteomics is also to reduce the complexity of the urinary proteome to allow low-abundance proteins of special pathophysiological significance to be detected. Urinary proteins can originate from glomerular filtration of low-molecular-weight plasma proteins or by the secretion of renal tubular soluble proteins. In addition, whole-cell shedding and apical plasma membrane shedding by nonspecific or apoptotic processes will lead to protein excretion in urine. Recent studies have demonstrated that small vesicles, so-called exosomes, which represent internal vesicles of multivesicular bodies are delivered to the tubular fluids and urine via fusion of the bodies with the apical plasma membrane of renal tubule epithelial cells. Exosomes were shown to contain numerous proteins of clinical importance that may also serve as markers of kidney function in health and disease [24].

Regarding the effects of nutritional factors and putative markers of diet-dependent diseases, there are only very few examples of proteome analysis being used as a discovery tool in human studies. In a controlled dietary intervention, MALDI-TOF spectra were generated from serum samples of 38 human volunteers. In a randomized controlled trial, the participants ate during separate feeding periods either a basal diet devoid of fruits and vegetables or a basal diet supplemented with cruciferous vegetables (broccoli). At the end of each 7-d feeding period, serum samples were obtained and large, abundant proteins removed. Bioinformatic analysis of MALDI-TOF spectra revealed two significant peaks that could classify participants based on diet with 76% accuracy. One of the peaks (at 2740 m/z) was identified as the B-chain of α-2-HS glycoprotein, a serum protein previously found to vary with diet and thought to be involved in insulin resistance and immune function [25].

The adipocyte fatty acid–binding protein (A-FABP) is considered to be a cytosolic fatty acid chaperone. However, mice with a targeted disruption of the A-FABP gene show protection from insulin resistance, hyperglycemia, and atherosclerosis, suggesting that A-FABP could have additional functions. 2D-gel-based separations of proteins from cultured adipocytes identified the cellular fatty acid-binding protein as a prominent secretion product. When obese patients were concomitantly screened for plasma levels of A-FABP, it was observed that concentrations of A-FABP were significantly higher in overweight and obese as compared to lean persons and after adjustment for age and sex, serum A-FABP concentrations correlated significantly with blood pressure, fasting insulin, waist circumference, and dyslipidemia. A-FABP therefore appears to be a new biomarker that is associated with obesity and the metabolic syndrome [26].

## 2.5 FUTURE PERSPECTIVES

The recent advancements in proteomic technologies, including improved two-dimensional gel electrophoresis, new mass spectrometric techniques, and convenient chip-based sample treatment techniques with simplified analysis combined with the advancements in bioinformatic tools should foster the discovery of new biomarkers that are both sensitive and specific to distinguish a healthy individual from a diseased one. The advantage of proteomics is that it assesses the abundance of proteins, which are the prime entities that carry out and mediate biological functions. This advantage, however, is currently counterbalanced by the expensive technologies and the rather difficult techniques. In view of proteome analysis as a tool for assessing health status in personalized nutrition concepts, simpler, faster and more convenient methods are needed. Protein microarrays are considered to meet these requirements for a simultaneous analysis of the abundance, function, and interaction of proteins on a systemwide scale [27]. The power of chip-based miniaturized protein assays lies in the potential to investigate in parallel large numbers of analytes in a variety of biological samples for innovative *in vitro* diagnostic applications. It can be expected that a range of customized and targeted equipment will become available in the next years for easy-to-use proteomics approaches in lifestyle monitoring and for the assessment of disease progression. As the field is rapidly developing with respect to the analysis of marker proteins in all kinds of body fluids (plasma, tears, saliva, urine, etc.), one can also expect that the consumers themselves will collect those fluids easily and send them via their doctors or specialized health-care providers to a proteomics laboratory for analysis. Initial applications will probably target the diagnostics of common diseases such as diabetes, arthrosclerosis, allergies, or autoimmune diseases. In diabetics, nonenzymatic glycosylation of target proteins may be measured routinely to assess the maintenance of healthy blood glucose profiles (similar to analysis of hemoglobin A1) or by monitoring the urine proteome, which may indicate disturbed kidney function at an early stage as the disease progresses. Detecting serum autoantibodies in autoimmune diseases or quantitative measurements of serum allergen-specific IgE levels in type I allergy are already possible via proteome analysis in chip formats with minute amounts of serum. A detailed analysis of the protein components of the lipoproteins of the LDL and HDL classes may provide better diagnostics for arthrosclerosis and heart disease, in particular, when different isoforms related to different organs of origin or because of genetic variations are taken into account. However, before proteomics moves into "the real world" and these new and more convenient assay systems become available, nutritional science needs to explore with existing technologies the "power of proteomics" in characterizing human metabolism and diet responses in well-defined studies.

## REFERENCES


1. Chambers, G. et al., Proteomics: a new approach to the study of disease, *J Pathol*, 192, 280, 2000.
2. Kussmann, M. et al., Proteomics in nutrition and health, *Comb Chem High Throughput Screen*, 8, 679, 2005.
3. Gorg, A. et al., The current state of two-dimensional electrophoresis with immobilized pH gradients, *Electrophoresis*, 21, 1037, 2000.
4. Cordwell, S.J. et al., Subproteomics based upon protein cellular location and relative solubilities in conjunction with composite two-dimensional electrophoresis gels, *Electrophoresis*, 21, 1094, 2000.
5. Corthals, G.L. et al., The dynamic range of protein expression: a challenge for proteomic research, *Electrophoresis*, 21, 1104, 2000.
6. Adam, G.C. et al., Profiling the specific reactivity of the proteome with non-directed activity-based probes, *Chem Biol*, 8, 81, 2001.
7. Conrads, T.P. et al., Utility of accurate mass tags for proteome-wide protein identification, *Anal Chem*, 72, 3349, 2000.
8. Chamrad, D.C. et al., Interpretation of mass spectrometry data for high-throughput proteomics, *Anal Bioanal Chem*, 376, 1014, 2003.
9. Wolters, D.A. et al., An automated multidimensional protein identification technology for shotgun proteomics, *Anal Chem*, 73, 5683, 2001.
10. Issaq, H.J. et al., The SELDI-TOF MS approach to proteomics: protein profiling and biomarker identification, *Biochem Biophys Res Commun*, 292, 587, 2002.
11. LaBaer, J. and Ramachandran, N., Protein microarrays as tools for functional proteomics, *Curr Opin Chem Biol*, 9, 14, 2005.
12. Qian, W.J. et al., Comparative proteome analyses of human plasma following *in vivo* lipopolysaccharide administration using multidimensional separations coupled with tandem mass spectrometry, *Proteomics*, 5, 572, 2005.
13. Rai, A.J. et al., Hupo plasma proteome project specimen collection and handling: towards the standardization of parameters for plasma proteome samples, *Proteomics*, 5, 3262, 2005.
14. Ping, P. et al., A functional annotation of subproteomes in human plasma, *Proteomics*, 5, 3506, 2005.
15. Richter, R. et al., Composition of the peptide fraction in human blood plasma: database of circulating human peptides, *J Chromatogr B Biomed Sci Appl*, 726, 25, 1999.

16. Garcia, A. et al., Applying proteomics technology to platelet research, *Mass Spectrom Rev*, 24, 918, 2005.
17. O'Neill, E.E. et al., Towards complete analysis of the platelet proteome, *Proteomics*, 2, 288, 2002.
18. Veenstra, T.D. et al., Biomarkers: mining the biofluid proteome, *Mol Cell Proteomics*, 4, 409, 2005.
19. Alaiya, A. et al., Clinical cancer proteomics: promises and pitfalls, *J Proteome Res*, 4, 1213, 2005.
20. Chatterjee, S.K. and Zetter, B.R., Cancer biomarkers: knowing the present and predicting the future, *Future Oncol*, 1, 37, 2005.
21. Liao, H. et al., Use of mass spectrometry to identify protein biomarkers of disease severity in the synovial fluid and serum of patients with rheumatoid arthritis, *Arthritis Rheum*, 50, 3792, 2004.
22. Davidsson, P. and Sjogren, M., Proteome studies of CSF in AD patients, *Mech Ageing Dev*, 127, 133, 2006.
23. Meier, M. et al., Identification of urinary protein pattern in type 1 diabetic adolescents with early diabetic nephropathy by a novel combined proteome analysis, *J Diabetes Complications*, 19, 223, 2005.
24. Pisitkun, T. et al., Identification and proteomic profiling of exosomes in human urine, *Proc Natl Acad Sci USA*, 101, 13368, 2004.
25. Mitchell, B.L. et al., Evaluation of matrix-assisted laser desorption/ionization-time of flight mass spectrometry proteomic profiling: identification of alpha 2-HS glycoprotein B-chain as a biomarker of diet, *Proteomics*, 5, 2238, 2005.
26. Xu, A. et al., Adipocyte fatty acid-binding protein is a plasma biomarker closely associated with obesity and metabolic syndrome, *Clin Chem*, 52, 405, 2006.
27. Kung, L.A. and Snyder, M., Proteome chips for whole-organism assays, *Nat Rev Mol Cell Biol*, 2006.

# 3 Metabolomics and the Personalized Metabolic Signature

*Michael J. Gibney, Marianne Walsh, and Lorraine Brennan*

## CONTENTS



## 3.1 INTRODUCTION

Whereas traditional nutrition and metabolism research sets out *a priori* the metabolites of interest in the hypothesis to be tested, nutritional metabolomics attempts to capture the presence of the maximum number of small chemicals regardless of their identity or relevance to any advance hypothesis. It is thus a hypothesis-generating exercise. The totality of all signals in a sample is reduced in a two-stage process to one point in two-dimensional space, and metabolic signatures that are comparable will cluster closely together and, as the metabolomic profiles differ, the points separate in proportion to the differences. Metabolomic profiles of many diseases have been studied, and distinct clusters have been identified. Similarly, metabolic profiles arising from pharmacological intervention have also been characterized and are found to cluster together for similar drugs. To date little or no serious work has been published on nutritional metabolomics, but a number of clear challenges exist. In nutrition, metabolic "noise" will be relatively high because food contains many nonnutrients, which are absorbed and which will be detectable in biofluids. This, coupled with the fact that the effect of diet on metabolomic profiles is likely to be milder than that of disease or drugs, makes the challenge of nutritional metabolomics very special. However, whether it is through targeted metabolomic profiles or universal metabolomic profiles, nutritional metabolomics offers great potential for nutrition research.

Traditionally, nutritional science has proceeded in a hypothesis-driven manner in which *a priori*, end points were known, were part of the hypothesis, and were the basis of experimental measure. Although that will remain so, new advances in biology have led to the development of a parallel strategy that is hypothesis generating rather than hypothesis testing. Metabolomics is part of that new biology. As ever in science, terminology becomes important, and two terms coexist in this field, *metabolomics* and *metabonomics*. For completeness we will present the original definitions of both and leave it to the reader to distinguish between the two. Metabonomics is defined as "the quantitative measurement of the time-related multiparametric metabolic response of living systems to pathophysiological stimuli or genetic modification." On the other hand, metabolomics has been defined in the literature as the "comprehensive and quantitative analysis of all metabolites…". Throughout this chapter we will use the term metabolomics exclusively but remind the reader that either term can be used.

In relation to human studies, metabolomics is the measurement of the maximum number of metabolites present in a biofluid. A range of analytical methods can be used to generate data. However, mass spectrometry (MS) in its various hyphenated derivations (LC-MS, GC-MS) and high-resolution $^{1}$H nuclear magnetic resonance spectroscopy ($^{1}$H NMR) are the dominant platforms. Both platforms have their advantages and disadvantages, and best practice is to apply both, if possible. For the purpose of this chapter we will focus more on NMR applications but in no way wish to claim it is a superior technique. In the case of $^{1}$H NMR, each biofluid has a characteristic spectroscopic fingerprint that reflects the metabolic composition (see Figure 3.1 for $^{1}$H NMR spectra of different biofluids). The intensities of peaks, in an NMR spectrum, belonging to a certain metabolite are determined by its concentration, and assignment can be made based on chemical shifts (position in spectra), spin multiplicities, and addition of authentic material. Typical metabolomic studies generate large amounts of data that cannot easily be analyzed in an unbiased way. To overcome this problem, a number of pattern recognition techniques have been applied to robustly analyze NMR spectra.

The most commonly used method to analyze metabolomics data is through principal component analysis (PCA). This statistical method reduces a large number of variables to a smaller number of variables, called *principal components*. The principles underlying the reduction of a complex multisignal NMR output to a single point in two-dimensional space through PCA is best illustrated with a 3-peak output rather than with the several hundred peaks normally found in NMR spectra. Figure 3.2A and Figure 3.2B show how these three "peaks" can be processed: first, the multipeak output is summarized by one point in multidimensional space and then reduced to a lower two-dimensional space. In the resulting scores plot, each point represents all the data contained in the spectrum belonging to one individual.

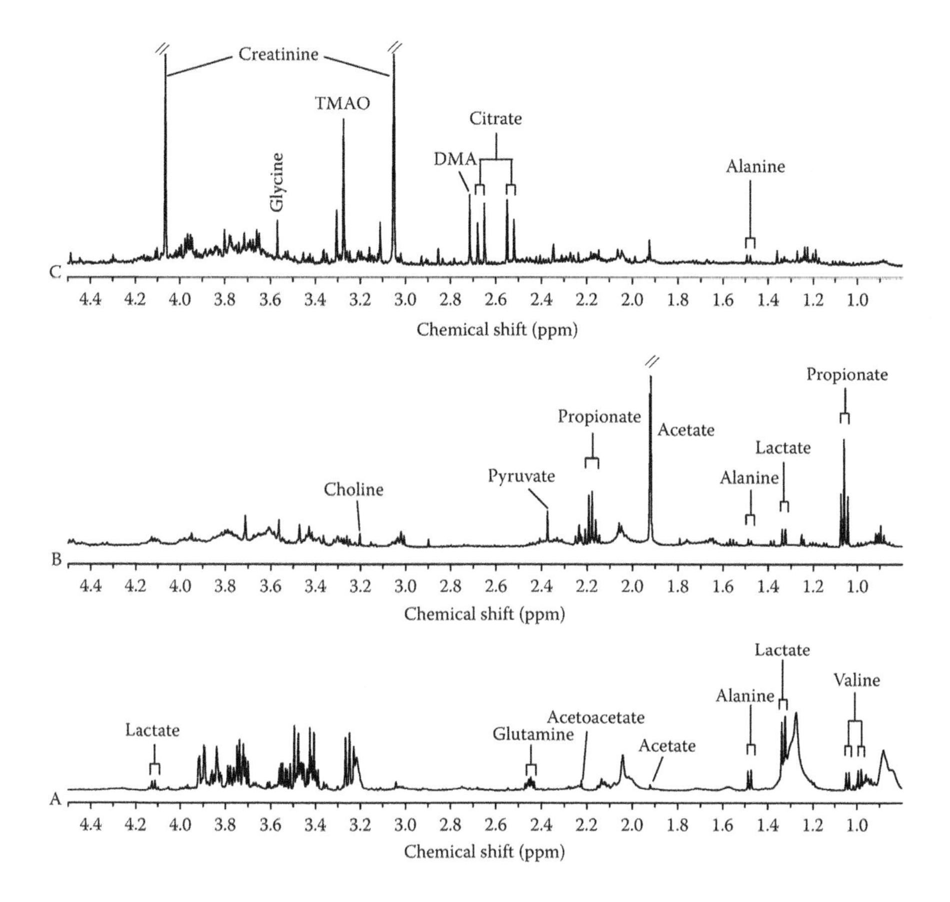


**FIGURE 3.1** Typical [1]H NMR spectra of biofluids obtained from a healthy volunteer: (a) plasma, (b) saliva, and (c) urine. TMAO, trimethylamine-*N*-oxide; DMA, dimethylamine. (From *Am J Clin Nutr*, 2006, 84:531–539. With permission.)

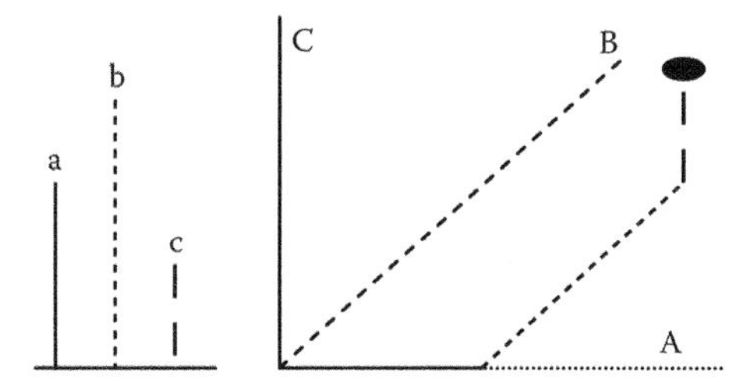


**FIGURE 3.2A** Three NMR or MS peaks *a*, *b*, and *c*, must be reduced to one point in multidimensional space. Three coordinates A, B, and C are used to achieve this. The signal strength of peak *a* is laid on coordinate A proportionate to the size of the signal. Peak *b* is now placed parallel to coordinate B, and similarly peak *c* is set parallel to coordinate C, each proportionate to the size of the relevant signal. The final point is the only position these three peaks can give in three-dimensional space, and the same holds true for *k* peaks in K-dimensional space.

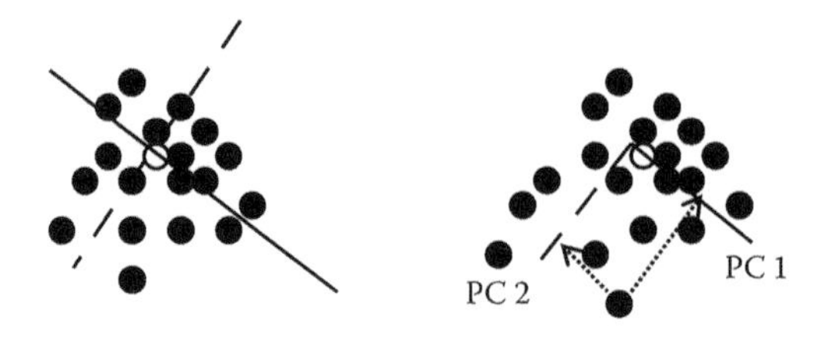


**FIGURE 3.2B** The figure on the left should be imagined as a bunch of grapes in multidimensional space. The center (nonfilled) grape is found, and a pencil is inserted into the bunch of grapes through the center multiple times from all possible angles until maximum variance to the bunch of grapes is found. A second pencil is similarly inserted at a right angle to the first. Half of each pencil is lost, and the distance each grape is from each pencil [principal components (PC) 1 and 2] is measured as shown for one point with an arrow on the right figure. Now, a two-dimensional plot retaining maximum information on multidimensional space is developed.

Hence, observation points that cluster close together have similar spectra, whereas those that are far apart will have very different spectra. The spectral variables responsible for the positioning of the observations in the scores plot can be obtained from the "loadings" plot. Although PCA is the initial unsupervised data analysis carried out in most metabolomic studies, it is usually followed by more sophisticated supervised techniques such as Partial Least Squares Discriminant Analysis (PLS-DA).

The power of these statistical techniques to reduce complex NMR profiles to single points in two-dimensional space is shown in Figure 3.3A and Figure 3.3B. Figure 3.3A gives typical NMR spectra for urine samples collected in the morning or in the evening by the same individual. Clearly, the samples taken at different time points exhibit differences in the NMR profiles which are clearly discernible to the

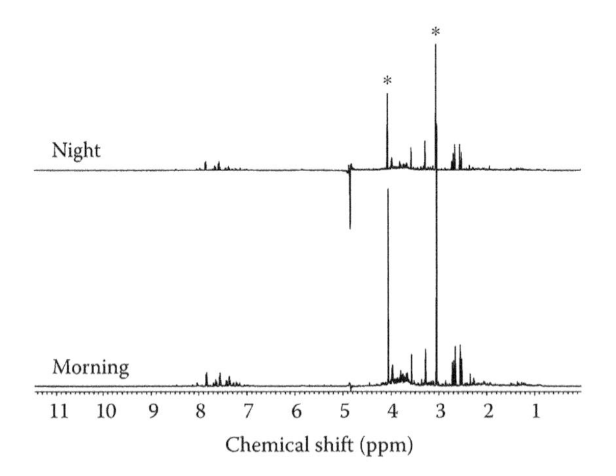


**FIGURE 3.3A** $^1$H NMR spectra of urine from the same subject sampled first thing in the morning and last thing in the evening.

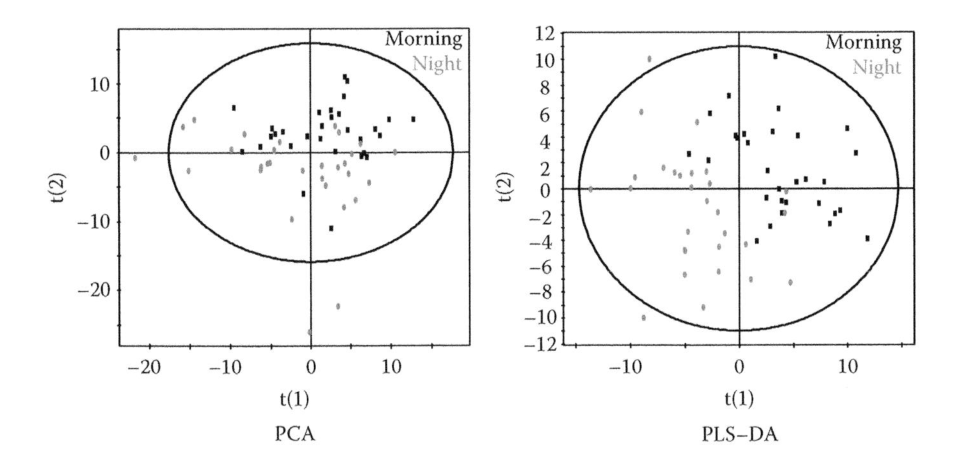


**FIGURE 3.3B** Principal component analysis (PCA) and partial least squares discriminant analysis (PLS-DA) of NMR data from human urine samples collected both in the early morning and late evening.

human eye, as shown by asterisks. When PCA and PLS-DA, in particular, are applied, quite clear separation of the night–morning samples is seen because the samples taken at each time point have comparable "signatures" but nighttime and morning-time signatures are quite different. To date, metabolomic profiling of biofluids have shown unique signatures for cases and controls in many chronic diseases such as cardiovascular disease, cancers, osteoarthritis, and several neurodegenerative diseases.

The metabolomic profiles of human biofluids are determined by a number of identifiable factors, although the quantitative effect of each individual factor remains, as yet, unknown. It is evident from later sections that the presence or absence of a disease or, if present, the severity of the disease is one determinant of a metabolic signature. However, for the purposes of this section of the chapter, the focus will be on physiological factors determining the nature of the metabolomic profiles in human biofluids. For clarity in what can be a rather confused landscape, environmental factors, including stress, will not be considered. This is not to say that these are unimportant but, rather, it is advantageous to focus on core determinants of metabolomic profiles that are amenable to dietary influence. Thus, this chapter will focus on the effects of phenotype and endogenous metabolism on food with an evaluation of the effects of both nutrients and nonnutrients, and also on the role of the colonic microflora.

### 3.1.1 Phenotype, Endogenous Metabolism, and Nutrients as Determinants of Metabolomic Signatures

It is the essence of life that biological systems turn over constantly with a simultaneous set of anabolic and catabolic pathways. The balance of these is determined by a variety of endocrine-based factors. The anabolic phase is dominant in growth, reproduction, and weight gain, whereas the catabolic factors are dominant in aging, illness, and weight loss. This constant entry and exit of metabolites from plasma plays a major role in determining the metabolic profile of that biofluid in the normal sampling state of fasting. Phenotype therefore must play a very significant role in shaping fasting plasma metabolomic profiles. For example, protein turnover is strongly related to lean body mass and, thus, per unit of plasma, the rate of exit and entry of amino acids into plasma will be far higher in individuals with a higher as compared to a lower lean body mass per unit weight. Height and girth will reflect skeletal differences, and greater skeletal mass will mean greater traffic of related metabolites in and out of plasma. Clearly, as percentage body fat increases, the constant anabolism and catabolism in adipose tissue determines the flow of nonesterified fatty acids, glycerol, glucose, and triacylglycerol-rich lipoproteins and their remnants to and from the liver via the plasma metabolome. Diet can clearly alter the nature of the plasma metabolome in the postprandial phase, and the nature of that effect will be dependent on the nature of the ingested meal. However, this is an acute event that in the short term will not influence the nature of the fasting plasma metabolome. If a modification to diet is sustained such that it can be described as chronic, then it will lead eventually to a readjustment of gene expression and to a redefining of the parameters of anabolic and catabolic pathways, and that will influence the fasting plasma metabolome. Thus, an acute change of the ratio of polyunsaturated to saturated fatty acids in the diet will have a transient effect on the postprandial metabolome, whereas a chronic change will lead to a sustained readjustment of the expression of many genes, resulting in altered fasting levels of plasma cholesterol fractions, haemostatic functions, insulin responsiveness, and the like. Phenotype will also influence urinary metabolomic profiles in that age, sex, height, weight, and the endocrine environment all shape the constituents of urine.

### 3.1.2 Food Nonnutrients as Determinants of Metabolic Signatures

There is no doubt from an extensive literature that chronic changes in the human diet significantly alter metabolic homeostasis and that the altered metabolic homeostasis will in turn alter the acute response to a nutrient load. There is, however, a major difference in the relative effects of food and nutrients on urinary and plasma metabolomic profiles. In the case of plasma, nutrients are preferentially retained unless fairly high renal thresholds are exceeded. In contrast, xenobiotics, which abound in the nonnutrient element of food, are preferentially secreted into urine. An extensive review of the metabolism of plant chemicals or phytochemicals shows an average half-life for excretion into urine of about 8 h, with a maximum of about 20 h. These phytochemicals do not enter normal metabolic pathways, but they do operate as receptor–ligands, triggering a number of metabolic responses such as is encountered with onion peeling, or the consumption of coffee, or the habit of cigarette smoking.

In effect, the plasma metabolomic profile is dominated by the body composition dimension of phenotype and by metabolites of a multitude of pathways. It can be altered by diet, but only after chronic exposure has adjusted gene expression and, thus, the management of metabolic pathways. In the case of urine, phenotypic characteristics will play a significant role, but they will be subject to considerable interference by recently ingested nonnutrients. In one study of urinary metabolomic profiles in subjects consuming chamomile tea, a significant number of outliers were characterized by high levels of trimethylamine oxide (TMAO) indicative of the recent consumption of seafood. A recent study by the authors has shown that strict and total control over food choice for 24 h prior to biofluid collection has no effect on reducing variability in plasma or saliva, but does have a very significant effect in reducing between-person variability in urinary metabolomic profiles. The authors speculated that this is best explained by the reduction in between-person variability in nonnutrient intake rather than any change in metabolic homeostasis. Thus, in human nutrition, urinary collections might have to be collected with strict control over the prior 24-h food choice, an issue for discussion by international groups setting standards for this area of research (www.nugo.org).

### 3.1.3 The Colonic Microflora as Determinants of Metabolic Signatures

A final diet-related factor to be considered is the large-bowel microflora. A case has been made that the continual production of metabolites by the colonic microflora will significantly influence the shape of the plasma and urinary metabolome. It is certainly the case from experimental studies that the transition from a gnotobiotic rodent status to a conventional rodent status is characterized by dramatic shifts in urinary metabolomic profiles. Equally, within established colonies of conventional animals, metabolomic subsets can be identified, which have been attributed to variation in the colonic microflora. However, to date, no human studies are available to ascertain whether the use of different prebiotics and probiotics would lead to detectable changes in the metabolomic profiles of different human biofluids.

## 3.2 CHARACTERIZING DIETARY PATTERNS USING METABOLOMICS

Although the early days of nutrigenomics heralded the dawn of personalized nutrition, literally at the level of the individual, it is becoming increasingly evident that such an approach is overambitious. Unquestionably, nutrigenomics will move us from the present paradigm where data at population epidemiology level is used to infer events at the individual level. However, it is more likely to move from whole population to subgroup rather than to the level of the individual. We have seen that metabolomics can be used to allocate an unknown metabolic signature to a given cluster of a clinical condition that has similar characteristics as the unknown signature. This is now moving from the individual to a similar subgroup of the population in terms of metabolomic profiles. Could the same be achieved for dietary patterns? One possibility to envisage would be to take population dietary patterns and to use cluster analysis to identify 8 to 12 dietary patterns that together explain 90% of dietary variability. Then, healthy volunteers varying in phenotype (age, sex, and body composition) could be employed to create reference metabolomic profile databases based on plasma and urinary samples. Then, "unknowns" could be run with the original databases appropriate for the given phenotype to ascertain where in the spectrum of dietary variability the unknown lies. Thus, the dietary profile of the subject would be characterized. This does not quantify food and nutrient intake patterns and will not replace such areas of investigation. However, it does overcome the enormous bottleneck that exists in dietary phenotyping, namely, energy underreporting, in which subjects misreport the consumption of a food or, if consumed, its frequency of consumption and portion size. In this scenario, the true overall pattern of food and nutrient intake will have been ascertained, and quantification at that point may lead to reduced manipulation of the truth, because the truth will have been ascertained by objective modern technologies.

A parallel question that will arise is whether, once a metabolomic profile has been established, any inference might be made as to the biological future of someone with that metabolic profile, such as their likely metabolic response, favorable or otherwise, to some change in diet. Until recently, this has been seen as belonging to the realm of nutrigenetics, which studies how common genetic variants (single-nucleotide polymorphisms) influence the responsiveness to dietary change. However, a recent study in rats has shown that knowledge of the metabolic profile of an animal prior to pharmacological intervention can accurately predict responsiveness to the test drug. At first this seems somewhat unexpected, but on reflection, the metabolomic profile is the ultimate signature of the product of phenotype as well as gene expression and single-nucleotide polymorphism and, as such, is the "universal biomarker."

## 3.3 BOTTLENECKS IN THE HUMAN NUTRITION METABOLOMICS RESEARCH ROAD MAP

Using metabolomics to characterize the human diet or to predict any biological consequence of a given metabolomic profile is at present within the realm of visionary thinking. In reality, many bottlenecks exist in this field that need to be addressed before that path can be realistically followed. Foundation studies that determine the relative strengths of the various determinants of the human nutrition metabolome need to be put in place in order to increase our confidence in interpreting the results of such studies. Such determinants include the acute, chronic, and acute-on-chronic effects of diet, including nutrients and nonnutrients, the role of phenotype and endogenous metabolism, and the role of the colonic microflora. There is also another major research challenge to human nutritional metabolomics. At present, most metabolomics research uses nontargeted approaches, that is, a total data capture approach. When two treatments or conditions are seen to differ using PCA, the relative importance of different parts of the NMR or MS spectra can be examined to ascertain which parts make the greatest contribution to the difference between treatments. Once the main differential compounds have been identified, a hypothesis can be generated to explain why these compounds might play such a role. In effect, this moves from the hypothesis-generating mode to the hypothesis-testing mode. Although this approach will continue to prosper, in human nutrition there is a commitment to a parallel approach in which the human nutrition metabolome is identified and in which there is an aspiration for the development of a new technology that would not only identify all the metabolites of this human nutrition metabolome but also quantify them in the various biofluids. The European Nutrigenomics Organisation (www.nugo.org) is committed to defining the human nutrition metabolome and to creating an open-source database on the biological details of all compounds in the human nutritional metabolome (www.nugowiki.org). This database will link with that of the Human Metabolome Database (www.metabolomics.ca), which is a major project of Genome Canada. The basic philosophy is that one day we will have access to a list of all nutrients present in plasma, for example, that are important in human nutrition and the pathways they regulate. Additionally, the factors controlling the balance of these nutrients, such as genetic factors, will be described in detail, and the normal and abnormal concentration ranges will be known. Thus, normal values for plasma cholesterol are well established, and so we can recognize low and high levels. In an ideal world we could recognize normality for the concentrations of the totality of plasma nutrients and related compounds in a metabolomic signature and, if that can be achieved, we should be able to recognize metabolic perturbations at an early stage.

## 3.4 WHAT IS THE FUTURE FOR METABOLOMICS IN PERSONALIZED NUTRITION?

Although metabolomics offers much potential for our understanding of diet and health, the subject is too immature at present to stake any special claim as a unique tool in personalized nutrition. Many basic foundation studies are needed to understand the relative strengths of the many determinants of the nutritional metabolome and its change with diet. Only when we have a firm understanding of these forces will we be able to plan and interpret the studies that will allow the true potential of metabolomics in personalized nutrition to be established. However, conceptually, metabolism is so close to nutrition that the likelihood that metabolomics will play a significant role in personalizing nutrition is significant. Recently, metabolomic profiling has been used to predict responsiveness to drug therapy in rodents. However, humans are far more heterogeneous than their rodent counterparts, and nutrient-based signals are much softer than those for pharma. However, the road map to test the role of metabolomics in personalized nutrition is clear and, thus far, uncluttered. The next 5 years will be critical.

## KEY READINGS

Bollard, M.E., Stanley, E.G., Lindon, J.C., Nicholson, J.K., and Holmes, E. NMR-based metabonomic approaches for evaluating physiological influences on biofluid composition. *NMR Biomed* 18: 143–62, 2005.

German, J.B., Hammock, B.D., and Watkins, S.M. Metabolomics: building on a century of biochemistry to guide human health. *Metabolomics* 1: 3–9, 2005.

Gibney, M.J., Walsh, M.C., Brennan, L., Roche, H.M., German, B., and van Ommen, B. Metabolomics in human nutrition: opportunities and challenges. *Am J Clin Nutr* 82: 497–503, 2005.

Keun, H.C. Metabonomic modeling of drug toxicity. *Pharmacol Ther* 109: 92–106, 2006.
Lamers, R.J., van Nesselrooij, J.H., Kraus, V.B., Jordan, J.M., Renner, J.B., Dragomir, A.D., Luta, G., van der Greef, J., and DeGroot J. Identification of a urinary metabolite profile associated with osteoarthritis. *Osteoarthritis Cartilage* 13:762–8, 2005.
Nicholson, J.K., Holmes, E., and Wilson, I.D. Gut microorganisms, mammalian metabolism and personalized health care. *Nat Review Microbiol* 3: 431–8, 2005.

# 4 Nutrition, Genomics, and Cardiovascular Disease Risk

*Jose M. Ordovas and Dolores Corella*

## CONTENTS



## 4.1 INTRODUCTION

The existence in the population of hyper- and hyporesponders to dietary modification and to any other therapeutic approach is a well-known phenomenon. Whereas some individuals are able to improve their plasma lipid profile or body weight using the current dietary guidelines, others are unable to gain any significant benefit. The basis for these interindividual differences are complex, and current knowledge suggests that it is partially genetic. During the last two decades, evidence of interaction between traditional lipid metabolism candidate genes, dietary components, and cardiovascular risk factors (i.e., plasma lipids and obesity-related traits) has been slowly gaining momentum. Several experimental approaches have been used for this research, including observational and interventional studies. However, the replication among studies is still limited, mostly driven by less-than-optimal experimental designs. Current studies are starting to incorporate experimental approaches (i.e., increased coverage of the genetic variation at each locus) that could provide more solid results. However, other limitations, such as small populations that limit the statistical power especially to examine higher-level interactions (gene–gene–diet–behavioral factors) have yet to be incorporated in nutrigenetic studies. Moreover, the current quality of the dietary and behavioral information adds another major limitation, specifically for observational studies. These needs can be met through the collaboration of experts in the different fields involved, ranging from basic scientists to computational biologists and behavioral scientists. Once more solid evidence is achieved, nutrigenomics could be applied toward primary prevention and treatment of cardiovascular diseases in the general population and subjects at high risk.

The effect of dietary changes on cardiovascular disease (CVD)-relevant traits (i.e., plasma lipid measures, glucose levels, body weight, and blood pressure) differs significantly among individuals [1]. Some individuals appear to be relatively insensitive (hyporesponders) to dietary intervention, whereas others display enhanced sensitivity (hyperresponders) [1]. This phenomenon has been more extensively researched in relation to changes in dietary fat and plasma lipid concentrations for the prevention of CVD compared to other pathological conditions. Although common knowledge associates low-fat diets with reductions in total and plasma low-density lipoprotein cholesterol (LDL-C), the clinical evidence shows dramatic interindividual differences in response and may be one of the underlying causes of the limited success of dietary recommendations in the prevention of diseases observed by recent randomized clinical trials [2].

A growing body of data supports the hypothesis that the interindividual variability in response to dietary modification is determined by genetic factors [3]. Indirect evidence comes from the general observation that the phenotypic response to diet is determined partly by the baseline value of the phenotype, which is itself affected by genetic factors [1]. Some of the main challenges are the following: (1) how to uncover and elucidate the many potential gene–diet interactions; (2) how to include in the experimental designs the ability to test for gene–gene–diet interactions; (3) how to investigate more complex and realistic scenarios, including the contributions of other behavioral factors (i.e., physical activity, smoking, socioeconomic status, traditions, and social environment); and (4) how to collect reliable and standardized information of relevant covariates [4]

Several studies have found specific candidate genes to be associated with the variability in response of LDL-C levels in response to changes in dietary fat, but so far, the humbling reality is that these findings have been highly inconsistent. These conflicting outcomes reflect both the complexity of the mechanisms involved in dietary responses and the limitations of the current experimental designs used to address these problems, some of which are due to the challenges listed in the previous paragraph. In addition, we need to keep in mind that the practical translation to the public of any nutrigenetic finding needs to be supported by a more holistic approach to health rather than applying the tunnel-vision approach of focusing exclusively on the changes in one particular risk factor. To this effect, it is true that low-fat diets can result in reduced plasma LDL-C levels, but also in lowering of HDL-C and increased triacylglycerol (TAG) concentrations, which may be particularly harmful for some persons. For example, it has been shown that individuals with a predominance of small, dense LDL particles (subclass pattern B), a phenotype that is associated with an increased risk of coronary heart disease, benefit more from a low-fat diet [5] than do those with the subclass pattern A (larger LDL). A significant proportion of the latter group unexpectedly exhibited a more atherogenic pattern B subclass after consuming a low-fat diet. Intervention studies are increasingly focusing on the interindividual differences in response to diet rather than on the mean effect analyzed for a population. Moreover, new evidence indicates that the variability in response is an intrinsic characteristic of the individual, rather than being the result of differing dietary compliance with the experimental protocols. Jacobs et al. [6] found that individual TAG responses to a high-fat or to a low-fat diet were vastly different, suggesting that many patients with hypertriglyceridemia are not treated optimally if general advice for either a low-fat or a high-fat diet is given. Understanding the mechanisms driving this variation will not only allow us to better grasp the biology of dietary response but also to identify individuals who can benefit from a particular dietary intervention.

## 4.2 HOW NUTRIENTS COMMUNICATE WITH GENES

There has been an ongoing debate about the correct term that would encompass the overarching goal of understanding the interaction between nutrients and genes and how different individuals may modulate the interaction according to their genome. Thus, the terms *nutrigenomics*, *nutrigenetics*, *nutritional genomics*, among others, have been used in the literature, and the ontology of each term has not been conclusively determined. In this work we will adhere to the convention used in the pharmacological field that we have previously described [7]. Therefore, before presenting some of the current nutrigenetic evidence in the area of lipid metabolism and CVD, it is helpful to gain an understanding of how nutrients and other chemicals in the diet may influence gene expression and drive gene–diet interactions, which covers, according to the previously indicated convention, the subject proper of nutrigenomics, which seeks to understand gene–diet interactions in the context of the total genetic makeup of each individual. Past technological limitations restricted investigators to a piecemeal approach: one gene, one gene product, and one nutrient at a time. Conceptual and technological advances are changing the playing field. For the first time, researchers can cast a wide net in the form of microarrays that can potentially capture the information about each one of the genes expressed in a specific cell or tissue of interest. Despite these advances, the challenges are not trivial, given the chemical complexity of food and our incomplete knowledge about the various bioactive components present in food grown in different climates at different times of the year. Moreover, our ability to carry out mechanistic studies in humans gets impaired by (1) our inability to assay gene expression in the most appropriate target tissues in humans and (2) the still-prohibitive cost of performing experiments using adequate number of samples, assay replicates, and time points or intervention levels.

Regulation of expression of genes involved in fatty acid metabolism may occur when a dietary fat or metabolite binds to and activates specific fatty acid transcription factors. These dietary chemical-regulated transcription factors are members of the nuclear receptor superfamily. This gene family consists of 48 mammalian transcription factors that regulate nearly all aspects of development, inflammation, and metabolism. Two subclasses, the peroxisome proliferator-activated receptors (PPARs) and liver X receptors (LXRs), are lipid-sensing receptors that have critical roles in lipid and glucose metabolism [8]. PPARs are among the best-studied fatty-acid-regulated nuclear receptors [9]. After uptake into target cells, a subset of them are transported to the nucleus in association with fatty acid binding proteins (FABPs), which facilitates their interaction with PPARs. Several PPAR subtypes have been described. PPAR-alpha (PPARA) plays a key role in lipid oxidation and inflammation, whereas PPAR-gamma (PPARG) is involved in cell (adipocyte) differentiation, glucose lipid storage, and inflammation. PPAR-delta (PPARD, also known as PPAR-beta) may play an important role in development, lipid metabolism, and inflammation [10].

Many of the previously published nutrigenetic [i.e., single-gene/single-nucleotide polymorphisms (SNPs)] studies focused on genes that are the subject of regulation by PPARs and other nuclear receptors [11]. Polymorphisms in promoter regions of these genes may disrupt, or at least alter, the communication with these transcription factors, which would have significant consequences in a person's response to dietary factors that are ligands (i.e., PUFAs) of the transcription factors. It is also obvious that polymorphisms within the transcription factors themselves will have a significant impact on the way each one of us responds to dietary components [12–14].

The quantitative evidence for gene–diet interactions between common SNPs at candidate genes and dietary factors related to lipid metabolism is increasing. However, we reiterate that caution is needed before applying these results to clinical practice for three primary reasons: (1) the meaning of "statistically significant results" is subject to differing interpretations and often depends on the study design, (2) many initial gene–nutrient–phenotypes associations were not replicated in subsequent studies, and (3) gene variations may influence phenotypes differently in individuals from different ancestral backgrounds owing to gene–gene (epistatic) interactions.

## 4.3 OBSERVATIONAL STUDIES: THE CURRENT WORKHORSE OF NUTRIGENETICS

Observational studies have the advantage of allowing the collection of data on large numbers of subjects and the ability to estimate long-term dietary habits. However, the level of evidence of the results obtained from these studies has traditionally been considered to be lower than that of experimental studies, and this topic has been extensively reviewed [7,15].

The median population size for recent observational studies is approximately below 1000. This sample size may be informative for traditional single genotype–phenotype association studies but, considering the higher measurement error of dietary intake in comparison with experimental studies, it may not have enough statistical power to address properly the complexity of gene–environment interactions, and the replication of results is still very low. The main reasons for the disparities are not much different from those already indicated previously; however, another factor to consider is that the interpretation of the studies may be much affected by differences in the analytic strategies and study populations. Investigators have reported different results for association of the Pro12 allele and T2DM by PUFA intake when they used different modeling methods (or statistical packages). If such differences are found within the same population, it is expected that different modeling methods may have an even more pronounced effect in diverse population groups. So, it is not surprising that when different study populations are combined with different analytical techniques, there are so many inconsistencies in the literature [14].

So far, most of the initial descriptions of gene–diet interactions have been based on observational studies; regardless of the apparent solidity of any initial reported finding, every gene–diet interaction needs to go through a series of verification steps, which should at least include (1) its replication on several other properly sized populations, (2) its testing on an interventional study in people preselected on the basis of their genotypes for the SNP under consideration, and (3) additional *in vitro* and *ex vivo* tests of functionality to provide the mechanistic knowledge that will support the reported statistical interactions. Moreover, genotype-nutrient-phenotype analyses may be improved by determining ancestral backgrounds of each study participant. These additional data are necessary because SNPs may be expressed differently among individuals of differing ethnicities because of varying gene-gene and gene-nutrient interactions.

The enumeration of those studies focusing on the interaction between genetic variants at candidate genes, nutrients, and CVD risk factors have been the subject of recent reviews [7,15,16], and we will not reproduce their contents in this chapter. Rather, we will focus on capturing the current trends in nutrigenetic research.

We will begin by focusing on one of the rising genes from the last few years: apolipoprotein A5 (*APOA5*). Totally unknown until 2001, APOA5 has become a major player in lipoprotein metabolism and specifically in triglyceride-rich lipoprotein (TRL) metabolism [17]. Five common *APOA5* SNPs have been reported in several populations: −1131T > C, −3A > G, 56C > G IVS3 + 476G > A, and 1259T > C, and these *APOA5* gene variants have been associated with increased TAG concentrations [18–21]. With the exception of the 56C > G SNP, the SNPs are reported to be in significant linkage disequilibrium [22]. Despite the relative good consistency with plasma TAG concentrations, the association between *APOA5* SNPs (or haplotypes) and CVD risk is still controversial [19,23,24]. Learning from previous experience, it is reasonable to implicate gene environment interactions modulating the association with CVD risk factors as well as with the disease risk itself. Consistent with this hypothesis, several intriguing interactions are beginning to emerge. In the Framingham Heart Study, we have reported a gene–diet interaction between the *APOA5* gene variation and the polyunsaturated fatty acids (PUFA) in relation to plasma lipid concentrations and lipoprotein particle size [25]. Furthermore, we have demonstrated that obesity modulates the effect of the *APOA5* gene variation in carotid intimal medial thickness (IMT), a surrogate measure of atherosclerosis burden. This association remained significant even after the adjustment for TG [26]. More recently, we have found a gene–diet interaction between the APOA5 gene and total fat intake in relation to body mass index (BMI), overweight, and obesity risk [27]. The homogeneity of this interaction was detected in both men and women and followed a dose-response relationship. In comparison with wild-type subjects, the carriers of the variant C allele at the −1131T > C SNP appeared to be protected from an increase in body weight when consuming more dietary fat. Interactions between BMI and *APOA5* had been previously reported by Aberle et al. [28]. Moreover, some interesting peculiarities are emerging that deserve further examination.

One relates to the specificity of the interactions in terms of the location of the *APOA5* tagging SNPs, one in the promoter region (−1131T > C) and the other affecting the primary structure of the protein (56C > G). We have reported that the complex interactions between *APOA5* SNPs, dietary intake, BMI, and IMT appear to be related to the promoter polymorphism, whereas the *APOA5* 56C > G SNP appears to associate with the different traits independently of environmental triggers [25–27]. The second aspect to consider is the specificity of the interactions in terms of dietary fat, being different for saturated, monounsaturated, and polyunsaturated n-6 and n-3. We investigated the interaction between these *APOA5* SNPs and dietary fat in determining plasma fasting TGs, remnant-like particle (RLP) concentrations, and lipoprotein particle size in Framingham Heart Study participants. Significant gene–diet interactions between the −1131T > C SNP and PUFA intake were found in determining fasting TGs, RLP concentrations, and lipoprotein particle size, but these interactions were not found for the 56C > G polymorphism [25]. The −1131C allele was associated with higher fasting TGs and RLP concentrations in only the subjects consuming a high-PUFA diet (>6% of total energy), regardless of gender. Interestingly, when we further analyzed the effects of n-6 and n-3 fatty acids, we found that the PUFA–*APOA5* interactions were specific for dietary n-6 fatty acids. Thus, higher n-6 (but not n-3) PUFA intake increased fasting TGs, RLP concentrations, and VLDL size and decreased LDL size in *APOA5* −1131C carriers, suggesting that n-6 PUFA-rich diets are related to a more atherogenic lipid profile in these subjects. This could shed some light into the data coming from postprandial studies [29–33] that will be discussed in the following text. Similar specificities in terms of SNP, exclusive for the −1131T > C, and dietary fat, primarily monounsaturated fat, were found in relation to the interaction between fat intake and BMI within the Framingham Study [27].

These observations suggest some new hypotheses regarding some of the observed geographical differences in CVD risk as well as the changes in risk observed following Westernization of lifestyles. In this regard, it is important to pay attention to the differences in allele frequencies of the *APOA5* SNPs identified so far. These frequencies appear to be higher in Asian compared to White populations [18]. If the interactions observed in Framingham apply to other geographical areas, we should expect that an increased fraction of the Asian population will be placed at higher CVD risk because of the current trend toward higher dietary fat intakes, especially if they are driven by increases in PUFA n-6. Moreover, we found in the Framingham Study that some individuals (carriers of the C allele at the −1131T > C SNP) may consume a high percentage of fat, especially MUFA, in their habitual diet without adversely affecting their BMI and their risk of overweight and obesity [27].

The studies described earlier provide evidence of the current transition from the traditional approach of studying one SNP per gene to a more comprehensive examination using multiple SNPs and haplotypes. Moreover, they represent a sample of the exploding interest for obesity-related phenotypes and their complications. Given the current public attention to this problem, it is not surprising that increasing number of researchers aim their focus on the investigation of gene–diet and obesity-related parameters.

Some of the recent reports examine obvious but previously ignored candidate genes. This is the case with the loci encoding the carnitine palmitoyltransferase I

(CPT1), a key enzyme in beta-oxidation of fatty acids. Robitaille et al. [34] screened the genes for CPT1A (11q13) and CPT1B (22qter) for common mutations in a French-Canadian population and selected nine variants within CPT1B and one variant within CPT1A for further analyses in relation with obesity based on the minor allele frequency (>10%) or on potential functional impact. A significant association between obesity phenotypes (BMI, weight, and waist girth) and CPT1B c.282-18C > T and p.E531K variants was observed. When subjects were divided into six groups according to p.E531K genotypes and further on the basis of fat using the median value as a cutoff point (34.4% of energy), BMI, weight, and waist girth were higher in E531/K531 on a high-fat diet compared to E531/K531 subjects under a low-fat diet. There was no difference among E531/E531 and K531/K531. This interaction is complex to interpret as the statistically significant interaction was driven by heterozygotes, and no differences were observed for the homozygous at each of the extremes. Similar results were obtained with the CPT1A p.A275T variant as BMI and waist girth were higher in A275/A275 on a high-fat diet compared to A275/A275 subjects on a low-fat diet. Among carriers of the T275 allele, obesity indices were not affected by fat intake. These findings suggest that obesity-related traits might be modulated by an interaction between CPT1 variants and fat intake, but their interpretation is not straightforward.

Other studies were initially designed to examine the genetics of obesity and to identify significant and valuable nutritional interactions. This was the case with NUGENOB [35]. This study examined 42 SNPs at 26 candidate genes for obesity in 549 adult obese women recruited from eight European centers in a case-only study. The nutritional variables assessed in this study were the dietary fiber intake (grams per day), the ratio of dietary polyunsaturated fat to saturated fat (P:S ratio), and the percentage of energy derived from fat in the diet as calculated from a weighed 3-d food record (%E). Some weak, confirmatory evidence for genotype-by-nutrient interactions in obesity was detected in this case-only study [i.e., hepatic lipase gene (LIPC); adiponectin (ADIPOQ) and PPARG3]. Although this design was initially considered useful for detecting interactions, the authors state that few genotype-by-nutrient interactions have been suggested in obese European women after completing the initial goals of the study.

Our own studies focused on the gene for human perilipin (PLIN), which is on chromosome 15q26, in the region of a linkage locus for diabetes, hypertriglyceridemia, and obesity. In a study to examine the regulation of lipolysis in obese and nonobese women [36], it was found that obese women exhibited two- to fourfold higher basal rates of lipolysis in fat cells obtained through a biopsy in the abdominal subcutaneous area. Similar differences in lipolysis rates were observed following noradrenaline induction. It was also noted that adipocyte perilipin content was reduced in obese women. This study also examined the effect of a polymorphism (11482G > A) in intron 6 of the perilipin locus in relation to perilipin content as well as the rates of lipolysis. Adipose tissue from women who were homozygous for the A allele at position 11482 exhibited 50 to 100% higher rates of lipolysis and 80% lower perilipin content. Following this study, several polymorphisms at the perilipin locus have been examined for potential associations with BMI or obesity risk. We have examined four SNPs (PLIN1: 6209T > C, PLIN4:11482G > A, PLIN5: 13041A > G, and

PLIN6:14995A > T) in several geographically and ethnically diverse populations to determine the patterns of linkage disequilibrium in the various populations and the associations between these polymorphisms with obesity-related traits. Our first report included 1589 white patient samples from a general Spanish population [37]. The aforementioned SNPs were common, with minor allele frequencies ranging from 0.26 to 0.38. Two of these (6209T > C and 11482G > A) were in strong linkage disequilibrium (D′ 0.96). The presence of one or both of these SNPs was associated with lower BMI and reduced risk of obesity in women. A significant gene–gender interaction was observed, however, and the effect was seen only in women. In addition, the 11482G > A polymorphism also showed significant associations with fasting glucose and triglyceride concentrations. Conversely, a trend was observed for the other two SNPs (13041A > G and 14995A > T) to be associated with increased BMI and risk of obesity. These same polymorphisms were then examined in 734 white patients (373 men and 361 women) who were attending a residential lifestyle modification program in California [38]. As with the study in Spain, the effects were seen primarily in women. As in Spanish women, the 6209T > C and the 11482G > A polymorphisms were associated with lower BMI. These associations, however, did not reach statistical significance. Instead, the presence of the rare alleles at positions 13041 and 14995 were associated with increased BMI. At this stage, it appeared that the rare alleles at positions 6209 and 11482 at the 5′ end of the perilipin locus had opposite effects on BMI when compared with the minor alleles at positions 13041 and 14995, at the 3′ end of the perilipin locus. Whereas the presence of the former was associated with reduced BMI, the latter were associated with increased BMI. In line with this notion, the haplotype that included the common alleles at the 6209T > C, 11482G > A SNPs and the rare alleles at the 13041A > G and 14995A > T SNPs had the greatest effect on obesity risk in the population in California. We subsequently proceeded to examine these SNPs in a multiethnic population living in Singapore comprising 2763 Chinese, 726 Malays, and 598 Asian Indians [39]. One interesting finding was that the intragenic linkage disequilibrium structure of the perilipin locus differed between populations that were white compared with populations of Asian extraction. Specifically, in whites, the 11482G > A polymorphism was in strong positive linkage disequilibrium with the 6209T > C polymorphism and negative linkage disequilibrium with the 13041A > G and 14995 A > T polymorphisms. In Chinese, Malays, and Asian Indians living in Singapore, the situation was reversed, with the 11482G > A polymorphism in negative linkage disequilibrium with the 6209T > C polymorphisms and in positive linkage disequilibrium with the 13041A > G and the 14995A > T polymorphisms. Given the differences in patterns of linkage disequilibrium observed, one would expect that the rare allele for the 11482G > A polymorphism, which was associated with lower levels of obesity in the white population, would be associated with increased levels of obesity in the Asian populations. In fact, this is exactly what was observed. Moreover, as in the two previous studies, the significant associations were observed only in females. They were only present in Malays and Asian Indians, however, not in Chinese. It is also worth noting that another study including 1120 individuals from France failed to find a statistically significant association between the 11482G > A polymorphism [40].

It is unclear at this time why no association was observed in French and Chinese ethnic groups despite being reasonably powered to detect an association, if present. If indeed complex traits such as obesity are a consequence of interactions between genetic and environmental factors [41], such gene–environment interactions could explain the discrepant findings among populations. It could simply be that the French and Chinese are exposed to different environments when compared with whites in Spain or California, and Malays and Asian Indians in Singapore. Do such gene–environment interactions operate in relation to the association between polymorphisms at the perilipin locus and obesity? In fact, the interaction between polymorphisms at this locus and gender has already been described in whites and some of the Asian groups. Recently, one study [42] has reported that individuals carrying the A allele for the 11482G > A polymorphism are resistant to weight loss with caloric restriction. Another [43] reported resistance to weight gain following treatment with the PPARG agonist rosiglitozone in individuals carrying this polymorphism. Therefore, overweight and obese individuals carrying this allele may not benefit from traditional dietary approaches to losing weight, and alternative approaches may be needed. In this regard, an interesting observation was made regarding the potential regulatory effects of a plant extract on perilipin, hormone-sensitive lipase, and other parameters of lipid metabolism in obese women [44].

Up to this point, we have dealt primarily with associations between polymorphisms at the perilipin locus and their associations with the degree of obesity *per se*, as opposed to the downstream effects of obesity, such as insulin resistance. Jang et al. [45] studied 177 obese Korean men and women who were treated with caloric restriction (–300 kcal per day) and found that the presence of the A11482 allele was associated with greater weight loss in response to caloric restriction and that this weight loss was primarily in the visceral fat compartment. Because visceral obesity is generally associated with increased plasma-free fatty acid concentrations, one may expect a greater reduction in plasma-free fatty acids in these individuals. Instead, these individuals experienced an increase in plasma-free fatty acids despite a greater reduction in visceral fat mass.

It is important to remember that fatty acids serve not only as a source of energy but also as signaling molecules. Free fatty acids result in impaired glucose homeostasis and may increase the risk of type 2 diabetes mellitus. To test the hypothesis that dietary fat may interact with polymorphisms at the perilipin locus to modulate diabetes-related traits, we reexamined data from the Singapore population, taking into consideration dietary macronutrient intake [46]. We found evidence of an interaction between dietary fat (specifically saturated fat) intake, polymorphisms at the perilipin locus (11482G > A and 114995A > T), and insulin resistance. Greater intake of energy from saturated fats was associated with increased insulin resistance among individuals who were homozygous for the rare alleles but not individuals who carried the common allele. This effect was independent of BMI and consistent with the associations with anthropometric measures; these interactions were observed only in women.

Overall, observational studies have provided substantial support to the concept of gene–diet interactions modulating cardiovascular risk factors; however, very few findings have been consistently replicated; among several concerns related to this approach, we want to underscore the need for more reliable assessment of dietary intake.

## 4.4 INTERVENTIONAL STUDIES IN NUTRIGENETICS

Interventional studies in which subjects receive a controlled dietary intake provide the best approach to conducting gene–nutrient–phenotype interaction studies. However, well-controlled feeding studies have several important logistical limitations, most importantly, the small number of participants and the brief duration of the interventions. Scores of interventional studies examining gene–diet interactions on different parameters of lipid metabolism have been published. However, similar to the situation described for observational studies, the level of replication among studies analyzing the same genetic variation tends to be low. The lack of replication is most likely due to the different characteristics (ethnicity, physical condition, age, and lifestyle differences) of study subjects, length of intervention, sample size, and heterogeneity in the design. In an initial systematic review, Masson et al. [47] identified 74 relevant articles, including dietary intervention studies, in which the lipid and lipoprotein response to diet in different genotype groups were measured and 17 reviews on gene–diet interactions. After a comparative analysis of the individual findings, they concluded that there is evidence to suggest that (1) variations in the *APOA1*, *APOA4*, *APOB*, and *APOE* genes contribute to the heterogeneity in the lipid response to dietary intervention and (2) all of these genes are regulated directly or indirectly by PPARA or other nuclear receptors. However, the evidence suggested by Masson et al. in relation to the foregoing genes comes from meta-analyses of the published data and described the average effect. The absence of total consistency of results among individual studies should be noted.

More recently, we [7,15,16] reviewed this topic extensively and included additional studies reported after 2002. The median for the sample sizes in these more recent studies was in the range of 60 subjects. These small sample sizes highlight one of the bases for the lack of reproducibility: the statistical power is very low, specially when the allele groups have not been balanced by *a priori* selection of the study subjects. In addition, the composition of the dietary intervention in these studies varied considerably. We propose that the design of future intervention studies be standardized for key dietary intake variables and phenotype measurements. A minimum set of variables would include patients' physical and genetic characteristics, medications, composition and length of the dietary treatment, and sample size. Such standardization would allow better comparison among studies and the possibility of conducting meta-analyses, which is not possible under current experimental conditions.

## 4.5 GENE–DIET INTERACTIONS IN THE POSTPRANDIAL STATE

Human beings living in industrialized societies spend most of the waking hours in a nonfasting state because of meal consumption patterns and the amounts of food ingested. Postprandial lipemia, characterized by a rise in TAG after eating, is a dynamic, non-steady-state condition [48]. Over 25 years ago, Zilversmit [49] proposed that atherogenesis was a postprandial phenomenon because high concentrations of lipoproteins and their remnants following food ingestion could deposit into the arterial wall and accumulate in atheromatous plaques. Several studies have investigated the potential interaction between some polymorphisms in candidate genes and diet on postprandial lipids (for a review see Reference 7). In postprandial studies, subjects usually receive a fat-loading test meal that has differing compositions depending on the nutrients to be tested. After the test meal, blood samples are taken to measure postprandial lipids to compare with preprandial levels [48]. Consistency among studies is still very low, and replication of findings is a major necessity. Postprandial studies often have low numbers of subjects (usually <50), with the added complexity that their designs may add even more bias than those seen in other experimental approaches [50].

Postprandial studies have also shown the specificity of the different dietary fat as drivers of gene–diet interactions. Thus, the slightly different outcomes regarding the interaction between postprandial metabolism and the *APOA5* SNPs [29–33] made us hypothesize that an impaired postprandial response in carriers of the C allele at the −1131T > C SNP could be triggered by PUFA n-6 rather than by saturated fatty acids.

This type of experimental approach faces some logistical problems, including standardization of the protocols (type of meals used for the fat load and time of sample collection). Moreover, it requires keeping the participating subjects for several hours at the study site. Conversely, a major advantage is that significant information might be gained in the space of 1 d of intervention vs. the weeks or months required to examine changes in lipids in the fasting state.

## 4.6 CONCLUSIONS AND STEPS FORWARD

Despite the excitement due to an increasing number of findings related to nutritional genomics, progress in the field is hampered by the inadequacy of the current experimental approaches to efficiently deal with the biological complexity of the phenotypes, the complexity of dietary intakes, differing genetic background among participants, and the limitations of low statistical power of the studies. We and others have proposed that only a comprehensive, international nutritional genomics approach [51,52] will yield short- and long-term benefits to human health by (1) revealing novel nutrient–gene interactions, (2) developing new diagnostic tests for adverse responses to diets, (3) identifying specific populations with special nutrient needs, (4) improving the consistency of current definitions and methodology related to dietary assessment, and (5) providing the information for developing more nutritious plant and animal foods and food formulations that promote health and prevent, mitigate, or cure disease. Achieving these goals will require extensive dialogue between scientists and the public about the nutritional needs of the individual vs. groups, local food availability and customs, analysis and understanding of genetic differences among individuals and populations, and serious commitment of funds from the public and private sectors. Nutritional genomics' researchers are seeking collaborations of scientists, scholars, and policymakers to maximize the collective impact on global poverty and health by advancing our knowledge of how genetics and nutrition can promote health or cause disease.

Although the current evidence from both experimental and observational nutrigenetics studies is not enough to start making specific personalized nutritional recommendations based on genetic information, there are a large number of examples of common SNPs modulating the individual response to diet as proof of concept of how gene–diet interactions can influence lipid metabolism. It is critical that these preliminary studies go through further replication and that subsequent studies be properly designed with sufficient statistical power and careful attention to phenotype and genotype. The many challenges that lie ahead are evident. This review has examined the vast world of nutrigenetics and nutrigenomics only through the small keyhole of lipid metabolism-related genes and dietary fat. These initial steps in understanding nutrigenomics will likely lead to fundamental breakthroughs that will both clarify today's mysteries and pave the way for clinical applications. However, to arrive at the point where it is possible to assess the modulation by specific SNPs of the effects of dietary interventions on lipid metabolism, well-designed, adequately powered, and adequately interpreted randomized controlled studies (or their equivalent) of greater duration than current studies are needed, with careful consideration given to which patients to include in such studies. Moreover, research must also investigate the potential mechanisms involved in the gene–diet interactions reported by nutrigenetic studies [51]. These imperative needs can be achieved only through the collaboration of experts in the different fields involved, which must include nutrition professionals [52]. In addition, a number of important changes in the provision of health care are needed to achieve the potential benefits associated with this concept, including a teamwork approach, with greater integration among physicians and nutrition professionals. Once more experience is gained from patients and individuals at high risk, these approaches could be applied toward primary prevention of CVD.

## ACKNOWLEDGMENTS

This work was supported by NIH grants HL72524, HL54776, and DK075030 and by contracts 53-K06-5-10 and 58-1950-9-001 from the U.S. Department of Agriculture Research Service. (JMO), and contracts 53-K06-5-10 and 58-1950-9-001 from the U.S. Department of Agriculture Research Service (JMO), and the Spanish Ministerio de Educación y Ciencia (PR2006-0258) and the Spanish Ministerio de Sanidad (CB06/03/0035).

## SUGGESTED LECTURES/URLS

www.nugo.org.
http://www.athero.org/.
http://www.isnn.info/.
http://www.nutragenomics.com.

## REFERENCES

1. Katan, M. B.; Beynen, A. C.; de Vries, J. H.; et al. Existence of consistent hypo- and hyperresponders to dietary cholesterol in man. *American journal of epidemiology* 123: 221–234; 1986.
2. Prentice, R. L.; Caan, B.; Chlebowski, R. T. et al. Low-fat dietary pattern and risk of invasive breast cancer: the Women's Health Initiative Randomized Controlled Dietary Modification Trial. *Jama* 295: 629–642; 2006.
3. Loktionov, A. Common gene polymorphisms and nutrition: emerging links with pathogenesis of multifactorial chronic diseases (review). *Journal of nutritional biochemistry* 14: 426–451; 2003.
4. Greenwood, D. C.; Gilthorpe, M. S.; Cade, J. E. The impact of imprecisely measured covariates on estimating gene-environment interactions. *BMC medical research methodology* 6: 21; 2006.
5. Krauss, R. M. Dietary and genetic effects on low-density lipoprotein heterogeneity. *Annual review of nutrition* 21: 283–295; 2001.
6. Jacobs, B.; De Angelis-Schierbaum, G.; Egert, S.; et al. Individual serum triglyceride responses to high-fat and low-fat diets differ in men with modest and severe hypertriglyceridemia. *The Journal of nutrition* 134: 1400–1405; 2004.
7. Ordovas, J. M.; Corella, D. Nutritional genomics. *Annual review of genomics and human genetics* 5: 71–118; 2004.
8. Jump, D. B. Fatty acid regulation of gene transcription. *Critical reviews in clinical laboratory sciences* 41: 41–78; 2004.
9. Clarke, S. D. The multi-dimensional regulation of gene expression by fatty acids: polyunsaturated fats as nutrient sensors. *Current opinion in lipidology* 15: 13–18; 2004.
10. Tobin, J. F.; Freedman, L. P. Nuclear receptors as drug targets in metabolic diseases: new approaches to therapy. *Trends in endocrinology and metabolism: TEM* 17: 284–290; 2006.
11. Mandard, S.; Muller, M.; Kersten, S. Peroxisome proliferator-activated receptor alpha target genes. *Cellular and molecular life sciences* 61: 393–416; 2004.
12. Soriguer, F.; Morcillo, S.; Cardona, F. et al. Pro12Ala polymorphism of the PPARG2 gene is associated with type 2 diabetes mellitus and peripheral insulin sensitivity in a population with a high intake of oleic acid. *The journal of nutrition* 136: 2325–2330; 2006.
13. Tai, E. S.; Corella, D.; Demissie, S.; et al. Polyunsaturated fatty acids interact with the PPARA-L162V polymorphism to affect plasma triglyceride and apolipoprotein C-III concentrations in the Framingham Heart Study. *The journal of nutrition* 135: 397–403; 2005.
14. Nelson, T. L.; Fingerlin, T. E.; Moss, L. K.; et al. Association of the peroxisome proliferator-activated receptor gamma gene with type 2 diabetes mellitus varies by physical activity among non-Hispanic whites from Colorado. *Metabolism: clinical and experimental* 56: 388–393; 2007.
15. Corella, D.; Ordovas, J. M. Single nucleotide polymorphisms that influence lipid metabolism: interaction with dietary factors. *Annual review of nutrition* 25: 341–390; 2005.
16. Ordovas, J. M.; Corella, D. Genes, diet and plasma lipids: the evidence from observational studies. *World review of nutrition and dietetics* 93: 41–76; 2004.
17. Pennacchio, L. A.; Olivier, M.; Hubacek, J. A.; et al. An apolipoprotein influencing triglycerides in humans and mice revealed by comparative sequencing. *Science* 294: 169–173; 2001.
18. Lai, C. Q.; Tai, E. S.; Tan, C. E.; et al. The APOA5 locus is a strong determinant of plasma triglyceride concentrations across ethnic groups in Singapore. *Journal of lipid research* 44: 2365–2373; 2003.

19. Lai, C. Q.; Demissie, S.; Cupples, L. A.; et al. Influence of the APOA5 locus on plasma triglyceride, lipoprotein subclasses, and CVD risk in the Framingham Heart Study. *Journal of lipid research* 45: 2096–2105; 2004.
20. Talmud, P. J.; Hawe, E.; Martin, S.; et al. Relative contribution of variation within the APOC3/A4/A5 gene cluster in determining plasma triglycerides. *Human molecular genetics* 11: 3039–3046; 2002.
21. Talmud, P. J. Rare APOA5 mutations-Clinical consequences, metabolic and functional effects: an ENID review. *Atherosclerosis*; 2007.
22. Pennacchio, L. A.; Olivier, M.; Hubacek, J. A.; et al. Two independent apolipoprotein A5 haplotypes influence human plasma triglyceride levels. *Human molecular genetics* 11: 3031–3038; 2002.
23. Talmud, P. J.; Martin, S.; Taskinen, M. R.; et al. APOA5 gene variants, lipoprotein particle distribution, and progression of coronary heart disease: results from the LOCAT study. *Journal of lipid research* 45: 750–756; 2004.
24. Dallongeville, J.; Cottel, D.; Montaye, M.; et al. Impact of APOA5/A4/C3 genetic polymorphisms on lipid variables and cardiovascular disease risk in French men. *International journal of cardiology* 106: 152–156; 2006.
25. Lai, C. Q.; Corella, D.; Demissie, S.; et al. Dietary intake of n-6 fatty acids modulates effect of apolipoprotein A5 gene on plasma fasting triglycerides, remnant lipoprotein concentrations, and lipoprotein particle size: the Framingham Heart Study. *Circulation* 113: 2062–2070; 2006.
26. Elosua, R.; Ordovas, J. M.; Cupples, L. A. et al. Variants at the APOA5 locus, association with carotid atherosclerosis, and modification by obesity: the Framingham Study. *Journal of lipid research* 47: 990–996; 2006.
27. Corella, D.; Lai, C. Q.; Demissie, S.; et al. APOA5 gene variation modulates the effects of dietary fat intake on body mass index and obesity risk in the Framingham Heart Study. *Journal of molecular medicine* 85: 119–128; 2007.
28. Aberle, J.; Evans, D.; Beil, F. U.; et al. A polymorphism in the apolipoprotein A5 gene is associated with weight loss after short-term diet. *Clinical genetics* 68: 152–154; 2005.
29. Martin, S.; Nicaud, V.; Humphries, S. E.; Talmud, P. J. Contribution of APOA5 gene variants to plasma triglyceride determination and to the response to both fat and glucose tolerance challenges. *Biochimica et biophysica acta* 1637: 217–225; 2003.
30. Kim, J. Y.; Kim, O. Y.; Koh, S. J.; et al. Comparison of low-fat meal and high-fat meal on postprandial lipemic response in non-obese men according to the −1131T > C polymorphism of the apolipoprotein A5 (APOA5) gene (randomized cross-over design). *Journal of the American College of Nutrition* 25: 340–347; 2006.
31. Jang, Y.; Kim, J. Y.; Kim, O. Y.; et al. The −1131T—>C polymorphism in the apolipoprotein A5 gene is associated with postprandial hypertriacylglycerolemia; elevated small, dense LDL concentrations; and oxidative stress in nonobese Korean men. *The American journal of clinical nutrition* 80: 832–840; 2004.
32. Masana, L.; Ribalta, J.; Salazar, J.; et al. The apolipoprotein AV gene and diurnal triglyceridaemia in normolipidaemic subjects. *Clinical Chemistry and Laboratory Medicine* 41: 517–521; 2003.
33. Moreno, R.; Perez-Jimenez, F.; Marin, C.; et al. A single nucleotide polymorphism of the apolipoprotein A-V gene −1131T>C modulates postprandial lipoprotein metabolism. *Atherosclerosis* 189: 163–168; 2006.
34. Robitaille, J.; Houde, A.; Lemieux, S.; et al. Variants within the muscle and liver isoforms of the carnitine palmitoyltransferase I (CPT1) gene interact with fat intake

to modulate indices of obesity in French-Canadians. *Journal of molecular medicine* 85: 129–137; 2007.

35. Santos, J. L.; Boutin, P.; Verdich, C.; et al. Genotype-by-nutrient interactions assessed in European obese women: a case-only study. *European journal of nutrition* 45: 454–462; 2006.
36. Mottagui-Tabar, S.; Ryden, M.; Lofgren, P.; Faulds, G.; Hoffstedt, J.; Brookes, A. J.; Andersson, I.; Arner, P. Evidence for an important role of perilipin in the regulation of human adipocyte lipolysis. *Diabetologia* 46: 789–797; 2003.
37. Qi, L.; Corella, D.; Sorli, J. V.; et al. Genetic variation at the perilipin (PLIN) locus is associated with obesity-related phenotypes in White women. *Clinical genetics* 66: 299–310; 2004.
38. Qi, L.; Shen, H.; Larson, I.; et al. Gender-specific association of a perilipin gene haplotype with obesity risk in a white population. *Obesity research* 12: 1758–1765; 2004.
39. Qi, L.; Tai, E. S.; Tan, C. E.; et al. Intragenic linkage disequilibrium structure of the human perilipin gene (PLIN) and haplotype association with increased obesity risk in a multiethnic Asian population. *Journal of molecular medicine* 83: 448–456; 2005.
40. Meirhaeghe, A.; Thomas, S.; Ancot, F.; et al. Study of the impact of perilipin polymorphisms in a French population. *Journal of negative results in biomedicine* 5: 10; 2006.
41. Manolio, T. A.; Bailey-Wilson, J. E.; Collins, F. S. Genes, environment and the value of prospective cohort studies. *Nature reviews* 7: 812–820; 2006.
42. Corella, D.; Qi, L.; Sorli, J. V.; et al. Obese subjects carrying the 11482G > A polymorphism at the perilipin locus are resistant to weight loss after dietary energy restriction. *The journal of clinical endocrinology and metabolism* 90: 5121–5126; 2005.
43. Kang, E. S.; Cha, B. S.; Kim, H. J.; et al. The 11482G > A polymorphism in the perilipin gene is associated with weight gain with rosiglitazone treatment in type 2 diabetes. *Diabetes care* 29: 1320–1324; 2006.
44. Abidov, M. T.; del Rio, M. J.; Ramazanov, T. Z.; et al. Effects of Aralia mandshurica and Engelhardtia chrysolepis extracts on some parameters of lipid metabolism in women with nondiabetic obesity. *Bulletin of experimental biology and medicine* 141: 343–346; 2006.
45. Jang, Y.; Kim, O. Y.; Lee, J. H.; et al. Genetic variation at the perilipin locus is associated with changes in serum free fatty acids and abdominal fat following mild weight loss. *International journal of obesity (2005)* 30: 1601–1608; 2006.
46. Corella, D.; Qi, L.; Tai, E. S.; et al. Perilipin gene variation determines higher susceptibility to insulin resistance in Asian women when consuming a high-saturated fat, low-carbohydrate diet. *Diabetes care* 29: 1313–1319; 2006.
47. Masson, L. F.; McNeill, G.; Avenell, A. Genetic variation and the lipid response to dietary intervention: a systematic review. *The American journal of clinical nutrition* 77: 1098–1111; 2003.
48. Ordovas, J. M. Genetics, postprandial lipemia and obesity. *Nutrition, metabolism, and cardiovascular diseases* 11: 118–133; 2001.
49. Zilversmit, D. B. Atherogenesis: a postprandial phenomenon. *Circulation* 60: 473–485; 1979.
50. Perez-Martinez, P.; Perez-Jimenez, F.; Bellido, C.; et al. A polymorphism exon 1 variant at the locus of the scavenger receptor class B type I (SCARB1) gene is associated with differences in insulin sensitivity in healthy people during the consumption of an olive oil-rich diet. *The journal of clinical endocrinology and metabolism* 90: 2297–2300; 2005.

51. van Ommen, B.; Stierum, R. Nutrigenomics: exploiting systems biology in the nutrition and health arena. *Current opinion in biotechnology* 13: 517–521; 2002.
52. Kaput, J.; Ordovas, J. M.; Ferguson, L.; et al. The case for strategic international alliances to harness nutritional genomics for public and personal health. *The British journal of nutrition* 94: 623–632; 2005.

# 5 Nutrigenomics and Chronic Inflammation

*Lynnette R. Ferguson and Martin Philpott*

## CONTENTS



## 5.1 INTRODUCTION: THE NATURE OF CHRONIC INFLAMMATION

Increased understanding of the basic pathologies of several noncommunicable diseases suggests that chronic inflammation may be a common underlying mechanism. Chronic inflammation has been linked with asthma, Alzheimer's disease, cardiovascular disease, and cancer and diabetes, among others. Inflammatory processes, including the release of proinflammatory cytokines and formation of reactive oxygen and nitrogen species, are an essential part of the immune system. Polymorphisms in the genes affecting immune response will have predictable effects on susceptibility to disease, while other genes affecting antioxidant effects, apoptosis, and cell signaling will interact. Each of the stages involved in inflammation is likely to respond to a different dietary intervention, and a complementary approach may be necessary to optimally reduce symptoms. Understanding the genetic polymorphisms involved may aid in developing more precise dietary strategies, in order to reduce chronic inflammation and its long-term implications.

Inflammatory processes lead to the release of proinflammatory cytokines and chemokines, growth and angiogenic factors, as well as formation of reactive oxygen species (ROS) and reactive nitrogen species (RNS). They provide an essential part of the immune system's response to a pathogen. Chronic inflammation is defined as "an inflammatory response of prolonged duration — weeks, months, or even indefinitely — whose extended time course is provoked by persistence of the causative stimulus to inflammation in the tissue"(medweb.bham.ac.uk/http/depts/path/Teaching/FOUNDAT/CHRONINF/chronic.html). This may occur through progression from *acute inflammation* because of persistence of the original stimulus, or following a number of episodes of acute inflammation.

Most cases of chronic inflammation are generally thought to occur through infectious agents that are somehow protected from host defenses, either through endogenous resistance mechanisms, or through being maintained in a protected environment. However, nonliving foreign material that cannot be broken down will have a similar effect. There are a number of examples of chronic inflammation being stimulated through a normal tissue component, because of a defect in the regulation of the body's immune response to its own tissues. Examples here are autoimmune diseases such as rheumatoid arthritis or lupus. There are also classes of diseases that have an underlying component of chronic inflammation, such as the inflammatory bowel diseases, Crohn's disease (CD) or ulcerative colitis (UC), where there is increasingly strong evidence for an interplay between genes and environment in the etiology.

A schematic depicting some of the known factors in inflammation is provided in Figure 5.1. ROS and NOS play a central role in enhancing the process, through the activation of stress kinases (including JNK, MAPK, and p 38), or redox-sensitive

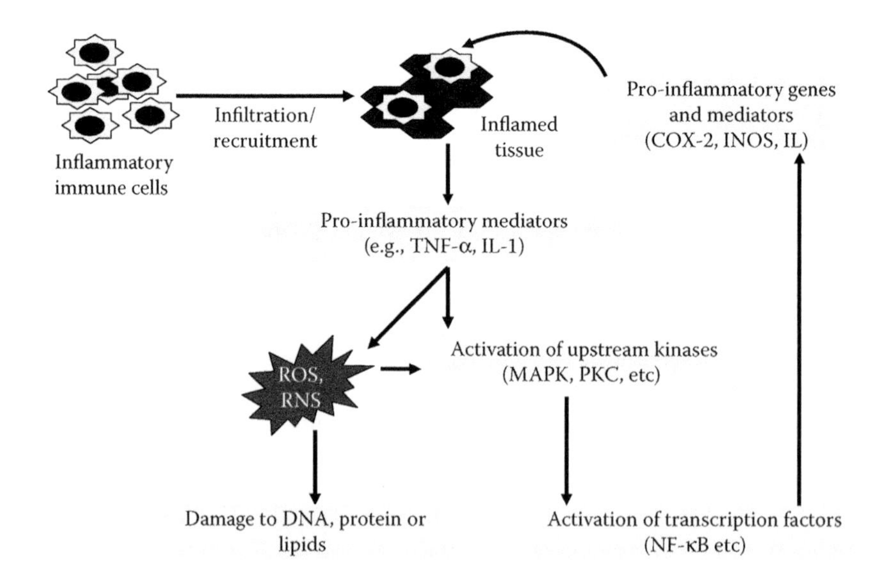


**FIGURE 5.1** Overview of the process of chronic inflammation, resulting in damage to host tissues and activation of proinflammatory genes.

transcription factors such as nuclear factor-κB (NF-κB) and AP-1. Although ROS and RNS may act directly to produce damage to DNA, lipid, or proteins, they also commonly act through secondary products such as the peroxidation product, 4-hydroxy-2-nonenal. NF-κB, a family of ubiquitously expressed transcription factors, regulates the expression of genes encoding proteins essential for stress response, maintenance of intercellular communication, cell cycle control, and apoptosis.

## 5.2 CHRONIC INFLAMMATION AND DISEASE

Chronic inflammation may be a common underlying mechanism of several noncommunicable diseases, including Alzheimer's disease (AD), cardiovascular disease, various types of cancer, diabetes, and rheumatoid arthritis.

Cancer may be the best studied of these examples, because chronic inflammation has long been considered to be a significant risk factor for a variety of epithelial cancers, including cancers of the prostate, cervix, esophagus, stomach, liver, colon, pancreas, and bladder.[1,2] A primary cause may be ROS and RNS, leading to DNA damage and mutation, hence contributing to cancer initiation. However, the release of growth factors and of proinflammatory cytokines from activated macrophages will also enhance cell growth and promote later stages of the process. NF-κB also acts in the tumor microenvironment, enhancing the survival of premalignant epithelial cells, thereby promoting tumor growth and vascularization.[3–5]

The release of cytokines not only drives inflammation, but may also lead to tissue destruction in diseases such as rheumatoid arthritis, psoriasis, chronic obstructive pulmonary disease, and atherosclerosis.[6] Two key cytokines, which have been targeted clinically for treatment of such diseases, are tumor necrosis factor-α (TNF-α) and interleukin-1 (IL-1). Toll-like receptors (TLRs), which recognize self vs. nonself molecular patterns, may also be pivotal in the regulation of cytokine-driven inflammation. Although there is still speculation as to whether targeting these or their downstream signaling pathways will be beneficial therapeutically, the action of each of these is likely to be impacted by nutrition.

The most common form of dementia is Alzheimer's disease (AD), whose pathology is characterized by activated microglia clustered around aggregated amyloid beta (Abeta1-42) peptide-containing plaques. This 42-mer peptide is associated with high levels of ROS, and is derived from the beta-amyloid precursor protein (APP).

## 5.3 GENES AND INFLAMMATION-PRONE DISEASES

Polymorphisms in the genes affecting immune response will have predictable effects on susceptibility to disease, while other genes affecting cell signaling, apoptosis, and antioxidant effects will interact. A review by Yamada and Ymamoto [7] summarizes some of the recent work, focusing on the postulated function of the genes and level of evidence of involvement in disease.

In keeping with the recognized importance of cytokines, a considerable number of genetic polymorphisms in genes associated with immune processes will be of obvious significance to the development and progression of inflammation-related disease. The bulk of functional polymorphisms thus far identified occur in upstream promoter sequences, leading to changes in the expression of the respective pro- or anti-inflammatory gene products. Interleukin Genetics is an example of a company that focuses attention on polymorphisms in a single gene. As pointed out by Kornman,[8] variants in the genes for the family of interleukin 1 (IL-1) proteins often lead to modified inflammatory response, and may result in increased susceptibility to a range of diseases, including coronary artery disease, AD, gastric cancer, and periodontitis. Similarly, they may modify the onset and progression of the deterioration associated with aging.

A number of other such loci have also been associated with multiple disorders. For example, polymorphisms in the cytotoxic T-lymphocyte-associated 4 (CTLA-4) gene have been associated with autoimmune thyroidosis[9] and type I diabetes mellitus,[10] and have been suggested as a general susceptibility factor in autoimmune disease.[11] Caspase recruitment domain-containing protein 15 (CARD15) functions as an intracellular receptor for bacteria, signaling the presence of pathogens by the production of NF-κB. Ogura et al.[12] provided evidence for certain polymorphisms in CARD15 significantly increasing susceptibility to Crohn's disease in humans, and others have more recently shown a key involvement in colorectal cancer.[13] The products of the HLA (human leukocyte antigen; HLA) family of genes play a critical role in regulation of the immune response.[14] There are recognized associations between several different HLA polymorphisms and a range of inflammatory diseases. Thus, individuals carrying the HLA-DQA1*0501, DQB1*0201 genotype show a more than 200-fold increased risk of developing celiac disease, whereas other related factors may be involved in the development of malignant lymphoma in individuals who already have celiac disease. Similar considerations pertain to the development of rheumatoid arthritis.[14]

The recognition of ROS involvement in chronic inflammation and tissue destruction suggests that either genes or nutrients involved in regulating antioxidant response will play a significant role in modulating the development and progression of inflammation. At a cellular level, redox homeostasis is generally achieved through the balance of ROS generation with mechanisms for their removal, including dietary antioxidants and intracellular antioxidant defense mechanisms. Chen and Kunsch[15] describe the antioxidant response element (ARE) as one of a class of cytoprotective regulatory genes. This element is located in the regulatory regions of a number of genes, including phase II detoxification enzymes proteins such as glutathione-*S*-transferases and gamma-glutamylcysteine synthase. It is bound by the transcription factor Nrf2, leading to activation of the expression of other leucine-zipper-containing transcription factors that have profound effects on immune and inflammatory responses. Factors that decrease expression of these genes enhance inflammatory responses to ROS, and also enhance the progression and development of autoimmune disease.

There are several polymorphisms in the PS-1 and APP genes that increase production of Abeta (1-42), and are likely to be the major causes of early onset familial AD.[16] High levels of ROS and RNS, and increased vulnerability to oxidative stress appear to be a consequence of elevated levels of Abeta (1-42), and may also contribute significantly to neuronal apoptosis and death in familial early-onset AD.[17]

The end point of a number of cell signaling pathways is apoptosis, or programmed cell death, which functions to remove cells from the body. It provides an essential function in growth and development, but also in disease processes such as cancer. PDCD1 (programmed cell death 1) is involved in the regulation of apoptosis, and is a strong candidate gene for systemic lupus erythematosus (SLE).[18] There is also evidence that this gene may be associated with diabetes mellitus I.[19]

## 5.4 OTHER GENES THAT IMPACT NUTRIENT REQUIREMENTS IN CHRONIC INFLAMMATION

As well as genes that are directly involved in chronic inflammation, polymorphisms in genes affecting uptake or efficacy of nutrient absorption will themselves play important roles in controlling the detrimental effects of inflammation-related disease processes.

An increasing range of genes affecting selenium uptake and selenoprotein function have been identified. A SNP at codon 593 of human Glutathione peroxidase-1 (hGPX1) changes a cytosine (C) to a thymine (T), resulting in a substitution of leucine for proline at position 198. Individuals carrying this variant show decreased activity of glutathione peroxidase, an antioxidant enzyme, in cell culture studies[20] and increased susceptibility to breast cancer, lung cancer, and prostate cancer.[21] Individuals carrying GPx proteins differing by a single amino acid at codon 198 respond differently to increasing selenium in the diet. They show different baseline levels of glutathione peroxidase activity per gram of hemoglobin, and these levels are not significantly affected by 6 months of selenium supplementation.[21]

Curran and coworkers[22] described different genetic polymorphisms in the gene for selenoprotein S that directly affected inflammatory response in two different population groups. Selenoprotein S (SEPS1, also called SELS or SELENOS) is a gene that appears to be involved in stress response in the endoplasmic reticulum, and in control of inflammation. They genotyped 13 SNPs in 522 individuals from 92 families, and considered whether groups of variants had increased or decreased evidence for inflammation, as measured by plasma levels of interleukin 6 (IL-6), interleukin 1L-1β (IL-1β), and TNF-α. They demonstrated a direct mechanistic link between the incidence of a variant allele in one particular SEPS1 and the production of inflammatory cytokines. From these data, they speculated that SEPS1 plays an important role in mediating inflammation. It is still unclear as to whether dietary supplementation with increased Se can overcome the defect in the group of individuals carrying the variant allele.

## 5.5 DIETARY MODULATION OF CHRONIC INFLAMMATION AND DOWNSTREAM EFFECTS

Different nutrients or nonnutrients, so called for their lack of a defined role in nutrition, particularly with respect to insufficiency disease, may modulate the various processes leading to chronic inflammation and to increased disease susceptibility (see Figure 5.2). These have been classified into three main groups, of which a few representative examples follow.

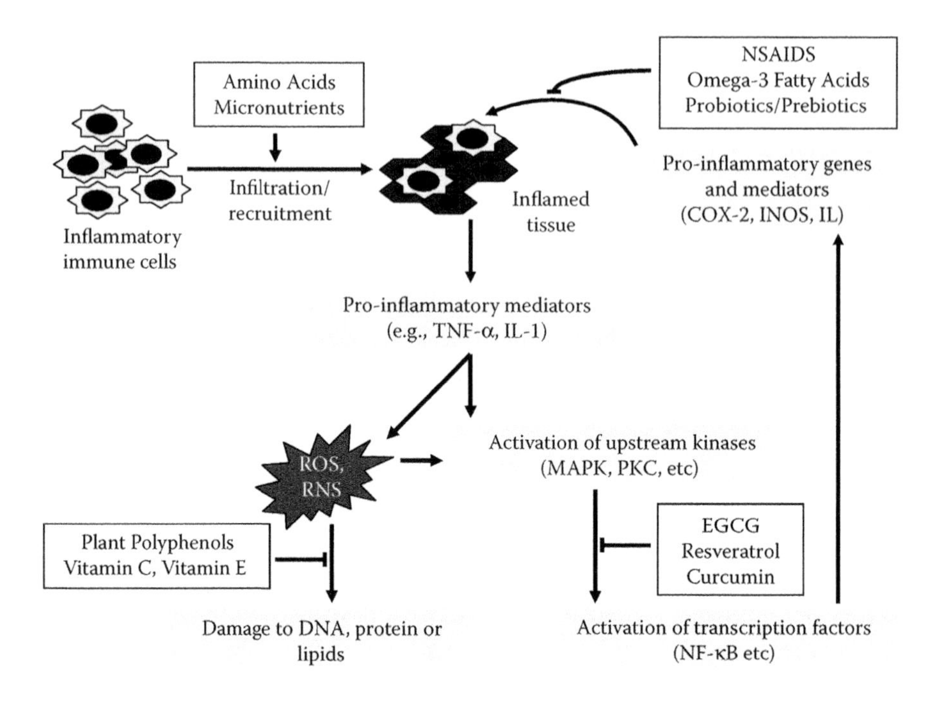


**FIGURE 5.2** Key points within the process of chronic inflammation where nutrients and nonnutrients interact, reducing the likelihood of chronic inflammation leading to a disease end point. Various micronutrients and amino acids are required for an essential early inflammatory response, whereas diverse nutrients and nonnutrients can inhibit later events and reduce concomitant damage to host tissues during chronic inflammation.

### 5.5.1 Recruitment and Growth Stimulation of Immune Cells

We have previously identified the role of various nutrients in immune response and cancer.[23] Various vitamins and minerals are particularly important to the immune system, as they are either preferentially used by the system or are rapidly consumed during an immune response, often because of enhanced transport and growth of certain cell types. For example, good cellular levels of selenium (Se) are important for effective antibody production by B-cells as well as for neutrophil chemotaxis and activity. In general, Se supplementation enhances T-cell responses by upregulation of the T-cell IL-2 receptor and increases antibody synthesis. Zinc is a component of proteins involved in signal transduction during T-cell activation and interaction with B-cells.[24] Although copper is essential for optimal immune function, little is known about the underlying mechanism. Copper deficiency results in decreased T-cell proliferation, possibly because of suppression of IL-2, and also in reduced numbers of circulating neutrophils. Iron deficiency leads to reduced neutrophil function, depression of T-cell numbers with thymic atrophy, defective T-cell proliferative response, and impaired IL-2 production by lymphocytes.

Amino acids are clearly important during cell growth. Although arginine and glutamine are generally considered nonessential amino acids, they may be depleted during an immune response. Nitric oxide (NO) is secreted by macrophages to kill pathogens, and arginine is the sole substrate for nitric oxide synthase. Glutamine is a specific fuel for the proliferation of lymphocytes.[24a] Many sulfur amino acids act as substrates for acute phase protein and immunoglobulin synthesis. Sulfur amino acid intake is particularly important for glutathione production, and insufficient levels will exert a proinflammatory influence.

### 5.5.2 Dietary Antioxidants

Much of the DNA and tissue damage associated with chronic inflammation occurs through formation of ROS and reactive nitrogen species (RNS), as well as DNA-reactive aldehydes, including *trans*-4-hydroxy-2-nonenal and malondialdehyde from lipid peroxidation (LPO).[25] There is evidence that individuals with chronic inflammatory conditions, including the inflammatory bowel diseases, ulcerative colitis and Crohn's disease, show elevated levels of oxidative damage compared to the normal population.[26] Several different ROS and RNS lead to a range of detrimental effects on different macromolecules. Enhancing the levels of dietary antioxidants (including free radical scavengers) or enhanced enzymatic cellular defense mechanisms has been suggested as an important therapeutic strategy for a range of inflammatory diseases, including lung diseases such as asthma and chronic obstructive pulmonary disease (COPD).[27]

Antioxidants that have effective wide-spectrum activity and good bioavailability and thiols or molecules that have dual antioxidant and anti-inflammatory activity may not only protect against the direct injurious effects of oxidants but may fundamentally alter the underlying inflammatory processes that play an important role in the pathogenesis of chronic inflammatory lung diseases. Many of the antioxidants in a normal Western diet are derived from plant foods. Important groups of free radical scavengers would include ascorbic acid (vitamin C), vitamin E, and carotenoids.[25] Although Se is an important component of the immune response, it also acts as an antioxidant, being a key component of glutathione peroxidase, which detoxifies the ROS hydroperoxide and hydrogen peroxide.

As well as known micronutrients, a large number of nonnutrients, particularly polyphenols such as tea catechins and anthocyanins from wine and some fruits and vegetables, have also been shown to act as powerful antioxidants *in vitro*.[28,29] It is less clear how well they function as antioxidants in humans,[30] although many studies have demonstrated a link between diets high in polyphenol antioxidants and reductions in inflammation-related degenerative diseases, including heart disease and cancer.[31–33] It is increasingly recognized, however, that many of these antioxidants have biological activity beyond their abilities to scavenge free radicals, and also have profound effects on signal transduction.[34,35]

### 5.5.3 Cell Signaling Molecules Mediating Inflammatory Response

Kundu and Surh[36] extensively surveyed the literature for dietary anti-inflammatory chemicals that disrupted signal transduction, as a rationale for chemoprevention. A range of nonnutrients or phytochemicals may play an important role. The available literature largely focuses on various plant polyphenols, including epigalocatechin galate (EGCG), curcumin, [6]-gingerol and resveratrol, whose effects have been identified at specific points in the pathways. These compounds have been shown to inhibit a variety of kinase cascade signal transduction pathways, including protein kinase C (PKC), I-κB kinase (IKK), mitogen-activated protein kinase (MAPK), and phosphoinositide-3 kinase (PI3K) pathways, resulting in reduced activation of proinflammatory transcription factors such as NF-κB, AP-1, and β-catenin. This has the downstream effect of reducing the production of proinflammatory enzymes, including COX-2 and iNOS, and proinflammatory mediators, such as TNF-α, IL-8, PGE2, and NO. Similar effects on cell signaling and inflammation are also reported for anthocyanins,[37] a variety of plant polyphenols common in highly colored foods such as sweet potatoes.[38]

## 5.6 GENE–DIET INTERACTIONS IN CHRONIC INFLAMMATION

The optimal levels of each of the various nutrients or phytochemicals will be governed by the nature and combination of SNPs in the various genes governing production of the relevant proteins.

Although companies such as Interleukin Genetics are focusing on pharmaceutical approaches to modulating the expression of genes such as IL-1, nutrition may actually provide a practical alternative.[8] This will not only be true for delaying the development and progression of chronic disease, but also for delaying the adverse consequences associated with aging. Given the number of nutrients affecting the immune response, a combined approach involving micronutrients and also a variety of lipids may be appropriate. However, a caution does also need to be sounded. An example is provided by intervention trials in AD. Walsh and Aisen[39] summarized the compelling set of available published information on a range of *in vitro* and animal studies suggesting a causal role for inflammation in development and progression of the disease. This background provided a strong rationale and justification for clinical trials to test the effect of anti-inflammatory drugs in this disease. However, such trials, despite testing a range of agents, have failed to show a consistent protective effect. The same is likely also to be true for anti-inflammatory dietary approaches.

Selenium provides an example of a nutrient whose desirable levels are impacted strongly by known genetic polymorphisms. Our own studies suggest that Se levels may be too low in approximately half of the Auckland population.[40] However, for those individuals with the codon 593 polymorphism in hGPX1, the activity of this enzyme saturates at lower Se levels than for the rest of the population, and increased Se does not improve this.[21] However, these individuals are highly susceptible to DNA damage, and this susceptibility may be counteracted by increased Se. They are also highly susceptible to prostate cancer, and it is not yet known if this risk can be overcome by supplementation with Se. Conversely, those individuals with the codon 718 polymorphism in hGPX4 may have decreased prostate cancer risk and decreased susceptibility to DNA damage. Increased Se may not decrease the risk of cancer in these individuals, and may actually be harmful (unpublished data; this laboratory).

## 5.7 FUTURE PERSPECTIVES

Susceptibility to chronic inflammation can occur through prolonged exposures to environmental pathogens or irritants, or through a combination of variant SNPs in certain key genes. It is suggested that nutrient combination approaches are essential if we are to find dietary approaches to overcoming susceptibility to chronic inflammation and its ensuing disease processes. Once the scientific barriers are overcome, there are still more hurdles. How do we put all this together? What do we tell the public? And what other work needs to be done? Network and collaborative approaches are essential if nutrigenomic approaches are to have a significant impact at the level of public health.

## ACKNOWLEDGMENTS

We thank the Auckland Cancer Society, The Cancer Society of New Zealand, and The Foundation for Research, Science and Technology (New Zealand) for funding support.

## KEY READINGS

Ferguson, L. R., Karunasinghe, N., and Philpott, M., Susceptibility to cancer and DNA damage to lymphocytes: can it be counteracted by dietary selenium?, in *Nutritional Biotechnology in the Feed and Food Industries: Proceedings of Alltech's Twenty Second Annual Symposium,* Lyons, T.P., Jacques, K.A., and Hower, J.M., Eds., Nottingham University Press, Nottingham, 2006, p. 143.

Kundu, J. K. and Surh, Y. -J., Breaking the relay in deregulated cellular signal transduction as a rationale for chemoprevention with anti-inflammatory phytochemicals, *Mutat. Res.,* 591, 123, 2005.

Philpott, M. and Ferguson, L. R., Immunonutrition and cancer, *Mutat. Res.,* 551, 29, 2004.

Yamada, R. and Ymamoto, K., Recent findings on genes associated with inflammatory disease, *Mutat. Res.,* 573, 136, 2005.

## REFERENCES

1. Dobrovolskaia, M. A. and Kozlov, S. V., Inflammation and cancer: when NF-kappaB amalgamates the perilous partnership, *Curr. Cancer Drug Targets,* 5, 325, 2005.
2. Ditsworth, D. and Zong, W. X., NF-kappaB: key mediator of inflammation-associated cancer, *Cancer Biol. Ther.,* 3, 1214, 2004.
3. Greten, F. R. et al., IKKbeta links inflammation and tumorigenesis in a mouse model of colitis-associated cancer, *Cell,* 118, 285, 2004.
4. Luo, J. L. et al., Inhibition of NF-kappaB in cancer cells converts inflammation-induced tumor growth mediated by TNFalpha to TRAIL-mediated tumor regression, *Cancer Cell,* 6, 297, 2004.
5. Pikarsky, E. et al., NF-kappaB functions as a tumour promoter in inflammation-associated cancer, *Nature,* 431, 461, 2004.
6. Andreakos, E., Foxwell, B., and Feldmann, M., Is targeting Toll-like receptors and their signaling pathway a useful therapeutic approach to modulating cytokine-driven inflammation?, *Immunol. Rev.,* 202, 250, 2004.

7. Yamada, R. and Ymamoto, K., Recent findings on genes associated with inflammatory disease, *Mutat. Res.,* 573, 136, 2005.
8. Kornman, K. S., Interleukin 1 genetics, inflammatory mechanisms, and nutrigenetic opportunities to modulate diseases of aging, *Am. J. Clin. Nutr.,* 83, 475S, 2006.
9. Yanagawa, T. et al., CTLA-4 gene polymorphism associated with Graves' disease in a Caucasian population, *J. Clin. Endocrinol. Metab.,* 80, 41, 1995.
10. Marron, M. P. et al., Insulin-dependent diabetes mellitus (IDDM) is associated with CTLA-4 polymorphisms in multiple ethnic groups, *Human Mol. Genet.,* 6, 1275, 1997.
11. Kristiansen, O. P., Larsen, Z. M., and Pociot, F., CTLA-4 in autoimmune diseases–a general susceptibility gene to autoimmunity? *Genes Immun.,* 1, 170, 2000.
12. Ogura, Y. et al., A frameshift mutation in NOD2 associated with susceptibility to Crohn's disease, *Nature,* 411, 603, 2001.
13. Roberts, R. L. et al., Caspase recruitment domain-containing protein 15 mutations in patients with colorectal cancer, *Cancer Res.,* 66, 2532, 2006.
14. Howell, W. M., Calder, P. C., and Grimble, R. F., Gene polymorphisms, inflammatory diseases and cancer, *Proc. Nutr. Soc.,* 61, 447, 2002.
15. Chen, X. L. and Kunsch, C., Induction of cytoprotective genes through Nrf2/antioxidant response element pathway: a new therapeutic approach for the treatment of inflammatory diseases, *Curr. Pharm. Des.,* 10, 879, 2004.
16. Walker, D. G. et al., Gene expression changes by amyloid beta peptide-stimulated human postmortem brain microglia identify activation of multiple inflammatory processes, *J. Leukoc. Biol.,* 79, 596, 2006.
17. Mohammad Abdul, H. et al., Mutations in amyloid precursor protein and presenilin-1 genes increase the basal oxidative stress in murine neuronal cells and lead to increased sensitivity to oxidative stress mediated by amyloid beta-peptide (1-42), HO and kainic acid: implications for Alzheimer's disease, *J. Neurochem.,* 96, 1322, 2006.
18. Prokunina, L. et al., A regulatory polymorphism in PDCD1 is associated with susceptibility to systemic lupus erythematosus in humans, *Nat. Genet.,* 32, 666, 2002.
19. Nielsen, C. et al., Association of a putative regulatory polymorphism in PDCD1 with susceptibility to type 1 diabetes, *Tissue Antig.,* 62, 492, 2003.
20. Hu, Y. J. and Diamond, A. M., Role of glutathione peroxidase 1 in breast cancer: loss of heterozygosity and allelic differences in the response to selenium, *Cancer Res.,* 63, 3347, 2003.
21. Ferguson, L. R., Karunasinghe, N., and Philpott, M., Susceptibility to cancer and DNA damage to lymphocytes: can it be counteracted by dietary selenium?, in *Nutritional Biotechnology in the Feed and Food Industries: Proceedings of Alltech's Twenty Second Annual Symposium,* Lyons, T.P., Jacques, K.A., and Hower, J.M., Eds., Nottingham University Press, Nottingham, 2006, p. 143.
22. Curran, J. E. et al., Genetic variation in selenoprotein S influences inflammatory response, *Nat. Genet.,* 37, 1234, 2005.
23. Philpott, M. and Ferguson, L. R., Immunonutrition and cancer, *Mutat. Res.,* 551, 29, 2004.
24. Bao, B. et al., Zinc modulates mRNA levels of cytokines, *Am. J. Phys. — Endo. Metab.,* 285, E1095, 2003.
25. Halliwell, B., Oxidative stress, nutrition and health. Experimental strategies for optimization of nutritional antioxidant intake in humans, *Free Rad. Res.,* 25, 57, 1996.
26. D'Odorico, A. et al., Reduced plasma antioxidant concentrations and increased oxidative DNA damage in inflammatory bowel disease, *Scand. J. Gastro.,* 36, 1289, 2001.
27. Rahman, I., Oxidative stress and gene transcription in asthma and chronic obstructive pulmonary disease: antioxidant therapeutic targets, *Curr. Drug Targets — Inflamm. Allergy,* 1, 291, 2002.

28. Rice-Evans, C., Plant polyphenols: free radical scavengers or chain-breaking antioxidants? *Biochem. Soc. Symp.,* 61, 103, 1995.
29. Dreosti, I. E., Antioxidant polyphenols in tea, cocoa, and wine, *Nutrition,* 16, 692, 2000.
30. Dragsted, L. O., Antioxidant actions of polyphenols in humans, *Int. J. Vit. Nutr. Res.,* 73, 112, 2003.
31. Das, D. K. et al., Cardioprotection of red wine: role of polyphenolic antioxidants, *Drugs Exp. Clin. Res.,* 25, 115, 1999.
32. Ferguson, L. R., Role of plant polyphenols in genomic stability, *Mutat. Res.,* 475, 89, 2001.
33. Bianchini, F. and Vainio, H., Wine and resveratrol: mechanisms of cancer prevention?, *Eur. J. Cancer Prev.,* 12, 417, 2003.
34. Scalbert, A., Johnson, I. T., and Saltmarsh, M., Polyphenols: antioxidants and beyond, *Am. J. Clin. Nutr.,* 81, 215S, 2005.
35. Williams, R. J., Spencer, J. P., and Rice-Evans, C., Flavonoids: antioxidants or signalling molecules? *Free Radical Biol. Med.,* 36, 838, 2004.
36. Kundu, J. K. and Surh, Y. -J., Breaking the relay in deregulated cellular signal transduction as a rationale for chemoprevention with anti-inflammatory phytochemicals, *Mutat. Res.,* 591, 123, 2005.
37. Wang, S. Y. et al., Antioxidant activity in lingonberries (*Vaccinium vitis-idaea* L.) and its inhibitory effect on activator protein-1, nuclear factor-kappaB, and mitogen-activated protein kinases activation, *J. Agric. Food Chem.,* 53, 3156, 2005.
38. Philpott, M. et al., Enhanced coloration reveals high antioxidant potential in new sweet potato cultivars, *J. Sci. Food Agric.,* 83, 1076, 2003.
39. Walsh, S. and Aisen, P. S., Inflammatory processes and Alzheimer's disease, *Expert Rev. Neurother.,* 4, 793, 2004.
40. Karunasinghe, N. et al., DNA stability and serum selenium levels in a high-risk group for prostate cancer, *Cancer Epidemiol. Biomarkers Prev.,* 13, 391, 2004.

# 6 Personalized Prevention of Type 2 Diabetes

*Hans-Georg Joost*

## CONTENTS



## 6.1 INTRODUCTION: TYPE 2 DIABETES IS A PREVENTABLE DISEASE

Type 2 diabetes mellitus is a complex, polygenic disease with a heterogeneous pathophysiology, mainly characterized by obesity-associated insulin resistance and a progressive failure of pancreatic β-cells. Its incidence can be lowered by reduction of the intra-abdominal fat mass and by pharmacological control of postprandial blood glucose levels. Several phenotypic risk factors and biomarkers (e.g., abdominal obesity, serum adiponectin, HbA1c, nutritional pattern, and physical activity) are known that determine the individual disease risk. Such a risk assessment can provide the basis for a personalized decision as to the quality and intensity of a preventive intervention. So far, genotyping for the presently known gene variants that confer an increased risk for type 2 diabetes adds relatively little to the information provided by the phenotypic risk factors. However, a risk assessment based on genetic information is necessary for a personalized intervention that begins before phenotypic risk factors are detectable. Furthermore, data from experimental animals indicate that the response to nutritional parameters, e.g., the dietary fat content, is determined by gene variants that modify disease risk and progression. Thus, identification of these genes and elucidation of their role in the human disease will allow a personalized, diet-based intervention.

During the last 30 years, a steady increase in the prevalence of type 2 diabetes has been observed in industrialized Western countries [1]. In Germany, approximately 5% of the population suffers from overt type 2 diabetes (fasting hyperglycemia), whereas prediabetes (IGT, impaired glucose tolerance) can be detected in 10 to 15% [2]. Thus, it has been estimated that the prevalence of overt type 2 diabetes in Germany will approach 10% in 2010. This development is associated with a marked increase in the prevalence of overweight and obesity. Consequently, the disease is detected in younger adults, adolescents, and even in children who are morbidly obese [3]. Thus, type 2 diabetes and its life-shortening secondary complications represent a substantial public health problem. The current trend, if it continues, will have adverse economic consequences for health-care systems [4,5], and will eventually even reduce the mean life expectancy [6]. Therefore, an effective prevention strategy is required to stop or even reverse the trend.

Type 2 diabetes develops by interaction of a polygenic basis with exogenous factors, e.g., nutrition and physical activity. There is ample evidence that a change in lifestyle leading to a reduction of intra-abdominal fat reduces the incidence of the disease [7]. Also, a pharmacological intervention with agents that reduce blood glucose levels, e.g., metformin [8] or the glucosidase inhibitor acarbose [9], reduces the incidence of diabetes in cohorts with impaired glucose tolerance. Thus, type 2 diabetes can be considered a largely preventable disease.

The decision to start drug therapy for prevention of type 2 diabetes has to be based on a risk-benefit assessment that takes into account the personal profile of a person potentially at risk. Indeed, the currently available data already allow a risk assessment based on phenotypic and, to a limited extent, also on genotypic data. Thus, personalized prevention of type 2 diabetes is a realistic concept. Furthermore, because its pathophysiology and genetics are heterogeneous, it is reasonable to assume that there are subtypes of individuals at risk who require different (personalized) intervention strategies. Along these lines, current research tries to identify nutritional factors predisposing for the disease in association with certain genotypes. Finally, the course of the disease is heterogeneous, and few factors, e.g., blood glucose control, are so far known predicting the onset of secondary complications. With a better prediction of these complications, personalized treatment is a realistic perspective for patients affected with type 2 diabetes.

## 6.2 PATHOGENESIS OF TYPE 2 DIABETES DATA FROM ANIMAL MODELS

### 6.2.1 GENETICS

Several strains of rodents exhibit a type 2 diabetes–like hyperglycemia closely resembling the human disease, e.g., the obese mouse strains *db/db* (monogenic deletion of the leptin receptor) and NZO (polygenic obesity). In these mouse lines, hyperglycemia is associated with morbid obesity and insulin resistance, and reflects a progressive failure of the pancreatic β-cells. The genetic basis of the diabetes can be dissected into adipogenic and diabetogenic (i.e., causing hyperglycemia) alleles [10–12]. Diabetes requires the presence of both types of predisposing alleles ("diabesity"). Consequently, in the absence of diabetogenic alleles, morbid obesity does not produce diabetes (e.g., in the *ob/ob*-mouse or the *fa/fa*-rat). Lean mouse lines (e.g., NON, SJL, or C57Ks/J) may carry diabetogenic alleles; these will become active as a diabetogenic background when the mice become obese either by a single obesity gene (e.g., in the *db/db* strain) or after crossbreeding with a polygenic obesity strain such as NZO [10–12].

### 6.2.2 Nutrition

Most mouse strains are sensitive to a high-fat diet in that they develop obesity and insulin resistance associated with impaired glucose tolerance [13]. Furthermore, in diabetes-susceptible mouse strains such as NZO, the development of diabetes can be accelerated by a high-fat diet [12]. Because diabetes in these mouse models reflects failure and destruction of insulin-secreting cells, the finding seems to indicate that the β-cell is sensitive against fatty acids and incorporated triglycerides (lipotoxicity; see later text). However, β-cell destruction appears to also depend on the dietary carbohydrates, because substitution of protein [14, 15] or fat [16] for carbohydrates delayed or prevented the diabetes in *db/db* or NZO mice, respectively. Interestingly, the effect of the high-fat diet on the development of diabetes can depend on certain genotypes. In NZO mice, the effect of a diabetogenic allele on chromosome 5 (tentatively designated Nob1) depend on the fat content of the diet, whereas the effect of a second QTL (Nidd/SJL) did not [12]. Such data provide proof of principle for the concept that gene variants may determine the quality of the response to nutrients. Identification of these variants in humans will allow the establishment of genotype-specific nutritional recommendations with regard to dietary fat and diabetes risk.

### 6.2.3 Mechanism of β-Cell Failure: Lipotoxicity and Glucotoxicity

The association of diabetes with obesity, and the diabetogenic effect of a high-fat diet, has lent support to the hypothesis that ß-cells incorporating excess triglycerides undergo apoptosis [17]. In mouse models of diabetes and insulin resistance, enhanced hepatic lipogenesis is a key pathophysiological feature [18,19]. When lipids accumulate in nonadipose tissues during overnutrition, fatty acids enter deleterious pathways such as formation of ceramide. Ceramide is probably the most damaging lipid and is a cause of lipoapoptosis [17]. Alternatively, it has been postulated that elevation of postprandial and postabsorptive blood glucose levels damage the pancreatic β-cell (glucotoxicity). According to this hypothesis, the β-cell is very sensitive to oxidative damage, or is sensitized by a low antioxidative capacity [20]. It was suggested that elevated blood glucose concentrations lead to formation of reactive oxygen radicals [21], which cause loss of essential transcription factors such as MafA and irreversible cell damage [22]. This hypothesis is supported by numerous experimental findings: Long-term culture of β-cells in the presence of high glucose concentrations affects their function [23]. In *db/db* [14,15] or NZO mice [16], diabetes (defined as histologically assessed β-cell damage) can be delayed or prevented by feeding a high-protein or high-fat, carbohydrate-free diet. Thus, carbohydrates are essential for β-cell destruction in mouse models of diabetes, and lipotoxicity appears to cooperate with glucotoxicity in this pathogenesis [24].

## 6.3 PATHOGENESIS OF HUMAN TYPE 2 DIABETES: RISK FACTORS

### 6.3.1 GENES

Type 2 diabetes is the paradigm of a complex disease that has a genetic basis but is precipitated by exogenous factors, e.g., lifestyle and diet [1]. The genetic component of its pathogenesis appears to be stronger than in type 1 diabetes: in identical twins, concordance of type 2 is approximately 80% for diabetes and even 96% for impaired glucose tolerance [25]. The genetic basis of type 2 diabetes is complex; a combination of numerous diabetogenic alleles appears responsible for development of the disease [26,27] (Table 6.1).

**TABLE 6.1**
**Anthropometric, Nutritional, Lifestyle, and Genetic Risk Factors for the Development of Type 2 Diabetes**

| | Risk Factors for the Development of Type 2 Diabetes |
|---|---|
| Anthropometry | Age ↑ |
| | Waist circumference ↑ |
| | Height ↓ |
| Nutrition | Whole grain bread (>50 g/d) ↓ |
| | Red meat (>100 g/d) ↑ |
| | Sugar-containing beverages (>300 ml/d) ↑ |
| | Coffee (150 ml/d) ↓ |
| | Moderate alcohol consumption (<40 g/d) ↓ |
| Lifestyle | Exercise (sport, hiking, biking, gardening) ↓ |
| | Smoking (>20/d) ↑ |
| Gene variants | Transcription factor PPARγ ↓ |
| | Potassium channel KIR 6.2 ↑ |
| | Transcription factor TCF7L2↑ |
| | Transcription factor HHEX ↓ |
| | Zn transporter SLC 30A8 ↓ |
| | CDKAL1 ↑ |
| | CDKN2 ↓ |
| | IGF2BP2 ↑ |
| | FTO ↑ |

*Note:* Arrows indicate increase or decrease of risk with the indicated factors or the rare allele of the indicated gene. A score based on these factors can be used to assess the individual diabetes risk, and can guide personalized prevention [61]. Interaction between a genotype and a nutritional variable has been suggested for the Pro12Ala polymorphism of PPARγ and the dietary fat content [62]. Details of nongenetic risk factors are described in Reference 34, and diabetogenic alleles are reviewed and described in references 26, 27, 31, and 64.

Considerable efforts have been made to identify genes that cause type 2 diabetes. In genomewide searches, chromosomal segments (quantitative trait loci, QTL) harboring alleles associated with hyperglycemia or other traits related with the disease were identified. In one of these QTL, positional cloning of the gene responsible for the effect, the calcium-dependent protease calpain-10, was successful [28]. In the original cohort, the diabetogenic haplotype of calpain-10 was associated with a threefold higher diabetes risk. Subsequent studies observed smaller effects, and a meta-analysis of 26 studies determined a mean effect of the allele of only 20% [29].

In addition, several gene variants associated with an elevated diabetes risk were identified in numerous case control studies by a candidate gene approach (e.g., the PPARγ Pro12Ala polymorphism and KIR6.2). These studies indicated that the contribution of each variant to the overall diabetes risk is small (20 to 30%), although statistically significant [26,27,30]. Thus, a single gene can predict only small increases of the risk for type 2 diabetes. More recently, the transcription factor TCF7L2 has been identified by positional cloning as a major diabetes gene in an Icelandic study population, giving rise to a 1.5- to 2.5-fold disease risk [31]. In addition, six other susceptibility genes (Table 6.1) have recently been identified in genome-wide association studies [64]. However, it appears reasonable to assume that many susceptibility genes have not been identified so far. Furthermore, it remains to be investigated whether the effect of the known susceptibility genes depends on nutritional or other environmental parameters, as has been demonstrated in mouse models.

### 6.3.2 Anthropometric Parameters

Excess adiposity is considered the most important risk factor of type 2 diabetes, because the anthropometric parameters body weight, body mass index (BMI), and waist circumference are major predictors of the individual disease risk [32–34]. The risk increase is mainly due to the intra-abdominal and intrahepatic fat depots [35,36], whereas subcutaneous fat appears not to play a causative role. Thus, waist circumference is the most precise anthropometric risk factor. Intrahepatic triglycerides are believed to cause insulin resistance and are therefore directly linked with the pathophysiology of diabetes; even a small reduction significantly lowers the diabetes risk [37]. The pathophysiological effect of insulin resistance is an increase and prolongation of postprandial blood glucose excursions, which enhances the exposure of β-cells to toxic glucose concentrations. Furthermore, intra-abdominal and intrahepatic fat stores might be a marker for the accumulation of triglycerides in β-cells, which has been suggested to produce islet cell failure (lipotoxicity).

### 6.3.3 Dietary Factors

Data from prospective cohort studies have indicated that the dietary carbohydrates — independent of the body weight — significantly modify diabetes risk. A diet rich in fibers and carbohydrates with a low glycemic index is associated with lower diabetes risk [38,39]. In contrast, the preferential consumption of carbohydrates with a higher glycemic index, giving rise to higher postprandial blood glucose excursions, is associated with a higher diabetes risk. In addition, the diabetes risk is increased by the consumption of sugar-sweetened soft drinks [40].

In addition to dietary carbohydrates, dietary fat seems to represent a major factor that determines diabetes risk. The consumption of saturated triglycerides and trans-fatty acids is associated with an increased, and the consumption of polyunsaturated fatty acids with a reduced risk [38]. These epidemiological associations may reflect direct effects of the different types of fat and fatty acids on the pancreatic β-cell, or indirect effects on insulin sensitivity, glucose tolerance and, consequently, on the postprandial blood glucose excursions. Thus, the data are consistent with a scenario in which blood glucose excursions, in particular under conditions of insulin resistance and a genetically determined susceptibility of the pancreatic β-cell, play a crucial role in the pathogenesis of diabetes.

In an attempt to identify nutritional patterns rather than single nutrients and food components associated with an increased diabetes risk, a "prudent" and a "western" dietary pattern were compared [41]. The prudent dietary pattern characterized by a higher consumption of vegetables, fruit, fish, poultry, and whole grains was associated with a lower diabetes risk, whereas the Western pattern (higher consumption of red meat, processed meat, French fries, high-fat dairy products, and refined grains) was associated with an increased risk (OR 1.6). More recently, the method of reduced rank regression (RRR) was applied for the first time to identify dietary patterns associated with a disease risk [42,43]. Using the risk factors serum adiponectin, HbA1c, HDL, and CRP, a nutritional pattern was identified in incident diabetics from the EPIC-Potsdam cohort that produced a maximal reduction of these risk factors. This nutritional pattern consists of a high consumption of fruits, a low consumption of meat, beer, soft drinks, and white bread, and is associated with an approximately 80% reduction of the diabetes risk [43]. Similar results were obtained independently in a Finnish cohort [44].

Moderate alcohol consumption, with the exception of beer [43], has consistently been observed to lower the diabetes risk [34]. This effect might reflect the inhibitory effect of alcohol on gluconeogenesis and hepatic glucose output, which could lead to a reduction of fasting blood glucose levels. A similar effect was observed in a study with the oral antidiabetic drug metformin, which exerts a blood-sugar-lowering effect by inhibition of hepatic glucose output [8]. Furthermore, the beneficial effect of blood sugar control on the incidence of progression of impaired glucose tolerance to overt diabetes (fasting hyperglycemia) has been shown with the glucosidase inhibitor acarbose, which blunts postprandial blood glucose excursions [9]. In the case of beer, the beneficial effect of the alcohol seems to be outweighed by its high carbohydrate content. Thus, the epidemiologic data as well as the results of different pharmacological intervention studies are consistent with a scenario in which blood glucose excursions play a major role in the pathogenesis of β-cell failure.

### 6.3.4 Lifestyle: Physical Activity and Smoking

In addition to genetic, anthropometric, and nutritional parameters, physical activity is a major factor determining diabetes risk [45]. Prospective cohort studies indicated that physical activity was significantly lower in diabetics before the onset of their disease than in healthy controls. Men who watched TV for more than 40 h per week had an approximately threefold higher diabetes risk than those who spent less than 1 h per week watching TV [46]. Furthermore, a protective effect of exercise as part of a weight reduction program including diet was observed in an intervention study [7]. As the intervention resulted in a minor weight reduction (approximately 4 kg) but a substantial (60%) reduction of diabetes risk, the authors suggested that exercise exerted an effect that was independent of the weight reduction. This effect may be due to an increased insulin sensitivity of muscle in response to exercise [47]. It should be noted, however, that at present there are no data from intervention studies directly comparing the effect of exercise with that of dietary intervention.

The majority of epidemiologic studies testing the effect of smoking have detected a moderate increase of the diabetes risk that was reversed after cessation of smoking [34]. It is noteworthy that the beneficial effect of smoking cessation apparently outweighs the adverse effect on weight gain. The pathophysiological mechanism of the effect of smoking is unclear. Nicotine stimulates sympathetic nervous activity and may therefore stimulate transient elevations of blood glucose; such an effect would be consistent with the concept that blood sugar excursions play a major role in the pathophysiology of the disease.

### 6.3.5 Biomarker of Blood Glucose, Insulin Resistance, and Inflammation

During the last few years, several serum factors have been identified that may indicate an increased risk of diabetes years before the actual onset of the disease. A small but significant increase of the glycosylated hemoglobin (HbA1c) has consistently been found to be associated with an increased risk of developing overt diabetes [48]. Type 2 diabetes is preceded by a prediabetic period in which glucose tolerance is impaired (IGT, impaired glucose tolerance). Fasting blood glucose is still normal, but increased postprandial blood glucose excursions are responsible for a small increase in HbA1c levels. There is a probability of 15 to 20% that IGT is converted to fasting hyperglycemia within the next year. In addition to HbA1c, it has been shown that a moderate elevation of fasting blood glucose levels predicts an increased risk of developing diabetes within a period of 6 years [49].

Serum parameters reflecting insulin resistance such as characteristic alterations of the lipoprotein profile (low HDL cholesterol and elevated triglycerides) and reduced levels of the cytokine adiponectin are associated with an increased diabetes risk [50]. Adiponectin is secreted from adipose tissue, and enhances insulin sensitivity of liver, muscle, and adipocyte [51]; its serum levels are reciprocal to body mass index and intrahepatic triglycerides [52].

Obesity is associated with a massive infiltration of adipose tissue with immune cells such as macrophages, and it has been suggested that the pathogenesis of type 2 diabetes has an immunologic component in that cytokines released from adipose tissue play a causal role in the insulin resistance and β-cell failure [53]. Consequently, serum levels of inflammatory cytokines or other biomarkers of inflammatory processes such as IL-6 and CRP are elevated long before the onset of overt type 2 diabetes [54,55].

## 6.4 INDIVIDUAL ASSESSMENT OF THE RISK OF DIABETES

Convincing evidence indicates that type 2 diabetes is to a large extent a preventable disease. In persons under the age of 60, with a BMI under 25, and without excess abdominal fat, the prevalence of the disease is very low. Intervention studies have demonstrated that weight reduction by lifestyle changes [7] or drug therapy [56], blood glucose control by oral antidiabetics [8,9], or bariatric surgery [57] significantly reduces the incidence of overt type 2 diabetes. Given the life-shortening and expensive secondary complications of the disease, it appears mandatory to intervene as early and as effectively as possible. However, the potential negative effects of the intervention have to be weighed against the benefits, the latter being a function of the disease risk. At present, there are no guidelines regarding a pharmacological therapy to reduce the diabetes risk [58], although intervention studies have shown its efficacy. Also, the decision regarding surgical therapy of obesity (gastric banding, gastric bypass) is currently based on the severity of the obesity rather on an assessment of the risk of secondary complications. A precise assessment of the individual diabetes risk would provide a rational basis for any decision as to intervene by drug or surgical therapy, but could also guide and support efforts to intervene by lifestyle changes.

The known risk factors described in this chapter allow an accurate assessment of the risk of developing overt type 2 diabetes within the next 5 to 10 years. Anthropometric parameters, dietary pattern, and physical activity can be determined with a simple questionnaire and be used for a simple, orientating risk assessment. In the next stage, clinical chemistry with parameters such as HbA1c, HDL, CRP, and adiponectin can be used to improve the precision of the risk assessment. Furthermore, genotyping for the known diabetogenic alleles (of PPARγ, calpain-10, Kir6.1, and TCF7L2) will add to the precision of the assessment in some individuals. As our knowledge of the diabetogenic genes advances, genotyping will become more important because it allows a much earlier risk assessment than the anthropometric, lifestyle, and serum parameters.

As a basis for an individualized prevention, simple risk scores such as the *Finnish Diabetes Risk Score* have been developed and validated [59]. These risk scores weigh the parameters age, abdominal obesity, activity, and nutritional profile. When applied to individuals in other countries, these risk scores appear to be less accurate: validation of the *Finnish Diabetes Risk Score* in a German study population resulted in a lower sensitivity and specificity of the test [60]. Thus, significant differences appear to exist between countries in the contribution of individual risk factors, presumably because of cultural and genetic differences. Consequently, an accurate risk score based on a German study cohort was developed recently [61]. In addition, specificity and precision of the scores can still be improved, because they are currently based on a relatively small number of incident cases. Furthermore, the quality of the scores could be improved by including known biomarkers such as HbA1c, HDL, CRP, adiponectin, and the known diabetogenic haplotypes.

## 6.5 FUTURE PERSPECTIVES: TOWARD A PERSONALIZED DIET IN THE PREVENTION AND THERAPY OF TYPE 2 DIABETES

Current dietary recommendations for the prevention of type 2 diabetes emphasize weight control, and advocate a "healthy diet" replacing saturated and trans fats with unsaturated fats, and refined grain products with whole grains [34]. Based on the assumption that subgroups with different sensitivity against nutritional variables (e.g., fat content, fat quality, and glycemic load) and a different response to a dietary intervention exist, the general recommendations could be personalized with parameters predicting the benefit of a particular diet in an individual. At present, there are few data from human studies indicating that such subgroups can be identified by genotyping. For instance, in the DPS study, carriers of the 12-Ala allele of PPAR$\gamma$ appeared to benefit more from the intervention (low-fat diet and exercise) with regard to their diabetes risk than the homozygous carriers of the 12-Pro allele [62]. Thus, further information regarding the interaction between diabetogenic alleles and nutritional variables may allow a personalized, diet-based prevention of type 2 diabetes.

As with a few other therapies, the treatment of diabetes requires regimens that are adapted to the individual patient. Of course, the therapeutic regimen is guided by the metabolic control accomplished as assessed with the parameters blood glucose and HbA1c. The different regimens of insulin therapy (conventional and intensive insulin therapy), and their combination with oral antidiabetic drugs are chosen and modified according to the personal characteristics of the patient. So far, there are almost no prognostic parameters other than the control of glycemia that could guide the therapy. Such additional parameters are desirable, because glycemic control is probably not the only parameter determining the course of secondary complications. At present, the only other parameter guiding therapy is the BMI, because there is evidence that suggests overweight diabetics particularly profit from therapy with metformin [63]. For further differentiation of the therapy, complex and expensive studies are required in which the course of the disease is monitored in patients under different therapeutic regimens. Furthermore, knowledge of the genetic basis of the disease will help not only to assess the diabetes risk but might also be useful for differentiation of the therapy. Implementation of such a genotype-based, personalized approach might still be some time away but seems entirely realistic, and type 2 diabetes could become a paradigm of the concept of individualized prevention and therapy of a complex disease.

## KEY READINGS


Diamond, J., The double puzzle of diabetes, *Nature*, 423, 599, 2003.

Hansen, L. and Pedersen, O., Genetics of type 2 diabetes mellitus: status and perspectives, *Diabetes Obes. Metab.*, 7,122, 2005.

Schulze, M.B. and Hu, F.B., Primary prevention of diabetes: what can be done and how much can be prevented? *Annu. Rev. Public Health*, 26, 445, 2005.

Stevenson, C., Barroso, I., and Wareham, N., The genetics of type 2 diabetes. In *Nutritional Genomics*, Eds. Brigelius-Flohé, R. and Joost, H.-G., Wiley-VCH, Weinheim, 223, 2006.

## REFERENCES

1. Diamond, J., The double puzzle of diabetes, *Nature*, 423, 599, 2003.
2. Hanefeld, M. and Kohler, C., Screening, prevention and early therapy of type 2 diabetics, *MMW Fortschr. Med.*, 146, 28, 31, 2004.
3. Wabitsch, M., Hauner, H., Hertrampf, M., Muche, R., Hay, B., Mayer, H., Kratzer, W., Debatin, K.M., and Heinze, E., Type II diabetes mellitus and impaired glucose regulation in Caucasian children and adolescents with obesity living in Germany, *Int. J. Obes. Relat. Metab. Disord.*, 28, 307, 2004.
4. Wolf, A.M. and Colditz, G.A., Current estimates of the economic cost of obesity in the United States, *Obes. Res.*, 6, 97, 1998.
5. Hauner, H., Landgraf, R., Schulze, J., Spranger, J., and Standl, E., Nationales Aktionsforum Diabetes mellitus, Prävention des Typ-2-Diabetes mellitus, Positionspapier des Nationalen Aktionsforum Diabetes Mellitus, *Dtsch. Med. Wochenschr.*, 130, 1053, 2005.
6. Manuel, D.G. and Schultz, S.E., Health-related quality of life and health-adjusted life expectancy of people with diabetes in Ontario, Canada, 1996–1997, *Diabetes Care*, 27, 407, 2004.
7. Tuomilehto, J., Lindstrom, J., Eriksson, J.G., Valle, T.T., Hamalainen, H., Ilanne-Parikka, P., Keinanen-Kiukaanniemi, S., Laakso, M., Louheranta, A., Rastas, M., Salminen, V., and Uusitupa, M., Finnish Diabetes Prevention Study Group. Prevention of type 2 diabetes mellitus by changes in lifestyle among subjects with impaired glucose tolerance, *N. Engl. J. Med.*, 344, 1343, 2001.
8. Knowler, W.C., Barrett-Connor, E., Fowler, S.E., Hamman, R.F., Lachin, J.M., Walker, E.A., and Nathan, D.M., Diabetes Prevention Program Research Group. Reduction in the incidence of type 2 diabetes with lifestyle intervention or metformin, *N. Engl. J. Med.*, 346, 393, 2002.
9. Chiasson, J.L., Josse, R.G., Gomis, R., Hanefeld, M., Karasik, A., and Laakso, M., STOP-NIDDM Trial Research Group. Acarbose for prevention of type 2 diabetes mellitus: the STOP-NIDDM randomised trial, *Lancet*, 359, 2072, 2002.
10. Leiter, E.H., Reifsnyder, P.C., Flurkey, K., Partke, H.J., Junger, E., and Herberg, L., NIDDM genes in mice: deleterious synergism by both parental genomes contributes to diabetogenic thresholds, *Diabetes*, 47, 1287, 1998.
11. Plum, L., Kluge, R., Giesen, K., Altmuller, J., Ortlepp, J.R., and Joost, H.G., Type 2 diabetes-like hyperglycemia in a backcross model of NZO and SJL mice: characterization of a susceptibility locus on chromosome 4 and its relation with obesity, *Diabetes*, 49, 1590, 2000.
12. Plum, L., Giesen, K., Kluge, R., Junger, E., Linnartz, K., Schurmann, A., Becker, W., and Joost, H.G., Characterisation of the mouse diabetes susceptibility locus Nidd/SJL: islet cell destruction, interaction with the obesity QTL Nob1, and effect of dietary fat, *Diabetologia*, 45, 823, 2002.
13. West, D.B., Boozer, C.N., Moody, D.L., and Atkinson, R.L., Dietary obesity in nine inbred mouse strains, *Am. J. Physiol.*, 262, R1025, 1992.
14. Leiter, E.H., Coleman, D.L., Eisenstein, A.B., and Strack, I., Dietary control of pathogenesis in C57BL/KsJ db/db diabetes mice, *Metabolism*, 30, 554, 1981.
15. Leiter, E.H., Coleman, D.L., Ingram, D.K., and Reynolds, M.A., Influence of dietary carbohydrate on the induction of diabetes in C57BL/KsJ-db/db diabetes mice, *J. Nutr.*, 113, 184, 1983.
16. Jürgens, H., Schmolz, K., Neschen, S., Ortmann, S., Blüher, M., Klaus, S., Tschöp, M., Joost, H.-G., and Schürmann, A., Development of diabetes in morbidly obese

New-Zealand Obese (NZO) mice requires dietary carbohydrates, Evidence for an essential role of glucose toxicity in ß-cell destruction, Submitted for publication, 2006.

17. Unger, R.H., Minireview: weapons of lean body mass destruction: the role of ectopic lipids in the metabolic syndrome, *Endocrinology*, 144, 5159, 2003.
18. Becker, W., Kluge, R., Kantner, T., Linnartz, K., Korn, M., Tschank, G., Plum, L., Giesen, K., and Joost, H.-G., Differential hepatic gene expression in a polygenic mouse model with insulin resistance and hyperglycemia: Evidence for a combined transcriptional dysregulation of gluconeogenesis and fatty acid synthesis. *J. Mol. Endocrinol.*, 32, 195 2004.
19. Lan, H., Rabaglia, M.E., Stoehr, J.P., Nadler, S.T., Schueler, K.L., Zou, F., Yandell, B.S., and Attie, A.D., Gene expression profiles of nondiabetic and diabetic obese mice suggest a role of hepatic lipogenic capacity in diabetes susceptibility, *Diabetes*, 52, 688, 2003.
20. Leahy, J.L., Natural history of beta-cell dysfunction in NIDDM, *Diabetes Care*, 13, 992, 1990.
21. Brownlee, M., A radical explanation for glucose-induced beta cell dysfunction, *J. Clin. Invest*, 112, 1788, 2003.
22. Harmon, J.S., Stein, R., and Robertson, R.P., Oxidative stress-mediated, post-translational loss of MafA protein as a contributing mechanism to loss of insulin gene expression in glucotoxic beta cells, *J. Biol. Chem.*, 280, 11107, 2005.
23. Robertson, R.P., Zhang, H.J., Pyzdrowski, K.L., and Walseth, T.F., Preservation of insulin mRNA levels and insulin secretion in HIT cells by avoidance of chronic exposure to high glucose concentrations, *J. Clin. Invest.*, 90, 320, 1992.
24. Poitout, V. and Robertson, R.P., Minireview: Secondary beta-cell failure in type 2 diabetes—a convergence of glucotoxicity and lipotoxicity, *Endocrinology*, 143, 339, 2002.
25. Medici, F., Hawa, M., Ianari, A., Pyke, D.A., and Lesile, R.D., Concordance rate for type II diabetes mellitus in monozygotic twins: actuarial analysis, *Diabetologia*, 42, 146, 1999.
26. Hansen, L., and Pedersen, O., Genetics of type 2 diabetes mellitus: status and perspectives, *Diabetes Obes. Metab.*, 7,122, 2005.
27. Stevenson, C., Barroso, I., and Wareham, N., The genetics of type 2 diabetes. In: Nutritional Genomics, eds. Brigelius-Flohé, R. and Joost, H.-G., *Wiley-VCH*, Weinheim, 223, 2006.
28. Horikawa, Y., Oda, N., Cox, N.J., Li, X., Orho-Melander, M., Hara, M., Hinokio, Y., Lindner, T.H., Mashima, H., Schwarz, P.E., del Bosque-Plata, L., Horikawa, Y., Oda, Y., Yoshiuchi, I., Colilla, S., Polonsky, K.S., Wei, S., Concannon, P., Iwasaki, N., Schulze, J., Baier, L.J., Bogardus, C., Groop, L., Boerwinkle, E., Hanis, C.L., and Bell, G.I., Genetic variation in the gene encoding calpain-10 is associated with type 2 diabetes mellitus, *Nat. Genet.*, 26, 163, 2000.
29. Song, Y., Niu, T., Manson, J.E., Kwiatkowski, D.J., and Liu, S., Are variants in the CAPN10 gene related to risk of type 2 diabetes? A quantitative assessment of population and family-based association studies, *Am. J. Hum. Genet.*, 74, 208, 2004.
30. Barroso, I., Luan, J., Middelberg, R.P., Harding, A.H., Franks, P.W., Jakes, R.W., Clayton, D., Schafer, A.J., O'Rahilly, S., and Wareham, N.J., Candidate gene association study in type 2 diabetes indicates a role for genes involved in beta-cell function as well as insulin action. *PloS. Biol.*, 1, E20, 2003.
31. Grant, S.F., Thorleifsson, G., Reynisdottir, I., Benediktsson, R., Manolescu, A., Sainz, J., Helgason, A., Stefansson, H., Emilsson, V., Helgadottir, A., Styrkarsdottir, U.,

Magnusson, K.P., Walters, G.B., Palsdottir, E., Jonsdottir, T., Gudmundsdottir, T., Gylfason, A., Saemundsdottir, J., Wilensky, R.L., Reilly, M.P., Rader, D.J., Bagger, Y., Christiansen, C., Gudnason, V., Sigurdsson, G., Thorsteinsdottir, U., Gulcher, J.R., Kong, A., and Stefansson, K., Variant of transcription factor 7-like 2 (TCF7L2) gene confers risk of type 2 diabetes, *Nat. Genet.*, 38, 320, 2006.

32. Colditz, G.A., Willett, W.C., Rotnitzky, A., and Manson, J.E., Weight gain as a risk factor for clinical diabetes mellitus in women, *Ann. Intern. Med.*, 122, 481, 1995.
33. Wang, Y., Rimm, E.B., Stampfer, M.J., Willett, W.C., and Hu, F.B., Comparison of abdominal adiposity and overall obesity in predicting risk of type 2 diabetes among men, *Am. J. Clin. Nutr.*, 81, 555, 2005.
34. Schulze, M.B., and Hu, F.B., Primary prevention of diabetes: What can be done and how much can be prevented? *Annu. Rev. Public Health*, 26, 445, 2005.
35. Bajaj, M., Suraamornkul, S., Pratipanawatr, T., Hardies, L.J., Pratipanawatr, W., Glass, L., Cersosimo, E., Miyazaki, Y., and DeFronzo, R.A., Pioglitazone reduces hepatic fat content and augments splanchnic glucose uptake in patients with type 2 diabetes. *Diabetes*, 52, 1364, 2003.
36. Stumvoll, M., Control of glycaemia: from molecules to men. Minkowski Lecture 2003. Diabetologia, 47, 770, 2004.
37. Petersen, K.F., Dufour, S., Befroy, D., Lehrke, M., Hendler, R.E., and Shulman, G.I., Reversal of nonalcoholic hepatic steatosis, hepatic insulin resistance, and hyperglycemia by moderate weight reduction in patients with type 2 diabetes, *Diabetes*, 54, 603, 2005.
38. Hu, F.B., Manson, J.E., Stampfer, M.J., Colditz, G., Liu, S., Solomon, C.G., and Willett, W.C., Diet, lifestyle, and the risk of type 2 diabetes mellitus in women, *N. Engl. J. Med.*, 345, 790, 2001.
39. Willett, W., Manson, J., and Liu, S., Glycemic index, glycemic load, and risk of type 2 diabetes, *Am. J. Clin. Nutr.*, 76, 274S, 2002.
40. Schulze, M.B., Manson, J.E., Ludwig, D.S., Colditz, G.A., Stampfer, M.J, Willett, W.C, and Hu, F.B., Sugar-sweetened beverages, weight gain, and incidence of type 2 diabetes in young and middle-aged women, *JAMA*, 292, 927, 2004.
41. van Dam, R.M., Rimm, E.B., Willett, W.C., Stampfer, M.J., and Hu, F.B., Dietary patterns and risk for type 2 diabetes mellitus in U.S. men, *Ann. Intern. Med.*, 5, 136, 201, 2002.
42. Hoffmann, K., Schulze, M.B., Schienkiewitz, A., Nothlings, U., and Boeing, H.. Application of a new statistical method to derive dietary patterns in nutritional epidemiology, *Am. J. Epidemiol.*, 159, 935, 2004.
43. Heidemann, C., Hoffmann, K., Spranger, J., Klipstein-Grobusch, K., Mohlig, M., Pfeiffer, A.F., and Boeing, H., A dietary pattern protective against type 2 diabetes in the European Prospective Investigation into Cancer and Nutrition (EPIC)-Potsdam Study cohort, *Diabetologia*, 48, 1126, 2005.
44. Montonen, J., Knekt, P., Harkanen, T., Jarvinen, R., Heliovaara, M., Aromaa, A., and Reunanen, A., Dietary patterns and the incidence of type 2 diabetes, *Am. J. Epidemiol.*, 161, 219, 2005.
45. Sigal, R.J., Kenny, G.P., Wasserman, D.H., and Castaneda-Sceppa, C., Physical activity/exercise and type 2 diabetes, *Diabetes Care*, 27, 18, 2004.
46. Hu, F.B., Leitzmann, M.F., Stampfer, M.J., Colditz, G.A., Willett, W.C., and Rimm, E.B., Physical activity and television watching in relation to risk for type 2 diabetes mellitus in men. *Arch. Intern. Med.*, 161, 1542, 2001.

47. Hawley, J.A., Exercise as a therapeutic intervention for the prevention and treatment of insulin resistance, *Diabetes Metab. Res. Rev.*, 20, 383, 2004.
48. Khaw, K.T., Wareham, N., Luben, R., Bingham, S., Oakes, S., Welch, A., and Day, N., Glycated haemoglobin, diabetes, and mortality in men in Norfolk cohort of European prospective investigation of cancer and nutrition (EPIC-Norfolk), *Br. Med. J.*, 322, 15, 2001.
49. Lyssenko, V., Almgren, P., Anevski, D., Perfekt, R., Lahti, K., Nissen, M., Isomaa, B., Forsen, B., Homstrom, N., Saloranta, C., Taskinen, M.R., Groop, L., and Tuomi, T., Botnia study group, Predictors of and longitudinal changes in insulin sensitivity and secretion preceding onset of type 2 diabetes, *Diabetes*, 54, 166, 2005.
50. Spranger, J., Kroke, A., Möhlig, M., Bergmann, M.M., Ristow. M., Boeing, H., and Pfeiffer, A.F., Adiponectin and protection against type 2 diabetes mellitus, *Lancet*, 361, 226, 2003, Erratum in: *Lancet*, 361, 1060, 2003.
51. Trujillo, M.E. and Scherer, P.E., Adiponectin — journey from an adipocyte secretory protein to biomarker of the metabolic syndrome, *J. Intern. Med.*, 257, 167, 2005.
52. Bajaj, M., Suraamornkul, S., Piper, P., Hardies, L.J., Glass, L., Cersosimo, E., Pratipanawatr, T., Miyazaki, Y., and DeFronzo, R.A., Decreased plasma adiponectin concentrations are closely related to hepatic fat content and hepatic insulin resistance in pioglitazone-treated type 2 diabetic patients. *J. Clin. Endocrinol. Metab.*, 89, 200, 2004.
53. Kolb, H. and Mandrup-Poulsen, T., An immune origin of type 2 diabetes? *Diabetologia*, 48, 1038, 2005.
54. Spranger, J., Kroke, A., Mohlig, M., Hoffmann, K., Bergmann, M.M., Ristow, M., Boeing, H., and Pfeiffer, A.F., Inflammatory cytokines and the risk to develop type 2 diabetes: results of the prospective population-based European Prospective Investigation into Cancer and Nutrition (EPIC)-Potsdam Study, *Diabetes*, 52, 812, 2003.
55. Sjoholm, A. and Nystrom, T., Inflammation and the etiology of type 2 diabetes, *Diabetes Metab. Res. Rev.*, 22, 4, 2006.
56. Torgerson, J.S., Hauptman, J., Boldrin, M.N., and Sjostrom, L., XENical in the prevention of diabetes in obese subjects (XENDOS) study: a randomized study of orlistat as an adjunct to lifestyle changes for the prevention of type 2 diabetes in obese patients, *Diabetes Care*, 27, 155, 2004.
57. Sugerman, H.J., Wolfe, L.G., Sica, D.A., and Clore, J.N., Diabetes and hypertension in severe obesity and effects of gastric bypass-induced weight loss, *Ann. Surg.*, 237, 751, 2003.
58. Costa, A., Conget, I., and Gomis, R., Impaired glucose tolerance: is there a case for pharmacologic intervention?, *Treat. Endocrinol.*, 205, 2002.
59. Lindstrom, J. and Tuomilehto, J., The diabetes risk score: a practical tool to predict type 2 diabetes risk, *Diabetes Care*, 26, 725, 2003.
60. Rathmann, W., Martin, S., Haastert, B., Icks, A., Holle, R., Lowel, H., and Giani, G., KORA Study Group. Performance of screening questionnaires and risk scores for undiagnosed diabetes: the KORA Survey 2000, *Arch. Intern. Med.*, 165, 436, 2005.
61. Schulze, M.B., Hoffmann, K., Boeing, H., Linseisen, J., Rohrmann, S., Möhlig, M., Pfeiffer, A.F.H., Spranger, J., Thamer, C., Häring, H.-U., Fritsche, A., and Joost, H.-G., An accurate risk score based on anthropometric, dietary and lifestyle factors to predict the development of type 2 diabetes, *Diabetes Care*, 30, 510, 2007.

62. Lindi, V.I., Uusitupa, M.I., Lindstrom, J., Louheranta, A., Eriksson, J.G., Valle, T.T., Hamalainen, H., Ilanne-Parikka, P., Keinanen-Kiukaanniemi, S., Laakso, M., and Tuomilehto, J.; Finnish Diabetes Prevention Study. Association of the Pro12Ala polymorphism in the PPAR-gamma2 gene with 3-year incidence of type 2 diabetes and body weight change in the Finnish Diabetes Prevention Study, *Diabetes*, 51, 2581, 2002.
63. U.K. Prospective Diabetes Study (UKPDS) Group: effect of intensive blood-glucose control with metformin on complications in overweight patients with type 2 diabetes (UKPDS 34), *Lancet*, 352, 854, 1998.
64. Zeggini, E., Weedon, M.N., Lindgren, C.M., Frayling, T.M., Elliott, K.S., Lango, H., Timpson, N.J., Perry, J.R., Rayner, N.W., Freathy, R.M., Barrett, J.C., Shields, B., Morris, A.P., Ellard, S., Groves, C.J., Harries, L.W., Marchini, J.L., Owen, K.R., Knight, B., Cardon, L.R., Walker, M., Hitman, G.A., Morris, A.D., Doney, A.S., McCarthy, M.L., and Hattersley, A.T., Replication of genome-wide association signals in U.K. samples reveals risk loci for type 2 diabetes, *Science*, in press, 2007.

# 7 Toward Personalized Nutrition for the Prevention and Treatment of Cancer

*John C. Mathers*

**CONTENTS**



## 7.1 INTRODUCTION

Cancers develop because of unrepaired genomic damage, causing aberrant gene expression that gives the tumor cell and its progeny a competitive advantage. For the majority of cancers, this genomic damage results from environmental influences, which supports the idea that if these influences were better understood, a large proportion of the significant, and growing, global burden of cancer is potentially preventable. There is strong support from epidemiologic studies that dietary (and lifestyle) factors play a substantial role in modifying risk for a number of the major cancers including breast, colon, and prostate. The exciting new information emerging from recent research on what determines personal cancer risk includes evidence for the influence of (1) individual genotype, (2) dietary factors on the acquisition and repair of genomic damage, and (3) interactions between polymorphisms in specific genes and food components. It also seems likely that diet will affect both quality of life and survival after cancer diagnosis. At present, the evidence base is too limited to justify personalized dietary advice based on knowledge of genotype and of diet–gene interactions in an attempt to reduce cancer risk. However, the limited evidence available to date is sufficiently promising to encourage research funders and researchers to adopt this area as a high priority for sustained research. It will also be important to undertake translational research to discover how best to deliver personalized dietary advice, products, or other services to elicit the desired behavioral changes.

In the year 2000, 6.2 million people died from cancer, and 4.7 million women and 5.3 million men were diagnosed with a malignant tumor [1]. Although mortality rates from cancer are twice as high in developed as in developing countries, the latter are catching up as the smoking epidemic spreads [1]. By 2020, it is anticipated that the global burden of cancer will have increased by 50% because of the prevalence of smoking and other unhealthy lifestyle choices, which are exemplified by the rising incidence of obesity [1,2]. Better screening and earlier diagnosis combined with more effective treatments and palliative care will all be important in management of the growing global cancer burden, but a strong case can be made for a greater focus on cancer prevention [1,3]. The evidence base for cancer prevention policies will include understanding of the biology of the disease and of the factors that contribute to risk for both populations and individuals.

## 7.2 CANCER BIOLOGY

At its most fundamental, cancer is a genetic disease in the sense that tumors result from genomic damage that causes aberrant gene expression (Figure 7.1). Loss of function of tumor suppressor genes (by mutation or epigenetic silencing) and gain of function by oncogenes are responsible for the "hallmark features" that characterize tumor cells [4]. The earliest genomic damage (the initiating event) provides the initiated

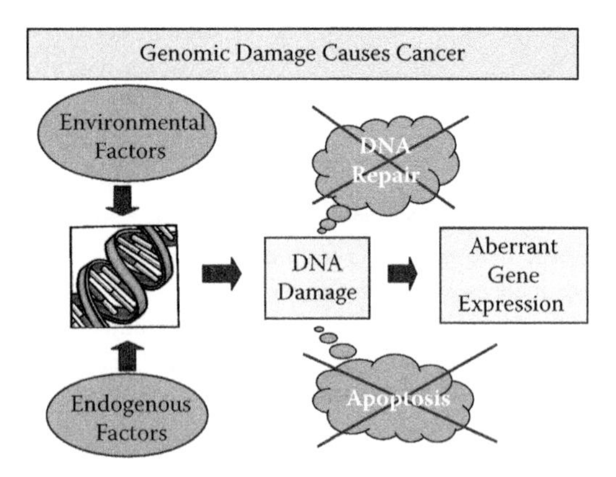


**FIGURE 7.1** Tumors arise in (stem) cells that have acquired genomic damage resulting in abnormal gene expression. Genomic damage can be repaired or damaged cells can be removed by apoptosis but, when these systems fail, cells that have a competitive advantage (in a Darwinian sense) may initiate tumorigenesis.

cell, and its progeny, with a selective advantage. In a Darwinian fashion, further "advantageous" genetic and epigenetic events enable the emerging neoplastic clone to grow through enhanced proliferation, evasion of apoptosis, disregard of differentiation signals, angiogenesis, and invasion [5]. Mutations of nuclear DNA, which result in expression of a disabled protein or no protein, are the best-known types of genomic damage, but mitochondrial DNA mutations, chromosomal abnormalities (loss, rearrangement, or duplication), loss of telomere function (which can lead to chromosomal instability), and aberrant epigenetic marking are also important features of tumors.

Epigenetics describes changes to the genome that result in altered gene expression, are heritable from one cell generation to the next, but do not involve changes to the primary sequence. The main epigenetic markings of the genome include (1) posttranslational modifications of the octet of histone proteins around which nuclear DNA is wrapped, causing alterations in chromatin structure and (2) the pattern of methylation of cytosine residues in CpG dinucleotides in DNA. Together, these epigenetic marks are believed to constitute an epigenetic code that regulates gene expression in particular cells under specific circumstances [6]. Over 20 years ago, Feinberg and Vogelstein provided early evidence that epigenetic events might be important in carcinogenesis when they reported that tumors had a lower level of DNA methylation than normal tissues [7]. It is now clear that epigenetic events play a critical role in most, if not all, cancers, and that they may be a mechanism through which environmental factors (including diet) influence stem cell biology and, thus, cancer risk [8,9]. "New" oncogenes and tumor suppressor genes whose expression is regulated by epigenetic events are being discovered, and it has been proposed that epigenetic changes might "addict" cancer cells to altered signal-transduction pathways early in tumorigenesis [10,11]. This evidence makes epigenetic markings an increasingly attractive target for identification of those at enhanced cancer risk and for chemoprevention [9,12,13].

## 7.3 GENETIC AND ENVIRONMENTAL INFLUENCES ON CANCER RISK

Studies of twins provide a powerful means of quantifying the contribution made by genetics to cancer risk. In a landmark analysis of 44,788 pairs of Swedish, Danish, and Finnish twins, Lichtenstein and colleagues concluded that inherited genetic factors make a relatively minor contribution (between one fifth and one third — see Table 7.1) to susceptibility to most types of cancer. [14] In this analysis, "nonshared," i.e., individual environmental factors accounted for about 60% of the variance in risk for most cancer [14]. This concurs with the earlier quantitative epidemiological analysis by Doll and Peto that concluded that about one third of the variation in cancer incidence between communities can be accounted for by variation in habitual diet and a similar proportion by smoking behavior [15]. The importance of eating patterns and nutrient intake in modifying cancer risk has been reviewed extensively and forms the basis for recommendations for dietary changes expected to reduce risk [16,17]. Although the evidence for diet as an etiological factor is much stronger for some cancer sites, e.g., the colorectum than for others, e.g., the testis, the lack of convincing evidence should not be interpreted as lack of a dietary effect, given the paucity of research on the role of diet in the development of many cancers [3,17].

**TABLE 7.1**
**Estimates of the Variance in Cancer Risk Accounted for by Heritable and Environmental Factors from Studies of Swedish, Danish, and Finnish Twins**

| Cancer Site | Heritable Factors | Shared Environmental Factors | Nonshared Environmental Factors |
|---|---|---|---|
| Stomach | 0.28 | 0.10 | 0.62 |
| Colorectum | 0.35 | 0.05 | 0.60 |
| Pancreas | 0.36 | 0 | 0.64 |
| Lung | 0.26 | 0.12 | 0.62 |
| Breast[a] | 0.27 | 0.06 | 0.67 |
| Ovary | 0.22 | 0 | 0.78 |
| Prostate | 0.42 | 0 | 0.58 |

[a] Data for women only.
*Source:* From Lichtenstein, P. et al., *N Engl J Med*, 343, 78, 2000. With permission.

### 7.3.1 Genetic Basis of Individual Cancer Risk

In most individuals, the genomic damage that causes neoplasia derives from genetic and epigenetic events experienced by individual somatic (stem) cells. However, for about 5 to 10% of all cancer cases, germ line defects are responsible for inherited cancer syndromes such as familial breast cancer (mutations in the *BRCA1* and *BRCA2* genes), familial bowel cancer [principally familial adenomatous polyposis (FAP) caused by mutations in the *APC* gene and hereditary nonpolyposis colon cancer (HNPCC) caused by mutations in a DNA mismatch repair gene], and retinoblastoma (*RB1* gene) and for greatly increased susceptibility to a number of other specific cancers (see Reference 18 for a review). Studies of these rarer syndromes have been highly informative about the biology of both inherited and sporadic tumorigenesis [19]. Although one copy of the tumor suppressor *APC* gene is mutated in every cell in the body of patients with a germ line *APC* mutation, loss of function of the second copy (by mutation, chromosomal loss, or epigenetic silencing) of this gatekeeper gene is required to initiate tumor development [19]. In contrast, damage to only one allele is sufficient to produce gain of function by oncogenes.

In so-called sporadic cancer cases, i.e., those in which there is little evidence of a familial condition, the genetic defects that are observed in tumors are similar to those occurring in the familial syndromes, but these defects have been acquired in somatic tissues [19]. Whereas a series of stochastic events is responsible for the genomic damage leading to sporadic neoplasia, individual genotype appears to contribute to individual susceptibility or resistance to tumorigenesis. The hypothesis that polygenic mechanisms are likely to be responsible for cancer susceptibility has stimulated the search for associations between genetic polymorphisms and cancer risk over the last two decades.

Although there is now a large literature on this topic, there are few robust genotype–cancer associations. Houston and Tomlinson carried out a systematic review of 50 studies, reporting relationships between common variants in 13 genes and bowel cancer risk [20].

They found significant associations in 16 of the 50 studies, but only 3 of these associations were reported in more than 1 study. After pooling data from a number of studies, they concluded that significant associations were seen for polymorphisms in three genes (Table 7.2) [20]. For the I307K polymorphism in *APC* (which is relatively common in the Ashkenazi population) and for the variable number tandem repeat polymorphism in *HRAS1*, those carrying the unusual versions of the gene had increased incidence of bowel cancer (Table 7.2). Conversely, those with TT at position 677 in the *MTHFR* gene had, on average, about 25% lower risk of bowel cancer. A more recent review by Sharp and Little of 10 studies involving more than 4000 bowel cancer cases showed that most studies suggested a lower, but not significantly so, risk for TT individuals [21]. Indeed, the relative risk of bowel cancer was clearly lower (0.45, 95% confidence interval 0.24 to 0.86) in TT compared with CC individuals only in the study of male physicians participating in the Physicians Health Study [21]. The authors concluded that the effect of the *MTHFR C677T* polymorphism *per se* is modest and emphasized the lack of understanding of gene–gene and of gene–environment interactions. [21] The *MTHFR* gene encodes the enzyme methylenetetrahydrofolate reductase, which catalyzes the remethylation of homocysteine to methionine. The TT version of the gene results in a protein with a valine rather than an alanine at amino acid position 222 and which has only about one third of the normal catalytic activity, because the mutant protein does not bind the cofactor FAD as strongly as does the wild-type protein [22]. As a consequence, individuals carrying the TT version of *MTHFR* require higher intakes of folate to maintain normal circulating concentrations of homocysteine.

Major mapping exercises such as those carried out by the International SNP Map Working Group and by the International HapMap Consortium have described the scale and nature of human genetic variability and provide tools for more extensive genetic association studies [23,24]. As an example, the Cancer Genetic Markers of Susceptibility Project (http://cgems.cancer.gov/index.asp), which began in 2005 and is expected to run for 3 years at a cost of $14 million, will use ultra-high-throughput genotyping to identify genetic variants that increase susceptibility to prostate and breast cancer. It is possible that such genomewide scans will identify either large numbers of gene variants each of which makes quite a modest contribution to risk or a much smaller number of larger-effect variants that, to date, have escaped detection. Some have urged caution about the potential benefits of such studies, arguing that (1) they overlook the importance of environmental factors, e.g., diet and lifestyle and that (2) even if the anticipated genetic variants are discovered, it is not clear how that knowledge can be translated into clinical benefit [25].

**TABLE 7.2**
**Polymorphisms Associated with Altered Risk of Bowel Cancer**

| Gene | Polymorphism | Odds Ratio | 95% Confidence Interval |
|---|---|---|---|
| APC | I1307K | 1.58 | 1.21–2.07 |
| HRAS1 | Variable number tandem repeat | 2.50 | 1.54–4.05 |
| MTHFR | C677T | 0.76 | 0.62–0.92 |

*Source:* From Houlston, R.S. and Tomlinson, I.P.M., *Gastroenterology*, 121, 282, 2001. With permission.

### 7.3.2 Diet–Gene Interactions and Cancer Risk

There is now ample support for the hypothesis that dietary factors interact with the genome to modify gene expression and that genotype influences responses to nutrients and, therefore, nutritional needs [26]. Given the evidence from epidemiologic studies and from animal models that diet can modify cancer risk, diet–gene interactions in cancer etiology would be anticipated. Note, however, that much of the evidence in this area comes from observational epidemiology (case control and cohort studies), which limits the ability to infer causality.

Genes encoding enzymes catalyzing one carbon transfer reactions and other folate-related transformations are among the most intensively studied for evidence of nutrient–gene interactions influencing cancer risk. Four out of five studies reviewed by Sharp and Little provided support for the notion that folate, methionine, and alcohol intake interacts with *MTHFR C677T* status to influence bowel cancer risk [21]. For example, the apparent protection against bowel cancer in men afforded by carriage of the TT version of *MTHFR* was highest in those with the highest folate and methionine intake but was abolished in those who reported consuming five or more alcoholic drinks per week [27]. Relationships between folate status and *MTHFR* genotype have been examined in respect of breast cancer risk in Chinese women [28]. Although there was no difference in the distribution of *MTHFR C677T* genotype among cases and controls, there was a significant inverse association of breast cancer risk with dietary folate intake for each of the genotypes that appeared to be stronger for those carrying the TT version of the gene (Table 7.3) [28].

The enzyme manganese superoxide dismutase (MnSOD) is a key component of the mitochondrial antioxidant defenses, where it dismutates the superoxide anion into oxygen and $H_2O_2$. A polymorphism at codon 16 in the mitochondrial targeting sequence of the *MnSOD* gene that results in an alanine (A) rather than a valine (V) appears to enhance transport of the protein to the mitochondrial matrix and may lead to greater MnSOD activity [29]. Several years ago, Ambrosone and colleagues reported that premenopausal women who were homozygous for the A allele and whose intakes of fruits and vegetables (good dietary sources of antioxidants) were low had increased risk of breast cancer [30]. Independent support for this association was provided subsequently from a study in Shanghai, China [31]. More recently, a large nested case control study within the

**TABLE 7.3**
**Apparent Interactions between *MTHFR C677T* Genotype and Folate Intake on Odds Ratio for Breast Cancer in Chinese Women**

| Genotype | Q4[a] | Q3 | Q2 | Q1 | *P* for trend |
|---|---|---|---|---|---|
| CC | 1.00[b] | 1.76 | 1.75 | 1.94 | 0.02 |
| CT | 1.16 | 1.50 | 1.73 | 2.17 | 0.06 |
| TT | 0.70 | 1.66 | 2.17 | 2.51 | 0.003 |

[a] Quartiles of dietary folate intake, Q4 = highest intake.
[b] Reference.
*Source:* From Shrubsole, M.J. et al., *Cancer Epidemiol Biomark Prev,* 13, 190, 2004. With permission.

Physicians Health Study investigated the association between *MnSOD* polymorphism and risk of prostate cancer. An important strength of this study was the fact that antioxidant status of the men had been determined prospectively, on average 8 years prior to cancer diagnosis [32]. Men with high antioxidant scores (based on plasma concentrations of lycopene, α-tocopherol, and selenium) had a 40% lower risk of all prostate cancer ($P_{trend}$ = 0.02) and a 60% lower risk of aggressive prostate cancer (defined as stage C or D, high-grade tumor (Gleason score 7 to 10) or prostate cancer death during follow up; $P_{trend}$ = 0.002) than those with low antioxidant status [32]. However, there was a significant interaction between antioxidant score and *MnSOD* polymorphism that affected prostate cancer risk. For men carrying one or more V alleles, there was no significant relationship between antioxidant status and prostate cancer risk. In contrast, men homozygous for the A allele showed a five and tenfold reduction in total and aggressive prostate cancer risk, respectively, between those with lowest and highest quartiles of antioxidant status [32]. Li and colleagues explained their findings by suggesting that the higher MnSOD activity associated with carriage of the AA allele may result in greater generation of $H_2O_2$ and a consequently greater need for catalase and the selenium-containing glutathione peroxidase [32]. When antioxidant status is low, the enhanced production of $H_2O_2$ may lead to antioxidant damage and to prostate cancer [32].

The major factors that are hypothesized to contribute to risk of cancer for any individual are summarized in the simple model known at the Health Pendulum (Figure 7.2). For each person, the fulcrum of the pendulum is determined by the

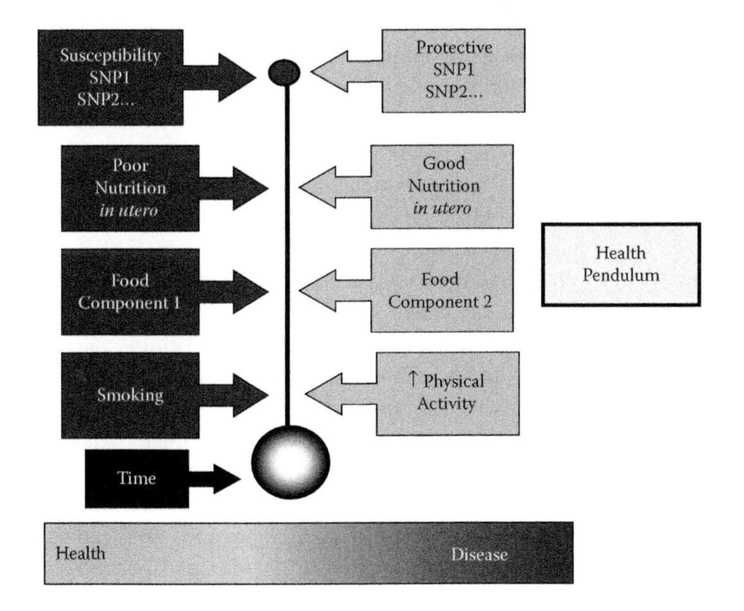


**FIGURE 7.2** The health pendulum. A simple model illustrating how key etiological factors influence cancer risk. For a given individual, the inherited collection of "susceptibility" and "protective" genes determines the position over the health–disease continuum from which the pendulum is suspended. Nutrition *in utero* and postnatal lifestyle factors interact with genetic makeup to further modify risk. For most common cancers, risk increases steeply with age. (Adapted from Mathers, J.C., *Br J Nutr,* 88 [Suppl. 3], S273, 2002.)

consortium of "susceptibility" and "resistance" genes that are inherited from the individual's parents. Throughout life, the pendulum is able to move being pushed to the right (further in the direction of cancer) or the left (better health) by a range of pre- and postnatal factors; i.e., a range of dietary and other factors interact with genotype to determine risk. A higher-risk lifestyle could include lack of physical activity, exposure to environmental mutagens, or a poor diet. For most common cancers, age is a potent carcinogen; i.e., risk rises steeply in old age.

## 7.4 NUTRITIONAL FACTORS IN SURVIVAL AFTER CANCER DIAGNOSIS; IS THERE AN OPPORTUNITY FOR PERSONALIZED NUTRITION?

In comparison with the wealth of literature investigating the role of diet in the etiology of cancer, much less effort appears to have been directed at determining whether, and how, dietary patterns can influence survival after cancer diagnosis. As with cancer etiology, most of the human data come from observational studies, with few examples of dietary interventions despite the experimental advantages in terms of timescales, subject targeting, and endpoints afforded by secondary prevention, quality-of-life, or survival studies.

Higher intakes of vegetables were associated with significantly longer [hazard ratio 0.75 (95%CI 0.57–0.99, $P_{Trend} = 0.01$ for highest vs. lowest third of intake)] survival after diagnosis with invasive epithelial ovarian cancer in a study of Australian women [33]. Although there were tendencies for better prognosis (time from diagnosis to death) with higher intakes of fruits and vegetables for those diagnosed with lung cancer in a Danish prospective cohort study, the opposite tendency was observed for higher consumers of potatoes, and none of the effects was statistically significant [34]. In a study of 1551 women previously treated for breast cancer, those with higher plasma total carotenoids concentrations had significantly reduced risk of breast cancer recurrence (hazard ratio = 0.57, 95% CI, 0.37–0.89 for highest vs. lowest quartile) [35]. Women diagnosed with breast cancer had reduced risk of death from causes other than breast cancer if they adopted a high "prudent dietary pattern" (characterized as higher amounts of fruit, vegetables, whole grains, and low-fat dairy products) [36]. In a recent review, Chan and colleagues concluded that there are limited data on diet and lifestyle factors that predict survival after prostate cancer diagnosis [37]. However, higher consumers of fish and tomato sauce appeared to have some protection against prostate cancer progression [38].

Among the few intervention studies is that by Sandler and colleagues, who used a double-blind randomized controlled trial to demonstrate that 325 mg aspirin/d reduced significantly ($P = 0.004$) the incidence of colorectal adenomas in a group of 635 patients with previous colorectal cancer [39]. In a much smaller intervention study of men with prostate cancer and rising prostate-specific antigen (PSA) that used a placebo-controlled crossover design, a soy-based dietary supplement reduced the rate of increase in PSA concentration [40].

It would be reasonable to hypothesize that the genotype of the individual patient might influence prognosis through modulation of both responses to cancer treatment and responses to diet post diagnosis. There is some evidence that *MTHFR* genotype may influence the effectiveness of 5-fluorouracil (5-FU; a common chemotherapy for bowel cancer) and the severity of side effects, but the studies to date have been small with conflicting outcomes (reviewed in Reference 41). A recent study of 52 advanced gastric cancer patients suggested that polymorphisms in both glutathione *S*-transferase and in thymidylate synthase predicted survival after 5-FU/cisplatin chemotherapy, and the authors concluded that such genotyping might be used to select those patients who are likely to benefit from this form of chemotherapy while sparing others the side effects of the treatment. [42].

It is now clear that individual tumors have distinct "molecular portraits" that can be observed as characteristic patterns of gene expression and which are a consequence of the particular types of genomic damage sustained in their development [43]. This is the basis for the development of the highly successful monoclonal antibody, Trastuzumab (herceptin®), which is targeted against HER2 (human epidermal growth factor receptor 2) overexpressing breast cancer cells. Two recent major trials have demonstrated that women with HER2-positive tumors treated with trastuzumab showed dramatic improvement in a range of clinical endpoints, including time to progression, response rate, duration of response and, most importantly, survival [44,45]. Such studies provide proof of principle for genetically targeted cancer therapy, and the challenge is to discover whether similar targeting can be used to personalize dietary treatments for those diagnosed with cancer to improve quality of life and survival.

## 7.5 MOTIVATION FOR BEHAVIOR CHANGE

The big questions for those working in the area of diet–gene interactions and cancer risk are: (1) will genotype-based intervention produce bigger health benefits than more generic advice and (2) will knowledge of one's genotype promote appropriate behavior change? In my view, it is much too early to answer the first of these questions. In the area of cardiovascular disease where understanding of diet–gene interactions is well established, Ordovas has commented recently that it is difficult to provide genotype-based dietary advice because of conflicting interactions between different genes [46]. The same is likely to be true for cancer. To date there have been rather few nutritional intervention studies with cancer as an endpoint [47], and none that has involved prospective genotyping. Research in the area of cancer prevention is hampered by the lack of robust surrogate endpoints [48].

It is often assumed that greater understanding of personal risk and of the modifiable factors that are likely to enhance, or reduce, risk will better motivate appropriate behavior change. In particular, the increasing availability of relatively cheap genotypic characterization coupled with information on gene–environment interactions associated with altered disease risk provides an opportunity for the development of novel personalized dietary advice or other personalized products. DNA-based information might enhance motivation for appropriate behavior change by strengthening belief (1) in the need for change and (2) that such changes will be beneficial. Alternatively, such genotype-based information might create a sense of fatalism because of the belief that genetic risk is immutable [49]. Because of the well-known difficulties in changing eating and other lifestyle behaviors, it cannot be assumed that provision of genotype-based information will elicit effective behavior change [50]. Although acknowledging the potential of genomic profiling to promote a healthy lifestyle, Haga et al. saw little reason for optimism concerning the potential for genetic test results to motivate behavior change [51]. The best evidence for the utility of such personalized advice will come from properly designed, powered, and conducted randomized controlled intervention trials. However, to my knowledge, no such trials have yet been attempted; such trials will present formidable design, ethical, and implementation issues.

## 7.6 FUTURE PERSPECTIVES FOR PERSONALIZED NUTRITION IN THE PREVENTION AND TREATMENT OF CANCER

Food choice plays a major role in the etiology of most common cancers and may do so through influencing the acquisition of genomic damage, which is fundamental to tumor development. There is fragmentary evidence that individual genotype may influence cancer risk directly and that this relationship may be modulated by dietary intake and nutritional status. However, as yet, the evidence base is insufficient to allow personalization of dietary advice for cancer prevention based on genotypic knowledge, although phenotypic information, e.g., identification of habitually low physical activity or raised adiposity, could be used to tailor advice. Advances in this area will require the development of robust surrogate endpoints that are prerequisites for genotype-specific dietary intervention studies (with prospective genotyping). It remains uncertain whether greater understanding of personal risk (based on genotype) and of the modifiable factors that are likely to enhance, or reduce, risk will better motivate appropriate behavior change. This is an important issue for the whole personalized nutrition field [53], including the development of public health strategies, and of products or services, that are intended to lower cancer risk.

There appear to be major opportunities to investigate the impact of diet, and of diet–gene interactions, on prognosis after cancer diagnosis. Because of (1) the greater motivation resulting from diagnosis with a life-threatening disease and (2) the potentially much greater individual support from health-care professionals following such a diagnosis, this might be a more fruitful area for eventual, personalization of dietary advice than primary prevention.

## ACKNOWLEDGMENTS

Research in my laboratory on cancer prevention is funded by the Medical Research Council (G0100496), the Biotechnology and Biological Sciences Research Council (D20173), and by the Food Standards Agency (N12015, N12016).

## KEY READINGS

Feinberg, A.P., Ohlsson, R., and Henikoff, S, The epigenetic progenitor origin of human cancer, *Nat Rev Genet,* 7, 21, 2006.

Joost, H.G., Gibney, M.J., Cashman, K.D., Gorman, U., Hesketh, J.E., Mueller, M., van Ommen, B., Williams, C.M., and Mathers, J.C., Personalized nutrition, *Br J Nutr* [in press], 2007.

Mathers, J.C., Nutrition and cancer prevention: diet-gene interactions, *Proc Nutr Soc,* 62, 605, 2003.
Rock, C.L. et al., Plasma carotenoids and recurrence-free survival in women with a history of breast cancer, *J Clin Oncol*, 23, 6631, 2005.
Stewart, B.W. and Kleihues, P., *World Cancer Report*, IARC Press, Lyon, 2003.

## REFERENCES

1. Stewart, B.W. and Kleihues, P., *World Cancer Report*, IARC Press, Lyon, 2003.
2. Calle, E.E. and Thun, M.J., Obesity and cancer, *Oncogene*, 23, 6365.
3. Mathers, J.C., Nutrition and cancer prevention: diet-gene interactions, *Proc Nutr Soc,* 62, 605, 2003.
4. Hanahan, D. and Weinberg, R.A., The hallmarks of cancer, *Cell*, 100, 57, 2000.
5. Ponder, B.A.J., Cancer genetics, *Nature*, 411, 336, 2001.
6. Jenuwein, T. and Allis, C.D., Translating the histone code, *Science* 293, 1074, 2001.
7. Feinberg, A.P. and Vogelstein, B., Hypomethylation distinguishes genes of some Human cancers from their normal counterparts, *Nature*, 301, 89, 1983.
8. Jones, P.A. and Baylin, S.B., The fundamental role of epigenetic events in cancer, *Nat Rev Genet,* 3, 418, 2002.
9. Feinberg, A.P., Ohlsson, R., and Henikoff, S, The epigenetic progenitor origin of human cancer, *Nat Rev Genet,* 7, 21, 2006.
10. Esteller, M., Epigenetics provides a new generation of oncogenes and tumour-suppressor genes, *Br J Cancer*, 94, 179, 2006.
11. Baylin, S.B. and Ohm, J.E., Epigenetic gene silencing in cancer — a mechanism for early oncogenic pathway addiction?, *Nat Rev Cancer,* 6, 107, 2006.
12. Belshaw, N.J. et al., Use of DNA from stools to detect aberrant CpG island methylation of genes implicated in colorectal cancer. *Cancer Epidemiol Biomark Control,* 13, 1495, 2004.
13. Mathers, J.C., Reversal of DNA hypomethylation by folic acid supplements: possible role in colorectal cancer prevention, *Gut,* 54, 579, 2005.
14. Lichtenstein, P. et al., Environmental and heritable factors in the causation of cancer, *N Engl J Med*, 343, 78, 2000.
15. Doll, R. and Peto, R., The causes of cancer: quantitative estimates of avoidable risks in the USA today, *J Natl Cancer Inst*, 66, 1191, 1981.
16. World Cancer Research Fund/American Institute of Cancer Research, *Food, Nutrition and the Prevention of Cancer: A Global Perspective*, World Cancer Research Fund/ American Institute of Cancer Research, Washington, D.C., 1997.
17. Department of Health, *Nutritional Aspects of the Development of Cancer, Report on Health and Social Subjects No. 48,* The Stationery Office, London, 1998.
18. Garber, J.E. and Offit, K., Hereditary cancer predisposition syndromes, *J Clin Oncol*, 23, 276, 2005.
19. Kinzler, K.W. and Vogelstein, B., Lessons from hereditary colorectal cancer, *Cell*, 87, 159, 1996.
20. Houlston, R.S. and Tomlinson, I.P.M., Polymorphisms and colorectal cancer risk, *Gastroenterology*, 121, 282, 2001.
21. Sharp, L. and Little, J., Polymorphisms in genes involved in folate metabolism and colorectal neoplasia: a HuGE review, *Am J Epidemiol,* 159, 423, 2004.
22. Guenther, B.D. et al., The structure and properties of methylenetetrahydrofolate reductase from *Escherichia coli* suggest how folate ameliorates human hyperhomocysteinemia, *Nat Struct Biol,* 6, 359, 1999.

23. Sachidanandam, R. et al., A map of human genome sequence variation containing 1.42 million single nucleotide polymorphisms, *Nature*, 409, 928, 2001.
24. International HapMap Consortium, A haplotype map of the human genome, *Nature*, 437, 1299, 2005.
25. Baker, S.G. and Kaprio, J., Common susceptibility genes for cancer: search for the end of the rainbow, *BMJ*, 332, 1150, 2006.
26. Mathers, J.C., Candidate mechanisms for interactions between nutrients and genes, in *Nutrient-Gene Interactions in Cancer,* Choi, S.-W. and Friso, S., Eds., CRC Press Taylor & Francis, Boca Raton, FL, 2005, chap. 2.
27. Chen, J. et al., A methylenetetrahydrofolate reductase polymorphism and the risk of colorectal cancer, *Cancer Res,* 56, 4862, 1996.
28. Shrubsole, M.J. et al., *MTHFR* polymorphisms, dietary folate intake, and breast cancer risk: results from the Shanghai Breast Cancer Study, *Cancer Epidemiol Biomark Prev,* 13, 190, 2004.
29. Sutton, A. et al., The Ala16Val genetic dimorphism modulates the import of human manganese superoxide dismutate into rat liver mitochondria, *Pharmacogenet,* 13, 145, 2003.
30. Ambrosone, C.B. et al., Manganese superoxide dismutase (MnSOD) genetic polymorphisms, dietary antioxidants, and risk of breast cancer, *Cancer Res*, 59, 602, 1999.
31. Cai, Q. et al., Genetic polymorphism in the manganese superoxide dismutase gene, antioxidant intake and breast cancer risk: results from the Shanghai Breast Cancer Study, *Breast Cancer Res,* 6, R647, 2004.
32. Li, H. et al., Manganese superoxide dismutase polymorphism, prediagnostic antioxidant status, and risk of clinical significant prostate cancer, *Cancer Res*, 65, 2498, 2005.
33. Nagle, C.M. et al., Dietary influences on survival after ovarian cancer, *Int J Cancer*, 106, 264, 2003.
34. Skuladottir, H. et al., Does intake of fruit and vegetables improve lung cancer survival?, *Lung Cancer*, 51, 267, 2006.
35. Rock, C.L. et al., Plasma carotenoids and recurrence-free survival in women with a history of breast cancer, *J Clin Oncol*, 23, 6631, 2005.
36. Kroenke, C.H. et al., Dietary patterns and survival after breast cancer diagnosis, *J Clin Oncol*, 23, 9295, 2005.
37. Chan, J.M., Gann, P.H., and Giovannucci, E.L., Role of diet in prostate cancer development and progression, *J Clin Oncol*, 23, 8152, 2005.
38. Chan, J.M. et al., Diet after diagnosis and the risk of prostate cancer progression, recurrence, and death (United States), *Cancer Causes Control*, 17, 199, 2006.
39. Sandler, R.S. et al., A randomised trial of aspirin to prevent colorectal adenomas in patients with previous colorectal cancer, *N Engl J Med*, 348, 1939, 2003.
40. Schröder, F.H. et al., Randomised, double-blind, placebo-controlled crossover study in men with prostate cancer and rising PSA: effectiveness of a dietary supplement, *Eur Urol*, 48, 922, 2005.
41. Little, J. et al., Colon cancer and genetic variation in folate metabolism: the clinical bottom line, *J Nutr*, 133, 3758S, 2003.
42. Goekkurt, E. et al., Polymorphisms of glutathione S-transferases (GST) and thymidylate synthase (TS) — novel predictors for response and survival in gastric cancer patients, *Br J Cancer*, 94, 281, 2006.
43. Perou, C.M. et al., Molecular portraits of human breast tumours, *Nature*, 406, 747, 2000.
44. Piccart-Gebhart, M.J. et al., Trastuzumab after adjuvant chemotherapy in HER2-positive breast cancer, *N Engl J Med*, 353, 1659, 2005.

45. Romond, E.H. et al., Trastuzumab plus adjuvant chemotherapy for operable HER2-positive breast cancer, *N Engl J Med*, 353, 1673, 2005.
46. Ordovas, J.M., Genetic interactions with diet influence the risk of cardiovascular disease, *Am J Clin Nutr,* 83, 443S, 2006.
47. Mathers, J.C., Food and cancer prevention: human intervention studies. In *Dietary Anticarcinogens and Antimutagens*, Johnson, I.T. and G.R. Fenwick, G.R., Eds., Royal Society of Chemistry, Cambridge, 2000, chap. 8.1.
48. Sanderson, P. et al., Emerging diet-related surrogate end points for colorectal cancer: U.K. Food Standards Agency diet and colonic health workshop report, *Brit J Nutr*, 91, 315, 2004.
49. Marteau, T.M. and Lerman, C., Genetic risk and behavioural change, *Br Med J*, 322, 1056, 2001.
50. Adamson, A.J. and Mathers, J.C., Effecting dietary change, *Proc Nutr Soc,* 63, 537, 2004.
51. Haga, S.B., Khoury, M.J., and Burke, W., Genomic profiling to promote a healthy lifestyle: not ready for prime time, *Nat Genet*, 34, 347, 2003.
52 Mathers, J.C., Pulses and carcinogenesis: potential for the prevention of colon, breast and other cancers, *Br J Nutr,* 88(Suppl. 3), S273, 2002.
53. Joost, H.G., Gibney, M.J., Cashman, K.D., Gorman, U., Hesketh, J.E., Mueller, M., van Ommen, B., Williams, C.M., and Mathers, J.C., Personalized nutrition, *Br J Nutr* [in press], 2007.

# 8 Nutrigenomics and Angiogenesis in Obesity

*Aldona Dembinska-Kieć*

## CONTENTS



## 8.1 INTRODUCTION

Development and maturation/plasticity of adipose tissue vascularity is critical for the function of this metabolic and the endocrine organ. The proangiogenic factors, as well as the endogenous inhibitors of angiogenesis, are synthesized locally in adipose tissue. It has been proved recently that treatment of animals with antiangiogenic factors (such as anti-VEGF or its receptor antibody) dose dependently, in a reversible manner, decreases adipose tissue depot and body weight. The involvement of basal nutrient (such as fatty acids, amino acids, carbohydrates, and polyphenols) availability and energy supply signals (i.e., caloric restriction) on the "nutrient sensors" such as the mammalian target of rapamycin (mTOR) or CHOP-10/gadd 153 and the other pathways regulating adipose tissue morphogenesis are reviewed on the basis of recent knowledge. Because transcriptomics applied to obesity, as well as caloric restriction studies in humans, point to the important changes in "pro- and anti-inflammatory" status, the essential role of personalized nutrition in regulation of the angiogenesis-driven remodeling of the stromal vascular fraction of adipose tissue is discussed.

Without appropriate blood supply from the capillary network, tissue cannot survive; the circulatory system is essential for oxygen and nutrient distribution between tissues and for the removal of by-products of metabolism. Vasculogenesis and angiogenesis play an essential role in a number of physiologic and pathologic events, such as fetal development, vascular and tissue remodeling in ischemia, inflammation, proliferative diabetic retinopathy, as well as in promotion of solid tumor growth and invasiveness (1,2).

The development and maturation/plasticity of adipose tissue vascularity is critical for the function of adipose tissue as the metabolic and the endocrine organ. It has also been demonstrated that fetal adipocyte development is spatially and temporally related to arteriolar development (3). Recent studies have evidenced that human endothelial progenitors and preadipocytes express similar patterns of genes and proteins [cellular markers and the proangiogenic factors such as CD34, AC133, vascular endothelial growth factor (VEGF) receptors, integrins, serine proteases, and others], which suggests a possible common origin from the stromal vascular progenitor cell fraction (SVF) (3,4,5).

In adolescence, the adipose tissue SVF releases only 6% of the main proangiogenic VEGF amount released by the differentiated adipocytes. Under the stimulus of insulin, the differentiated adipocytes rather than the stromal vascular fraction are a source of VEGF released by visceral adipose tissue (6), pointing to the stimulation of angiogenesis by the growing mass of tissue.

## 8.2 THE MAIN PRINCIPLES OF ANGIOGENESIS

The multistep process of angiogenesis is organized by a sensitive balance of activators and inhibitors of recruitment of endothelial cells and their progenitors. It includes induction of various growth factors, production of proteolytic enzymes to digest the basement membrane and extracellular matrix, endothelial cell migration, proliferation and tube formation, and differentiation of pericytes/vascular smooth muscle with reconstruction of basement membranes. Ischemia, blood shear stress forces, and cytokine-driven induction of the sequence certain genes are responsible for the outgrowth and maturation of the new capillary network (1) (Figure 8.1).

There are several proangiogenic growth factors and cytokines induced in ischemic tissue, such as VEGF, tumor necrosis factor (TNFα), basic fibroblast growth factor (bFGF), interleukin-8, (IL-8), platelet-derived growth factor (PDGF), angiopoietins, ephrins, proangiogenic vasoconstrictors such as angiotensin II (AngII), endothelin (End), thromboxan (TxA2), and a plethora of others acting by its specific receptors, or other angiogenic modulators, such as nitric oxide (NO) (1). VEGF is the main, most important proangiogenic factor. It exists in several isoforms (VEGF-A, -B, -C, -D, and -E) that are derived from the alternative splicing of the same gene. These isoforms transduce their signals to the nucleus mainly through three receptors. The VEGFR-1(Flt) induces the activation of EC, vessel wall permeability, EC fenestration, and pathological angiogenesis seen in cancer vasculature (1). VEGFR-3 is involved in lymphangiogenesis. VEGF–2 (Flk/KDR) receptor has thyrosine kinase activity, thus regulating EC proliferation (cell cycle) by activation of extracellular signal-regulated kinase (ERK)1/2 mitogen-activated protein kinases

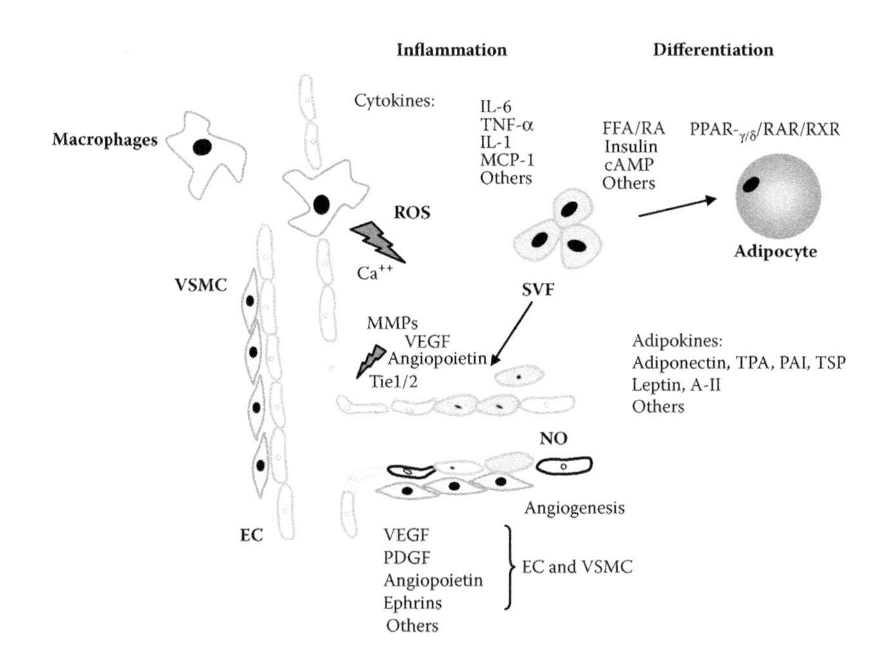


**FIGURE 8.1** Multistep process of angiogenesis.

(MAPKs) and p70S6 kinase (S6K), migration of ECs by the stress-activated protein kinase 2/p38 pathway, and survival (antiapoptotic effect) by Akt activation (7). VEGF-A induces genes of the main metalloproteinases: MMP-2 and MMP-9, as well as integrins (VE-cadherin or $\alpha_v\beta_3$). The IL-8-induced activation of CXCR-2 receptor is necessary for matrix remodeling, adhesion, and EC differentiation during tubulogenesis. The VEGF gene expression is induced by several factors such as hypoxia (by the involvement of the hypoxia-inducible-factor, HIF-1), insulin, insulin growth factors (IGFs), cytokines, as well as by nitric oxide (NO) (1,2,7).

Angiopoietin (Ang)-1 and Ang-2 with their receptors, Tie-1 and Tie-2, are considered to be the most important partners of VEGF in the maturation of capillary networks, especially in branching of the sprouts and modifying apoptosis to be not redundant for capillary-sprouting cells. VEGF signaling is initiated through the assembly of a multicomponent complex composed of the vascular endothelial (VE)-cadherin, β-catenin, VEGF-R2, and PI3-kinase. This complex then stimulates Akt, leading to the downstream activation and nuclear translocation of the transcription factor NF-κB, antiapoptotic Bcl-2 protein synthesis, induction of IL-8, and monocyte chemoattractant protein-1 (MCP-1) gene expression. This is followed by infiltration of macrophages and tubulogenesis of the growing capillary network (1,7,8). Ephrin B (EphB2) and its receptor EphB4 expressed on endothelial cell membranes determine arteriovenous shifting of capillary differentiation (8). Transforming growth factor (TGFβ) with tumor necrosis factor (TNFα), or platelet-derived growth factor (PDGF) are induced in ischemic tissue or are released from activated macrophages or platelets. They establish the lengthening of capillaries by regulating endothelial cell quiescence, cell-to-cell interactions, and differentiation of fibroblast-like progenitors to pericytes or vascular smooth muscle cells (9). Nitric oxide (NO) synthesized by the endothelial nitric oxide synthase (eNOS) is induced by several proangiogenic factors (including VEGF, TNFα, angiotensin II (AII), insulin, leptin, adiponectin, and others). Nitric oxide plays an essential role in angiogenesis. It protects endothelial cells against apoptosis by stimulation of Akt, and induction of Bcl-2 and other antiapoptotic proteins (IAPs). By inhibition of platelet aggregation and adhesion of inflammatory cells (macrophages, leukocytes, and lymphocytes), NO inhibits penetration of cells generating pro- and antiangiogenic factors (VEGF, PDGF, TNFα, AII, metalloproteinases, IL-8, IL-1, INF-γ, etc.). By inhibition of vascular wall smooth muscle cell (VSMC) proliferation and basement membrane protein synthesis, NO is responsible for the maturation of the capillary network and inhibition of pathological remodeling of the vessel wall (1,7–9).

Simultaneously with the proangiogenic factors, the endogenous inhibitors of angiogenesis are synthesized locally. Examples are thrombospondins (TSP-1 and TSP-2) with their receptor CD36, which is also the long-chain fatty acid scavenger-type receptor, or the other inhibitory products deriving from the protein digestion such as the angiostatin, endostatin, maspin, and others (1,2,9).

### 8.2.1 Angiogenesis and Adipose Tissue Plasticity

Primitive fat cell clusters resembling vascular structures without any or only a few preadipocytes were observed in fetuses of several species (10). There is also some evidence for overlap of autocrine/paracrine developmental relationship between the preendothelial/preadipocyte cells (reviewed by Hausmann and Richardson (3). Both type of cells express the $\alpha_v\beta_3$ integrin, release PAI-1 that supports coordination of angiogenesis and adipogenesis (10). Both the adipose as well as the stromal vascular (non-fat-containing cell) fraction (SVF) release VEGF; however, adipocytes are the main source of the proangiogenic VEGF, IL-8 and PAI-1 (but not IL-6), released from differentiated adipocytes under stimulation with insulin (6). Interestingly, VEGF induction and release from adipocytes is also activated by factors promoting lipolysis such as norepinephrine, forskolin, and dibutyryl-cAMP, but not dexamethasone (6). Angiopoietin 2 (Ang-2) gene expression, which supports proangiogenic VEGF activity, was found in preadipocytes as well as *ob/ob* mice fat tissue under stimulation with leptin. Leptin and adiponectin exert regulatory effects on angiogenesis directly or by inducing the infiltration of macrophages (the important source of VEGF and metalloproteinases, or by activation of endothelial NO release (1,3,4,10). The long-form leptin receptor is expressed in endothelial cells and adipocytes in human and mouse adipose tissue. Its activation promotes the Erk1/2 and STAT3 phosphorylation mediating EC proliferation, migration, and survival, and also (similar to VEGF) increases permeability of endothelium by the formation of endothelial gaps. Additionally, leptin increases VSMC proliferation and migration necessary for maturation and remodeling of the vessel wall (3,11).

There is evidence suggesting that angiogenesis is a pivotal factor for adipogenesis. During fetal development, arteriolar differentiation and synthesis of extracellular matrix proteins precedes the differentiation of adipocytes (3). The undifferentiated vessel wall fibroblasts, pericytes, as well as circulating stromal progenitory cells, may serve as the early preadipocytes, and the adipocyte tissue stromal vascular fraction (SVF) secrete several factors necessary for angiogenesis and modulation of the capillary network (4,5,12). Thus, during the postnatal period, VEGF expression and resulting angiogenesis may precipitate adipogenesis (3). VEGF (as well as leptin) are induced by ischemia (mediated by HIF-1) or insulin, and the exposure to cold induces VEGF expression in the brown adipose tissue (1,6,8).

Using several experimental models of genetically modified mice (knockout or transgenic), it has been demonstrated that the manipulation of the tPA, uPA/PAI-1, or plasminogen gene expression deeply influences adipose tissue mass and weight gain of mice fed a high-fat diet. Remodeling of extracellular matrix proteins by endothelial, adipocyte, or macrophage-derived MMP-2 and MMP-9 is necessary for angiogenesis and adipogenesis (1,3), and the TIMP-3 deficient mice exhibit increased adipogenicity during mammary gland involution.

It has been proved recently that treatment of animals with antiangiogenic factors, (such as anti-VEGF or its receptor antibody) dose dependently, in a reversible manner, decreases adipose tissue deposition and body weight (13).

### 8.2.2 Nutrients and Differentiation of Adipose Tissue

Manipulation of dietary factors with the aim of decreasing adipose tissue mass attenuate the "inflammatory" response in adipose tissue and improve insulin sensitivity. It is an important event for prevention and treatment of metabolic syndrome and type 2 diabetes. Moloney et al. (14) have demonstrated that that a subgroup of fatty acids known as conjugated linoleic acid (CLA), in particular, the *cis-9, trans-11*-CLA isomer, markedly improves insulin sensitivity and lipid metabolism as well as inflammatory cytokine biosynthesis by lowering of nuclear P65 levels and decreasing NFκB DNA binding.

The developing blood vessels in fat tissue represent a potential target for regulating adipose tissue mass showing metabolism and substrate-fuel buffering properties. With the microarray method, it has been demonstrated that the expression of many adipogenic genes (SREBP-1, C/EBPα, or PPARγ) was significantly decreased in adipose tissue from obese animals, indicating a process of dedifferentiation, i.e., loss of adipocyte phenotype similar to the response seen after treatment of adipose tissue with TNFα. Voros et al. (15) reported that treatment of *ob/ob* as well as C57Bl/6 mice on high-fat diet for 15 weeks increases adipo- and angiogenesis in subcutaneous and gonadal fat pads. It was accompanied (dependent on the duration of feeding) by downregulation of Ang-1 and elevation of TSP-1, pointing to changes in angiogenesis. In *ob/ob* mice the placental growth factor (PIGF) and Ang-2 expression was increased in subcutaneous fat, when TSP-2 in subcutaneous and gonadal fat (15).

The early phase of preadipocyte differentiation is induced by the sequence of the genes regulated by the two groups of transcriptional factors: the CCAAT/enhancer binding protein (C/EBP) and peroxisome proliferator-activated receptors (PPARs). PPAR-δ and PPARα/γ heterodimerize with the other nuclear receptors (RAR/RXR, LXR, etc.) and regulate the expression of the multiple genes of differentiated adipocytes such as an adipocyte-specific fatty-acid-binding protein (FABP), FAT/CD36 (scavenger receptor for long-chain FFA and thrombospondin), perilipin, adipsin, stearoyl-CaA desaturase (SCD-1), GLUT-4, phosphenolpyruvate carboxykinase (PEPECK), and leptin (16). Expression of these genes in progenitor undifferentiated cells (SVF) is connected with inhibition of expression of the genes related to angiogenesis. Exogenous PPARγ ligands cause reduction of VEGF-R1 and VEGF-R2 expression in endothelial cells, thus inhibiting angiogenesis by inhibition of endothelial cell migration and proliferation, as well as by the inhibition of the important-for-angiogenesis infiltration of macrophages. However, the induction of VEGF gene and protein by PPARγ ligands (glitazones) in adipocytes and vascular smooth muscle cells was reported. Blocking the PPARγ pathway by transfecting the preadipocytes with the PPARγ-dominant negative construct abrogates not only adipose tissue differentiation but also reduces angiogenesis (17). Similarly, inhibition of angiogenesis by blocking of VEGF-R2 activity by the specific antibody inhibited the preadipocyte differentiation *in vivo* and *in vitro*, in spite of the fact that preadipocytes do not express the VEGF-R2 (17). This results in strong support of the parallel, reciprocal regulation of angio- and adipogenesis in not well recognized but involving fatty acids and its derivatives paracrine manner (3,11,16,17).

The involvement of basal nutrient availability and energy supply signals (i.e., amino acid, glucose sufficiency) on the "nutrient sensors" such as the mammalian target of rapamycin (mTOR) or CHOP-10/gadd 153 pathways regulating adipose tissue morphogenesis remains to be investigated (18). Moreover, the fact that the transcriptomics applied to obesity as well as the caloric restriction study in humans points to the important changes in the pro- and anti-inflammatory status, and thus to the regulation of the angiogenesis regulating factor gene expression in the stromal vascular fraction of the adipose tissue (19). For example, the Wnt family of proteins, which are the paracrine growth factors highly expressed in preadipocytes, are the potent inhibitors of angiogenesis (reviewed in Reference 29). Depending on the local conditions, Wnt signaling causes precursor cell proliferation, apoptosis, differentiation, or maintenance in undifferentiated status. The inhibition of adipogenesis is connected with Wnt/fizzled cooperation, which results in downregulation of C/EBPα and PPARγ, and inactivation of glycogen synthase kinase 3 (GSK3) by preventing it from phosphorylating β-catenin with subsequent degradation. The stabilization of β-catenin may be responsible for the maintenance of the precursor cells (satellite cells) in tissues, such as the SVF of adipose tissue. This may be the clue event for adipose tissue plasticity and adipose tissue accumulation, as well as the "jo-jo" effect in patients (18–20).

GSK3 modulation by a large number of growth factors (including insulin) and nutrients is an important regulator of cell differentiation. Disruption of Forkhead box C2 (FOXC2) gene expression linking cell cycle with glucose sensitivity causes embryonic or perinatal death with severe vascular and skeletal defects (20). Also, the sprouty proteins (Spry), which may both activate or inhibit activity of several receptor tyrosine kinase (RTK) signaling, are involved in the early progenitor cell fate decision, and thus also in angiogenic vs. adipogenic differentiation of SVF. Sprouty proteins were found to suppress the MAPK signaling induced by EGF, VEGF, or PDGF (20). The importance of polymorphisms of "nutrient sensors" in metabolic disorders remains to be established. For that the new scientific approach, i.e., "systems biology," is necessary to understand the nutrient–metabolism–genotype dependence.

### 8.2.3 Polyphenols and Other Naturally Occurring Nutrients in Angiogenesis and Adipogenesis

Polyphenols, especially flavonoids, are claimed to act as active components in prevention of cancer, cardiovascular diseases, or metabolic disorders, including diabetes. Flavonoids are plant phytochemicals that cannot be synthesized by humans. The six classes of flavonoids (flavanones, flavones, flavonols, isoflavonoids, anthocyanins, and flavans) vary in their structural characteristics. Flavanones occur predominantly in citrus fruits, flavones in herbs, isoflavonoids in legumes, anthocyanins and catechins in fruits, and flavonols in all fruits and vegetables. Grains and oilseeds, honey, and chocolate have flavonoids; however, the flavonoid content may be destroyed by food processing. Fresh green tea contains large amounts of catechin and caffeine polyphenols, whereas resveratrol, myricetin, and quercetin are rich in grapes, black currants, cranberry, and red wine. Phytic acid [inositol hexaphosphate(IP6)] is present in most legumes (corn, soy beans, wheat bran, and nuts).

In adipose tissue, polyphenols (i.e., epigallocatechin gallate) have been shown to exert a thermogenic effect, suppress adipogenesis by reduction of C/EBP-$\alpha$, PPAR-$\gamma$, and SREBP-1 gene expression, promote apoptosis of adipocytes, and influence weight control in rodents as well as in humans (21).

Antiangioprevention and antiangiogenic therapy (preventive/therapeutic inhibition of tumor angiogenesis) are considered efficient strategies for controlling the growth and metastasis of solid tumors as well as for other diseases involving pathological angiogenesis such as atherosclerosis, rheumatoid arthritis, psoriasis, and diabetic retinopathy (1,2,9). The broad spectrum of the chemopreventive and antiangiogenic mechanisms of the natural compounds has been suggested to explain this activity. They include the antioxidant, anti-inflammatory, antiproliferative (directly by the cell cycle inhibition or by the growth factors and hormone intracellular signaling inhibition), proapoptotic, immune-enhancing, and modification of xenobiotic phase I/II enzyme induction properties. In addition to, and independently of, their antioxidant effects, plant polyphenols enhance the production of vasodilating factors [NO, prostacyclin, and endothelial hyperpolarizing factor (EDHF)], and inhibit the synthesis of vasoconstrictory, proangiogenic endothelin-1 (ET-1). The inhibitory effect on the prostate, breast, colon, lung, and the other tumor angiogenesis and tumor progression, correlates with the inhibition of metalloproteinases (MMP-2, MMP-9), as well as inhibition of VEGF and its receptor gene and protein induction in experimental models. Recent studies indicate that VEGF expression and release are prevented by red wine polyphenols at concentration as low as 3 mg/l. It has been also reported that flavones: 3,4 dihydroxyflavone, resveratrol, and luteolin are among the most potent antiendothelial polyphenols in suppression of cell proliferation with $IC_{50}$ of 1.4 to 2 $\mu M$ (22).The effect of polyphenols (including resveratrol, a polyphenolic phytoestrogen found in some grapes and wines, or epigallocatechin-3-gallate, found in green tea) is mediated by the prevention of the growth factors or ischemia-induced redox-sensitive activation of polyvalent intracellular signaling, including Stat3, NF$\kappa$B, PI3-kinase/Akt, p38 MAPK, pathways regulating the endothelial homeostasis, and intracellular $Ca^{2+}$ concentration (22,23). Genistein and luteolin, with regard to its antimitotic activity, inhibits the VEGF-induced phosphorylation of p70 S6 kinase (S6K), a downstream effector of PI3K responsible for G1 phase progression of cell cycle, but not the VEGF-induced phosphorylation of the extra-cellular signaling-regulated kinase $^{1}/_{2}$ (ERK1/2) in endothelial cells (23).

Resveratrol and the soybean isoflavones bind and increase the transcriptional activity of estrogen receptors (ERs) α and β on endothelial cells. Similar to estradiol ($E_2$), they rapidly increase eNOS gene expression as well as direct NO release by increasing eNOS activity. Genistein, daidzeoin, and biochanin A, a soy isoflavone, inhibit the growth and reduce angiogenesis of transplantable bladder cancer in mice (24–28). Genistein is currently in clinical trials as an angiogenesis inhibitor for the treatment of breast and prostate cancer (24).

However, clinical evidence to support many of the currently claimed health benefits of this drugs remains to be confirmed. Despite the advantageous effects of some of these agents demonstrated *in vitro* and in experimental animal models, their mostly dosage-related, possible toxic effects must also be of concern at the same time (25). The presence of different numbers of -OH moieties on the B-ring of the flavonols may contribute to their antioxidant activity, as well as to their toxicity and antiangiogenic activity measured by the proliferation, migration, and the primitive capillary tubular structure formation (24).

Some studies have also demonstrated pro-oxidant activity of flavonoids. Bleomycin-dependent DNA damage was accelerated by quercetin and kaempferol (but not naringin), especially in the presence of $Fe^{+3}$ and the high concentrations of flavonoid (23). It has been reported that endothelial response to the red wine polyphenols is critically dependent on a redox-sensitive mechanism involving the formation of superoxide anions by a flavin-dependent enzyme (22). In chemoprevention of lung cancer, as well as antiatherogenic beta-carotene was unexpectedly found to increase the risk of lung cancer among the high-risk groups of patients.

The beta-carotene-induced expression of genes in endothelial as well as endothelial progenitor cells *in vitro* measured by microarray pointed to the activation of chemotaxis, homing, decrease of connexin 43, induction of the stress, and xenobiotic phase I and II metabolizing enzymes' groups of genes as well as genes involved in proangiogenic activity (26).

The inhibition of tumorigenesis by caffeine or tea was shown to be closely related to the reduction of body fat (25). The mechanism of the flavone-induced antiadipogenic effect was documented to be connected with the blocking insulin receptor substrate (IRS) from phosphorylation (thus inhibiting glucose uptake by decrease of GLUT-4), and with increasing lipolysis by the hormone-sensitive lipase in adipose tissue. Quercetin, catechin, and kaempferol flavonoids inhibit the terminal differentiation of preadipocytes by decrease of the C/EBP-α, PPAR-γ, and SREBP-1 gene expression (21). Oral administration of green tea and epigallo-catechin galleate (EGCG) decreases adipose mass, stimulates thermogenesis and fat oxidation, and decreases lipemia in animals and humans, but at a rather high dose level. In humans drinking green tea according to Chinese traditions, serum levels of the most abundant tea catechin compound EGCG are in the range of 0.1 to 0.3 $\mu M$ (21). The intake of soy proteins (source of genistein and daidzen) by Chinese and Japanese populations is considerable higher (30 to 35 g/d) than in Western populations (5 to 10 g/d), and the concentration of genistein in the urine of humans eating a plant-based diet is 30-fold higher compared to those consuming a traditional Western diet. Thus, the beneficial effect may be related also to the ethnic diet.

Interestingly, ferrets receiving the high dose of beta-carotene (the source of retinoic acid) gained more weight than control animals, which is consistent with the proadipogenic PPAR/RXR/RAR-induced pathway. No such effect was seen with the low dose of beta-carotene (27). The size of the subcutaneous–inguinal fat depot in animals treated with the high dose of beta-carotene was significantly higher than that of animals treated with the low dose and slightly higher than that of controls. This study also showed that chronic treatment with beta-carotene induced a dose-dependent hypertrophy of white adipocytes and increased neoangiogenesis in subcutaneous WAT in all treated ferrets. It is in accordance with the suggested proangiogenic activity of beta-carotene observed by the gene expression in endothelial cells measured by microarray (26,27).

Beta-carotene treatment reduced the UCP1 protein levels in the interscapular BAT as well as in the inguinal and retroperitonal WAT depots, pointing to the accumulation of WAT-type tissue. Interestingly, rodents with knockout β,β-carotene-15,15′-mono-oxygenase (*Bcmo1*$^{-/-}$) gene accumulate beta-carotene in adipose tissue and have increased body fat mass, which is consistent with the previously described possible proangiogenic and proadipogenic effect of beta-carotene (28).

## 8.3 PERSONALIZED NUTRITION AND ANGIOGENESIS IN ADIPOSE TISSUE REMODELING

Diet, with its composition (nutrients) and caloric density, is the pivotal regulator of angiogenesis, which decides fetal tissue development and tissue remodeling during the whole period of life. Thus, the individual genotype determining the phenotype also affects angiogenesis-dependent tissue, including tumor, remodeling (29). Thus, at the present time polymorphisms of the VEGF, MMP, TPA/PAI, and TNF genes seem to be of great interest among the markers influencing the magnitude of angiogenesis.

Thus, parallel to mechanistic, the epidemiologic (with the appropriately matched number of participants and case control) studies aim to prove association between the nutrient/angiogenesis cooperation in regulation of the accumulation of adipose tissue mass. The application of quantitative trait locus (QTL) analysis and the more advanced bioinformatic methods may be helpful for the identification of the gene/chromosomal localization of the genetic background and genotype/nutrient relation of metabolic and vascular disease interrelationship (30).

## KEY READINGS

Carmeliet, P. Angiogenesis in health and disease. *Nat Med* 9(2003), 653–60.

Hausman, G.J. and Richardson, R.L. Adipose tissue angiogenesis. *J Anim Sci* 2004; 82, 925–934.

Rupnick, M.A., Panigrahy, D., Zhang, C.Y., Dallabrida, S.M., Lowell, B.B., Langer, L., and Folkman, M.J. Adipose tissue mass can be regulated through the vasculature. *Proc Natl Acad Sci USA* 2002; 99, 10730–10735.

Voros, G., Maguoi, E., Demeulemeester, D., Clerx, N., Collen, D., and Lijen, H.R. Modulation of angiogenesis during adipose tissue development in murine models of obesity. *Endocrinology* 2005; 146, 4545–4554.

Wang, S., Yehya, N., Schardt, E.E., Wang, H., Drake, T.A., and Lusis, A.J. Genetic and genomic analysis of a fat mass trait with complex inheritance reveals marked sex specificity. PLoS Genetics /www.plosgenetix.org; 2006; 2, 0148–0153.

## REFERENCES

1. Carmeliet, P. Angiogenesis in health and disease. *Nat Med* 9(2003), 653–60.
2. Folkman, J., Merler, E., Abernathy, C., and Williams, G. Isolation of a tumor factor responsible of angiogenesis. *J Exp Med* 1971; 133, 275–288.
3. Hausman, G.J. and Richardson, R.L. Adipose tissue angiogenesis. *J Anim Sci* 2004; 82, 925–934.
4. Rodriguez, A.M., Elabd, C., Amri, Ez-Z., Alhaud, G., and Dani, C. The human adipose tissue is a source of multipotent stem cells. *Biochemistry* 2005; 87, 125–128.
5. Prunet-Marcassus, B., Cousin, B., Caton, D., Andre, M., Penicaud, L., and Casteilla, L. From heterogeneity to plasticity in adipose tissues: site-specific differences. *Exp Cell Res* 2006; 312, 727–736.
6. Mick, G.J., Wang, X., and McCornick, K. White adipocyte vascular endothelial growth factor; regulation by insulin. *Endocrinology* 2002; 143, 948–953.
7. Dembinska-Kiec, A., Dulak, J., Partyka, Huk, I., and Malinski, T. VEGF-nitric oxide reciprocal regulation. *Nat Med* 1997; 3, 11–77.
8. Jośko, J. and Mazurek, M. Transcription factors having impact on vascular endothelial growth factor (VEGF) gene expression in angiogenesis. *Med Sci Monit* 2004; 10, RA89–98.
9. Crandall, D.L., Hausman, G.J., and Kral, J.G. A review on the microcirculation of adipose tissue: anatomic, metabolic and angiogenic perspectives. *Microcirculation* 1997; 4, 211–232.
10. Park, H.Y., Kwon, H.M., Lim, H.J., Hong, B.K., Lee, J.Y., Park, B.E., Jang, Y., Cho, S.Y., and Kim, H.S. Potential role of leptin in angiogenesis; Leptin induces endothelial cell proliferation and expression of metaloproteinases *in vivo* and *in vitro*. *Exp Mol Med* 2001; 33, 95–102.
11. Planat-Benard, V., Silvestre, J.S., Cousin, B., Andre, M., Nibbelink, M., Tamarat, R., Clerque, M., Manneville, C., Saillan-Barreau, C., Duriez, M., Tedgui, A., Levy, B., Penicaud, L., and Casteilla, L. Plasticity of human adipose lineage cells toward endothelial cell: physiological and therapeutic perspectives. *Circulation* 2004; 109, 656–663.
12. Rechman, J., Tractuev, D., Li, J., Merfeld-Clauss, S., Temm-Grove, C.J., Bovenkerk, J.E., Pell, C.L., Johnstone, B.H., Considine, R.V., and March, K.L., Secretion of angiogenic and antiapoptotic factors by human adipose stromal cells. *Circulation* 2004; 109, 1292–1298.
13. Rupnick, M.A., Panigrahy, D., Zhang, C.Y., Dallabrida, S.M., Lowell, B.B., Langer, L., and Folkman, M.J. Adipose tissue mass can be regulated through the vasculature. *Proc Natl Acad Sci USA* 2002; 99, 10730–10735.
14. Moloney, F., Noone, E., Loscher, C., Gibney, M.J., and Roche, H.M. *Cis-9, trans 11* conjugated linoleic acid improves metabolic and molecular markers of insulin sensitivity in adipose tissue and liver. *Proc Nutr Soc* 2004; 64,58A.
15. Voros, G., Maguoi, E., Demeulemeester, D., Clerx, N., Collen, D., and Lijen, H.R. Modulation of angiogenesis during adipose tissue development in murine models of obesity. *Endocrinology* 2005; 146, 4545–4554.

16. Rosen, ED. and Spiegelman, B.M. Molecular regulation of adipogenesis. *Annu Rev Cell Dev Biol* 2000; 16, 145–171.
17. Fukumura, D., Ushiyama, A., Duda, D.D., Xu, L., Tam, J., Chatterjee, V.K.K., Garkavtsev, I., and Jain, R.K. Paracrine regulation of angiogenesis and adipocyte differentiation during *in vivo* adipogenesis. *Circ Res* 2003; 93, e88–e97.
18. Kim, J.E. and Chen, J. Regulation of peroxisome proliferator-activated receptor-γ activity by mammalian target of rapamycin and amino acids in adipogenesis. *Diabetes* 2004; 53, 2748–2756.
19. Viguerie, N., Poitou, C., Cancello, R., Stich, V., Clement, K., and Langin, D. Transcriptomics applied to obesity and caloric restriction. *Biochemie* 2005; 87, 117–123.
20. Novakofski, J. Adipogenesis: usefulness of in vitro and in vivo experimental models. *J Anim Sci* 2004; 82, 905–915.
21. Dulloo, A.G., Duret, C., Rohrer, D., Girardier, L., Mensi, N., Fathi, M., Chantre, P., and Vandermander, J. Efficacy of a green tea extract rich in catechin polyphenols and caffeine in increasing 24-h energy expenditure and fat oxidation in humans. *Am J Clin Nutr* 1999; 70, 1040–1045.
22. Stoclet, J.C., Chataigneau, T., Ndiaye, M., Oak, M.H., Bedoui, J.E., Chataigneau, M., and Shini-Kert, V.B. Vascular protection by dietary polyphenols. *Eur J Pharmacol* 2004; 500, 299–313.
23. Bagli, E., Stefaniotou, M., Morbidelli, L., Ziche, M., Psillas, K., Murphy, C., and Fosis, T. Luteolin inhibits vascular endothelial growth factor-induced angiogenesis; inhibition of endothelial cell survival and proliferation by targeting phosphatidilinositol 3′-kinase activity. *Cancer Res* 2004; 64, 7936–7946.
24. Cao, Y. and Cao, R. Brakenhielm Antiangiogenic mechanism of diet-derived polyphenols. *J Nutr Biochem* 2002; 13, 380–390.
25. Mennen, L.I., Walker, R., Bennetau-Pelissero, C., and Scalbert, A. Risk and safety of polyphenol consumption. *Am J Clin Nutr* 2005; 81, 326S–329S.
26. Dembinska-Kiec, A., Polus, A., Kiec-Wilk, B., Grzybowska, J., Mikolajczyk, M., Hartwich, J., Razny, U., Szumilas, K., Banas, A., Bodzioch, M., Stachura, J., Dyduch, G., Laidler, P., Zagajewski, J., Langman, T., and Schmitz, G. Proangiogenic activity of beta-carotene is coupled with the activation of endothelial cell chemotaxis. *Biochim Biophys Acta* May 30, 2005; 1740(2): 222–39.
27. Luisa Bonet Murano, I., Morroni, M., Zingaretti, M.C., Oliver, P., Sanchez, J., Fuster, A., Pico, C., Palou, A., and Cinti, S. Morphology of ferret subcutaneous adipose tissue after 6-month daily supplementation with oral beta-carotene. *Biochim Biophys Acta* May 30, 2005; 1740(2): 305–12. Epub November 17, 2004.
28. von Lintig, J., Hessel, S., Eichnger, A., Isken, A., Oberhauser, V., Vogt, K., Goralczyk, R., and Wyss, A. Analysis of *Bcmo1* knock-out mouse model uncovers a role of β-carotene for the regulation of lipid metabolism. In *Oxidants and Antioxidants in Biology*. Abstract book of the Oxygen Club of California. Santa Barbara; March 15–18, 2006, p 21.
29. Balasubramanian, S.P., Brown, N.J., and Reed, M.W.R. Role of genetic polymorphisms in tumor angiogenesis. *Br J Cancer* 2002; 87, 1057–1065.
30. Wang, S., Yehya, N., Schardt, E.E., Wang, H., Drake, T.A., and Lusis, A.J. Genetic and genomic analysis of a fat mass trait with complex inheritance reveals marked sex specificity. PLoS Genetics /www.plosgenetix.org; 2006; 2, 0148–0153.

# 9 Metabolic Programming during Pregnancy: Implications for Personalized Nutrition

*Simon C. Langley-Evans*

## CONTENTS



## 9.1 INTRODUCTION

This chapter will introduce the concept that nutritional factors before birth impact disease risk in later life. Evidence from epidemiologic and experimental studies demonstrates that variation in nutrition during fetal development exerts a programming effect on tissue development and metabolic/physiological status in adult life. These programming effects have profound implications for the attainment of metabolic phenotypes that promote the development of the metabolic syndrome and associated disease outcomes. There is growing evidence of interactions between the genotype and indicators of fetal growth and nutrition in determining this disease risk phenotype. For example, a well-characterized association between low birth weight and risk of type 2 diabetes in adult life is dependent on the pro12ala polymorphism of the peroxisome proliferators activated receptor $\gamma 2$. Similarly, the established association between the Bsm1 polymorphism of the vitamin D receptor and degenerative disease of bone appears to be modified by fetal growth-related factors. In considering how this knowledge might be applied to the development of personalized nutrition, the identification of simple markers of nutritionally programmed disease phenotypes may be an important adjunct to screening for genotypic biomarkers. The development of sensitive biomarkers of programmed events using nutrigenomics approaches should be an important priority for future research in the metabolic programming field.

## 9.2 NUTRITIONAL PROGRAMMING OF HEALTH AND DISEASE

The environment encountered during fetal life and infancy is strongly related to risk of noncommunicable diseases in adult life. This association of early life factors with conditions that may not develop for another four decades or more may be explained in terms of adaptations during critical phases of growth and development that ensure the maintenance of homeostasis and hence survival when the environment is compromised. The means through which events in early life trigger permanent responses have been described as nutritional or metabolic programming. These terms describe the process through which a stimulus or insult during a critical window of fetal or infant development elicits permanent responses that produce long-term changes in tissue structure or function (Langley-Evans, 2004).

There may be a number of potential insults that initiate such intrauterine adaptations. Maternal stress, infection, exposure to toxins, and hypoxia have all been suggested as agents that may promote long-term physiological change to fetal physiology. For most of the human population, however, the most likely insult will be variation in nutrient supply during early development. Whatever may drive the process, programming occurs because of the innate capacity of developing tissues to adapt to the environment they encounter. For almost all cell types, in all organs, this plasticity is a characteristic that is present for only a short period before the time of birth (Gluckman and Hanson, 2004). As a result the prenatal period represents a unique life-stage in which exposure to suboptimal nutrition may shape the lifelong capacity of the organism to respond to the environment and, consequently, the long-term disease risk phenotype.

### 9.2.1 Evidence from Epidemiologic Studies

The concept that human disease states may arise, at least in part, through exposure to adverse programming *in utero* arose from the findings of a broad range of epidemiologic studies indicating associations between disease risk and infant characteristics at birth. Many cohort studies have demonstrated that there are inverse associations between birth weight and risk of coronary heart disease, stroke, hypertension, glucose intolerance, type 2 diabetes, and the metabolic syndrome (Barker, 2004). These relationships are also observed in relation to body proportions at birth. For example, babies with low ponderal index at birth have significantly greater risk of insulin resistance and diabetes in adulthood, whereas babies born with a large head circumference relative to body length appear to be at greater risk of later atopy

(Table 9.1). Low birth weight and disproportion at birth are essentially simple markers of constrained growth *in utero*. Such growth impairment is therefore proposed to be central to programming of disease risk, but the effects of intrauterine growth restriction are also modulated by postnatal growth rates. Thus, the individual at greatest risk of metabolic syndrome is likely to have been born small but undergone rapid catch-up growth in infancy, attaining an increased body mass index in adolescence (Eriksson et al., 2003a).

The relationship between risk of coronary heart disease, non-insulin-dependent diabetes, and birth weight has been attributed to the effects of variation in maternal nutritional status on fetal growth. However, this explanation at first glance appears tenuous as in human populations the association between maternal nutrient intake and birth weight is difficult to demonstrate (McMillen and Robinson, 2005). It is estimated that maternal nutrient intake only explains approximately 6% of the variation in birth weight. In extreme situations, such as the wartime Dutch Hunger Winter and siege of Leningrad, starvation had only minor effects on birth weight. In well-nourished populations, although isolated studies show that intakes of animal protein or sucrose are related to birth weight and placental weight, the majority of studies find no significant relationships between maternal diet and weights of either baby or placenta.

Although the lack of clear associations between maternal nutrient intake and birth weight, or proportions at birth, appears to undermine the nutritional programming hypothesis, there are important studies that directly demonstrate associations between maternal nutritional status in pregnancy and disease-risk markers in the resulting offspring. A Jamaican study showed that higher blood pressure in prepubescent boys was predicted by low maternal hemoglobin, weight gain, and triceps skin fold thicknesses in pregnancy (Godfrey et al., 1994). A study of men born in Aberdeen in the 1950s found that blood pressure was related to maternal intakes of animal protein and of carbohydrate (Campbell et al., 1996). Data from the ongoing

**TABLE 9.1**
**Associations between Anthropometric Indices at Birth and Markers of Disease Risk in Human Populations**

| Birth Characteristic | Associated Disease State | Associated Risk Factor |
|---|---|---|
| Low birth weight | Coronary heart disease, type 2 diabetes, asthma, COPD, osteoporosis, depression, schizophrenia, stroke, cataracts | Obesity, hypertension, insulin resistance, poor response to vaccination, metabolic syndrome, raised clotting factors, raised LDL-cholesterol |
| Low ponderal index[a] | Type 2 diabetes, schizophrenia | Insulin resistance, hypertension, hypercortisolism |
| Reduced abdominal circumference | | Hypertension, raised LDL-cholesterol, hyperinsulinemia |
| Large head circumference[b] | Asthma, eczema | Raised IgE |

[a] Ponderal index is a marker of relative thinness at birth (birth weight, kg/length, $m^3$).
[b] Corrected for crown-heel length. COPD = chronic obstructive pulmonary disease.

Project Viva study in the U.S. also appear to support the concept of nutritional programming. For example, higher maternal calcium intakes in pregnancy result in lower blood pressure in 6-month-old babies (Gillman et al., 2004).

The inconsistencies in the literature relating to maternal diet and birth weight almost certainly arise because of the lack of appropriate methodology to assess the nutrient supply the fetus actually gets. This is partly determined by maternal intake, but will also depend on maternal stores going in to pregnancy, the metabolic demands of the mother, and the perfusion of the placenta. These are all problems that are best addressed by experimental animal models. These have been widely used to investigate the plausibility of the programming concept and to consider the mechanistic basis of nutritional programming.

### 9.2.2 Evidence from Experimental Studies

In addition to the epidemiologic evidence suggesting that human cardiovascular disease may be programmed by the intrauterine environment, a number of animal models have been developed to study the process and its underlying mechanisms. It has been consistently noted in rats, mice, and guinea pigs that fetal exposure to undernutrition produces elevated blood pressure (Langley-Evans, 2006). For example, the feeding of a protein-restricted diet in rat pregnancy results in elevations to systolic blood pressure in the resultant offspring that are of the order of 15 to 30 mm Hg. The elevation of blood pressure occurs despite the fact that the maternal dietary manipulation is sufficiently mild to produce offspring that are of normal weight at birth. Blood pressure is elevated from the age of weaning, and the magnitude of increase depends on the timing of undernutrition during pregnancy (Figure 9.1). Similar

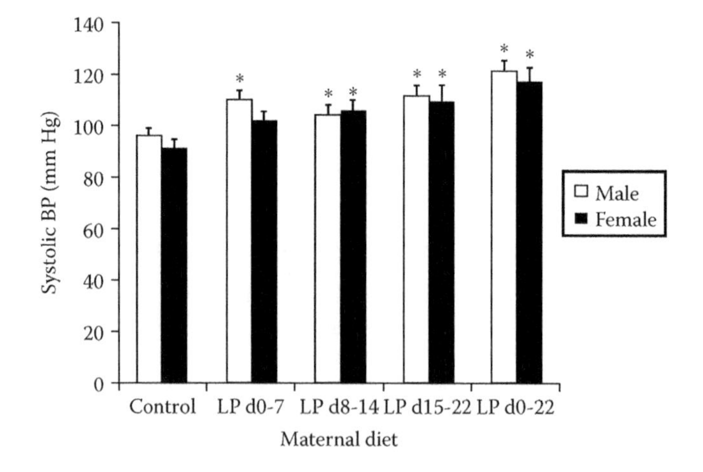


**FIGURE 9.1** Systolic blood pressure in 4-week-old rats exposed to low-protein diet during specific periods of pregnancy. Undernutrition at any stage of gestation increases later blood pressure, and these effects persist into adulthood. Figure reproduced from data published in Langley-Evans et al. (1996). LP = low-protein diet. Full rat gestation is 22 d (d 0 to 7 represents targeting of protein restriction to early gestation, d 8 to 14 to midgestation, d 15 to 22 to late gestation). * denotes $P < 0.05$ compared to control group.

observations in large animal species, such as the sheep, suggest that programming of cardiovascular function occurs in all mammals.

A broad spectrum of nutritionally programmed disorders have been reported from animal studies, but in general such experiments uncover blood pressure, glucose intolerance, insulin resistance, and increased adiposity as common endpoints of nutritional interventions targeted at pregnancy, or specific periods in pregnancy (Table 9.2). It is becoming increasingly apparent that in addition to programming disease states or their direct risk factors (glucose intolerance, adiposity, and hypertension), alterations to the quality or quantity of rodent diets in pregnancy determine behavioral antecedents of metabolic risk. For example, food restriction and protein

**TABLE 9.2**
**Programming Effects of Maternal Undernutrition in Animal Models**

| Observed Phenotype in Offspring | Maternal Diet Manipulation in Pregnancy | Species |
|---|---|---|
| Hypertension | Food restriction | Rat, sheep, and guinea pig |
| | Low-protein diet | Rat and mouse |
| | Uterine artery ligation | Rat |
| | High saturated fat | Rat |
| | Iron deficiency | Rat |
| | Calcium deficiency | Rat |
| Insulin resistance | Food restriction | Rat and guinea pig |
| | Low-protein diet | Rat |
| Disordered lipid metabolism | Low-protein diet | Rat |
| Obesity | Postnatal overfeeding | Rat |
| | Food restriction | Rat, sheep, and guinea pig |
| | High saturated fat | Rat |
| | Low-protein diet | Rat and mouse |
| | High-protein diet | Rat |
| Altered appetite | Postnatal overfeeding | Rat |
| | Low-protein diet | Rat |
| Bone disorders | Low-protein diet | Rat |
| Renal injury | Low-protein diet | Rat |
| | Food restriction | Rat, sheep |
| Shorter life span | Low-protein diet | Rat, mouse |
| Impaired immune function | Low-protein diet | Rat |
| | Zinc deficiency | Mouse |
| | High saturated fat | Rat |

restriction in rat pregnancy have both been shown to impact feeding and locomotor behavior in the offspring (Vickers et al., 2003).

Working with species that have relatively short life span and gestation allows evaluation of intergenerational effects and consideration of interactions between dietary exposures at different developmental stages in pre- and postnatal life. Using this approach, it has been possible to show that although the combination of undernutrition before birth combined with overnutrition in adulthood does not increase risk of obesity, the introduction of overnutrition in the early postnatal (suckling and weaning stages) following prenatal restriction can induce extreme central adiposity (Langley-Evans et al., 2005). Such animal models, although varying in the detailed approaches adopted, importantly underpin the nutritional programming hypothesis, demonstrate that programming of cardiovascular changes can occur even in the absence of fetal growth retardation, and provide useful tools with which to study the mechanisms involved in nutritional programming.

### 9.2.3 Mechanistic Basis of Programming

The developmental origins of health and disease hypothesis is a concept that raises interesting possibilities in terms of the prevention and treatment of disease. One of the simplest approaches may be to intervene in pregnancy, identifying women most at risk of bearing children who are programmed for later disease and providing appropriate advice for dietary change. Alternatively, given appropriate markers to indicate that adverse programming has occurred, it may be possible to target at-risk individuals with guidance for nutritional change, or with early pharmaceutical intervention to counteract programmed effects. All of these strategies will require an understanding of the mechanistic basis of programming.

At the simplest level, nutritional programming in early life is likely to involve remodeling of key organs and tissues. All tissues develop as a consequence of proliferation and differentiation of progenitor cell lines. Disruption of these processes will result in tissues with either a reduced cell number, with altered cell types, or both of these outcomes. Evidence of this can be seen in the offspring of animals fed low-protein diets in pregnancy, which exhibit reduced numbers of nephrons in the kidney, reduced number and vascularization of Islets of Langerhans in the pancreas, and altered neuronal densities in the hypothalamus (Langley-Evans, 2006). All of these tissue-remodeling effects could explain many of the observed disease risk phenotypes due to nutritional programming.

For most species, and in particular for humans, relatively mild variations in maternal nutritional status are unlikely to significantly perturb fetal nutritional status. Release of maternal stores along with adaptive responses to increase placental blood flow and nutrient transfer will buffer the fetus against all but the most severe fluctuations in maternal nutrition. It is difficult, therefore, to see how changes in nutrient intake lead to the development of major disease in the adult offspring. In the search for mechanisms that may drive nutritional programming effects, attention has focused on the contribution of relatively subtle shifts in metabolic pathways and on the actions of stress hormones as vehicles for programming effects. In both cases, the true drivers of programming are environmentally triggered changes in fetal gene expression.

Variation in nutritional status may act as a physiological stressor. Stress responses mediated via the hypothalamic–pituitary–adrenal axis may impact the developing fetal tissues, resulting in permanent programmed responses. In most species there is a gradient in concentrations of active glucocorticoid hormones across the placenta. For example, in the rat, maternal corticosterone concentrations are between 100- and 1000-fold greater than in the fetal compartment. This gradient is maintained by the activity of 11ß-hydroxysteroid dehydrogenase type 2 (11ßHSD2), which converts active glucocorticoids to inactive forms (Seckl and Meaney, 2004). Animal studies show that 11ßHSD2 is subject to nutritional regulation. Undernutrition in pregnancy therefore leads to downregulation of this gatekeeper enzyme in placenta and, consequently, overexposure of the fetal tissues to active glucocorticoids of maternal origin (Langley-Evans, 2006).

Glucocorticoids are potent regulators of gene expression, and it is proposed that exposure of the fetal tissues to inappropriate hormone concentrations disrupts the normal developmental patterns of gene expression and resets homeostatic processes in the long term through tissue remodeling and modifications to cell–cell signaling pathways. Experiments in which pregnant animals are treated with synthetic glucocorticoids that are not substrates for 11ßHSD2 or with inhibitors of 11ßHSD2 largely duplicate the programmed phenotypes that result from variation in maternal nutrition (Seckl and Meaney, 2004; Langley-Evans, 2006). This strengthens the argument that at least some of the long-term effects of suboptimal nutrition in pregnancy are mediated by glucocorticoids.

Gene silencing through processes such as DNA methylation and histone acetylation may also provide mechanisms through which early life nutrition exerts long-term programming effects. Waterland and Jirtle (2003) demonstrated using the Agouti mouse that the expression of transposable elements controlling coat color could be switched on or off by varying the supply of methyl donors during pregnancy. The postnatal period also represents a period of plasticity during which dietary or other environmental stimuli may determine the methylation status of genes and, hence, their long-term expression (Weaver et al., 2004).

The rat model of maternal low-protein feeding has been one of the most widely studied and best-characterized experimental protocols used for the study of nutritional programming (Langley-Evans, 2006). It has been demonstrated that the deleterious effects of fetal exposure to protein restriction can be, at least in part, prevented by the addition of folic acid or glycine to the maternal diet. Folic acid, or more specifically tetrahydrofolate, is the major donor of methyl groups for DNA methylation, whereas glycine plays a critical role in folate metabolism during pregnancy. Maternal protein restriction increased hepatic expression of glucocorticoid receptor (GR) and the peroxisome proliferator-activated $\alpha$ receptor in young rats, and these increases were associated with reduced DNA methylation of these genes (Lillycrop et al., 2005). However, nutritional modulation of DNA methylation during fetal life does not explain all aspects of early programming, as some phenotypic effects of maternal protein restriction are not ameliorated by glycine and folate supplementation, and some long-term changes in gene expression are not associated with DNA hypomethylation.

## 9.3 PROGRAMMING AND THE FETAL NUTRITION–GENOTYPE INTERACTION

Unfortunately, there are no studies that have been able to consider the interaction of maternal nutrient intakes or specific nutrient deficiencies in human pregnancy with known polymorphisms that associate with disease states in adulthood. Thus, all literature in this field depends on the use of infant anthropometry, either at birth, or at 1 year of age, as a proxy for the fetal and infant environment. Although weight at birth or markers of disproportion at birth (for example, a large head circumference in relation to overall stature) may be seen as rather crude, insensitive indicators of fetal nutritional status, weight at 1 year provides a reasonable proxy for nutritional status during infancy, although this will always be confounded by the lack of information on genetic growth potential.

These caveats notwithstanding, there are a number of interesting studies that indicate there are strong interactions between the fetal or infant environment and the genotype. Thus, programming effects can modulate disease risk associated with a particular genotype and *vice versa*. The association of low birth weight with disease may be observed only in individuals carrying particular alleles. Most of the studies considering these issues have investigated genotype-programming interactions in relation to either type 2 diabetes or bone health.

### 9.3.1 Type 2 Diabetes

The peroxisome proliferator-activated receptor γ (PPARγ) is a ligand-dependent transcription factor that is predominantly expressed in adipose tissue and plays an important role in adipogenesis, fat, and energy metabolism. To date, three isoforms of PPARγ (γ-1, γ-2, and γ-3) have been identified, and each is expressed by different tissues. PPAR γ-2 is predominantly expressed in adipose tissue and contains a polymorphic region in the isoform specific exon B (Eriksson et al., 2002). The Ala allele of this pro12ala polymorphism has been proposed to have a protective role in type 2 diabetes, but the association of this allele with improved insulin sensitivity and lower diabetes risk is somewhat variable and is likely to depend on unidentified lifestyle factors. Eriksson and colleagues, working with unique cohorts of men and women born in Helsinki between 1924 and 1933, have assessed the interaction of the pro12ala polymorphism with markers of prenatal growth in determining adult insulin sensitivity, cholesterol metabolism, and risk of cardiovascular disease.

These studies demonstrated that the Ala12 allele was associated with significantly lower fasting insulin and HOMA-IR index, but that this beneficial effect of the polymorphism was isolated to individuals who had been of lower weight at birth (Eriksson et al., 2002). In other words, the detrimental effect of the Pro12Pro genotype was only seen if weight at birth was low. The genotype–fetal environment interaction worked both ways, and the association between weight at birth and insulin resistance, which has been so frequently reported in other cohorts (Barker, 2004), was only seen in individuals with a Pro12Pro genotype (Figure 9.2). The same genotype was shown by Eriksson et al. (2003b) to associate with total and HDL- and LDL-cholesterol concentrations in the same subjects. Individuals with the Pro12Pro genotype were also more likely than individuals with at least one Ala12

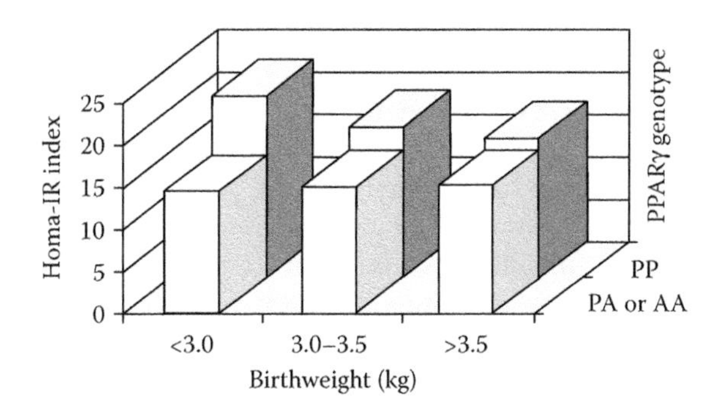


**FIGURE 9.2** The interaction of genotype for PPARγ with birth weight in determining adult insulin sensitivity. Subjects genotyped according to the Pro12Ala polymorphism in the PPARγ gene were grouped according to weight at birth. The Pro12Pro (PP) variant was associated with raised HOMA-IR only in subjects in the two lowest birth weight groups ($P < 0.005$ comparing PP and PA or AA genotype for birth weight less than 3.0 kg, $P = 0.03$ for birth weight 3.0 to 3.5 kg). Birth weight was only related to adult HOMA-IR ($P = 0.002$) in the population subset with the PP genotype. Figure produced from data reported by Eriksson et al., 2002.

allele to have higher blood pressure and to require hypertensive medication, but once again this detrimental effect of the genotype was observed only in individuals who had been of lower weight or shorter stature at birth (Yliharsa et al., 2004).

Overall, these studies of the Pro12Ala polymorphism in PPARγ suggest that a single genotype can give rise to different phenotypes because of variation in early life experience. This evidence of programmed modulation of the effects of disease-related alleles is of great importance when considering strategies for personalized nutrition.

The same considerations are clearly indicated by studies of the interaction between early life characteristics and the effects of the K121Q polymorphism of plasma cell glycoprotein 1 (PC1). This is a strong candidate gene for non-insulin-dependent diabetes, as PC1 is an inhibitor of insulin signaling downstream from the insulin receptor. The K121Q polymorphism in exon 4 of this gene is associated with variation in the inhibitory effects of PC1. The 121K variant lowers the inhibitory action, whereas 121Q enhances the inhibition and is consequently associated with insulin resistance, raised plasma glucose, and hyperinsulinemia. In the study of Kubaszek et al. (2004) no variation in insulin concentrations or HOMA-IR index was noted between individuals with a K121K genotype and those with at least one 121Q allele. However, once grouped by weight at birth, it was apparent that the 121Q allele had adverse effects. Adults that had the lowest weights at birth had greater insulin concentrations and HOMA-IR index if they carried the 121Q variant. Most importantly, although there was no variation in prevalence of diabetes or hypertension that could be attributed solely to PC1 genotype, in individuals who were of short stature at birth (birth length below 49 cm), the 121Q allele increased prevalence of hypertension by threefold and type 2 diabetes by twofold. In this study there was no apparent effect of the genotype until the interaction with a proxy of fetal growth was considered in the analysis. Thus, without anthropometric data from birth, genotyping for the PC1 polymorphism would be of little use in the application of personalized nutritional advice.

Human angiotensin converting enzyme (ACE) has an insertion/deletion (I/D) polymorphism that appears to impact both circulating and tissue activities of the enzyme. The insertion is a 287 bp fragment, the presence of which lowers ACE activity and apparently increases risk of vascular injury in diabetic subjects (Kajantie et al., 2004). However, the effects of this very common allele (the ID form predominates in populations, whereas II is the rarest variant) are inconsistent and, as with the PPARγ Pro12Ala polymorphism, this is probably explained by gene–environment factors. Kajantie et al. (2004) found that the DD variant was associated with lower weight, smaller head circumference, and shorter length at birth, implying that this variant of ACE plays a role in regulation of fetal growth. In adult life, subjects with the II variant exhibited greater insulin responses to a glucose tolerance test than those with DD, but this difference was only observed in those of lower weight at birth. In this case the polymorphic allele may confound the association between birth weight and disease, because the I allele is itself associated with shorter gestation and increased weight at birth. However, this study is a further example of how the effects of a polymorphism on a diabetes risk marker are modulated by early growth.

### 9.3.2 Osteoporosis

Mapping of the genetics of bone metabolism is well advanced, and a number of putative risk-determining genes have been identified, including the vitamin D receptor (VDR), the estrogen receptors, and the type 1 collagen A1 gene (Walker-Bone et al., 2002). Polymorphisms at these loci have been identified, including 22 separate polymorphisms of VDR, but population studies suggest that these explain only a small proportion of variation in bone mass. For example, it is estimated that the BB variant of the Bsm I restriction site in VDR can reduce site-specific bone mineral density by at most 2%.

The influence of genotype on bone health is clearly modulated by lifestyle and environmental factors. As with diabetes, any consideration of such factors has to include some assessment of proxies for early life nutrition and growth. Several studies have suggested that growth *in utero* and in the first year of infancy determine osteoporosis and osteoarthritis (Walker-Bone et al., 2002). In a study of the Bsm 1 polymorphism of VDR, Jordan and colleagues (2005) reported that the B allele increased severity of osteophytosis (the outgrowth of immature bony processes, reflecting the presence of degenerative disease) in the lumbar region. In men, but not women, there was an interaction of the VDR genotype with weight at birth in determining the severity of the lumbar degeneration. Thus, fetal factors modified the risk associated with this particular VDR genotype.

The tt variant of the Taq1 polymorphism of VDR is also associated with disease risk. Individuals with a tt genotype have lower bone mineral density and greater prevalence of fractures. Adult bone mineral density is strongly a function of the peak bone mass attained in the third decade of life, and this to some extent depends on earlier rates of growth. Keen et al. (1997) reported that the tt variant of VDR was associated with weight at 1 year, suggesting that patterns of skeletal growth even in the very early years are determined by the VDR genotype. The early environment may therefore interact with genotype to determine rates of skeletal growth, and the two factors together program adult bone characteristics.

SNPs have also been identified in the growth hormone gene cluster, which in addition to the growth hormone (GH1) gene, includes placental lactogen, placental growth hormone, and the chorionic somatomammotrophin genes. Polymorphisms of GH1 are associated with variability in bone mineralization. Dennison et al. (2004) found that over a 4 year period, the loss of bone from the lumbar spine and proximal femur was greatest in individuals with the 2 allele of the GHV1 and GHV4 loci. Individuals with these unfavorable allele variants also exhibited blunted growth hormone secretory profiles. However, these effects depended entirely on an interaction with weight at age 1 year. Individuals in the lowest tertile of infant weight showed a strong association between GHV1 genotype and rates of bone loss, whereas in adults who had been heavier infants, GHV1 genotype had no effect on bone loss. These data show that the environment encountered in infancy can modulate the effect of GH1 genotype on bone health up to seven decades later.

## 9.4 FUTURE PERSPECTIVES FOR PROGRAMMING AND PERSONALIZED NUTRITION

The developmental origins of health and disease hypothesis, and more specifically the concept that variation in maternal nutritional status can program disease risk, has important implications for the future management of the health of individuals and populations. Future goals that arise from research in this area will include appropriate dietary interventions in pregnancy, early screening and selective treatment of individuals with programmed disease risk, and the development of new drugs to counteract programming.

With an improved understanding of the life-course basis of disease, it is becoming clear that disease-causing metabolic disturbances do not just arise as a consequence of accumulated experience of fetal and postnatal nutrition and the environment. At the heart of the balance between health and disease lies a complex genetics–programming–mature environment interaction (Figure 9.3). The data from the studies of the ACE and PPARγ polymorphisms described earlier clearly suggest that certain genotypes may make the impact of programming more powerful. The converse will also be true, as programming may exacerbate the impact of a polymorphism, and could just as likely nullify the impact of the polymorphism. Findings of this nature should lead us to question whether measuring polymorphisms is of any value in determining personalized nutrition strategies.

In any future development of personalized nutrition strategies, it will be necessary to make assessments of markers of programming, just as effectively as assessing biomarkers of the genotype. In the programming field we currently lag behind in this regard as generally the only data that are routinely available are crude anthropometric estimates of fetal growth. The combination of poor intrauterine growth and childhood catch-up is, however, clearly a warning sign that could already be factored into personalized nutrition advice for individuals with high-risk genotypes.

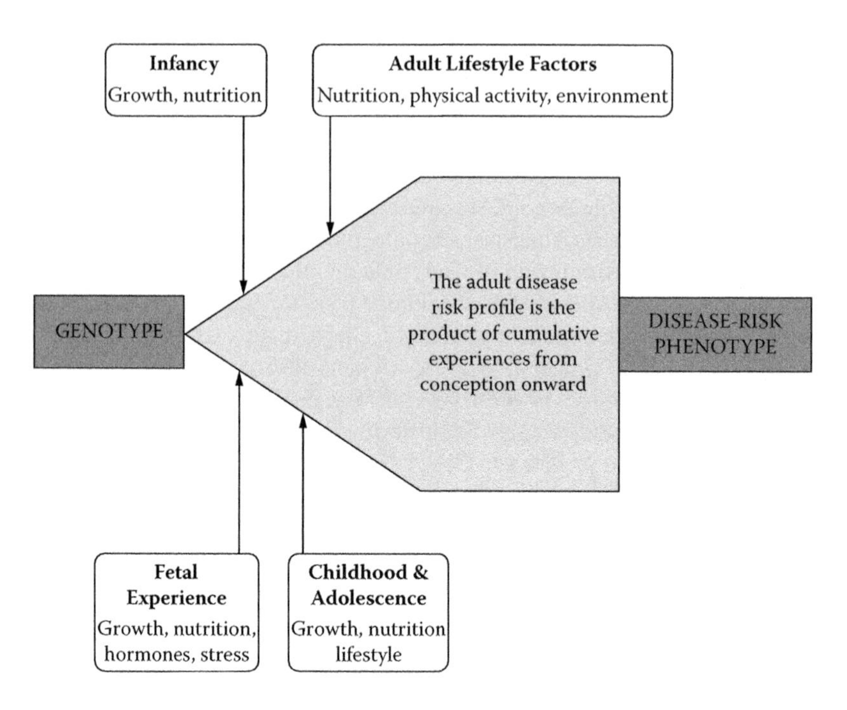


**FIGURE 9.3** Disease risk in adult life is a product of cumulative experience across the life course. Gene–environment interactions occur at all stages of life. The product of this interaction in early life will determine the strength and nature of such responses in adulthood.

To date the emphasis of the research agenda in the field of metabolic programming has been on demonstrating the biological principle and defining the mechanistic basis of programming. The time has come to consider the possible nutritional interventions that might reverse adverse programming effects. To construct appropriate personalized nutrition interventions, we require better-quality information about the characteristics of a programmed disease-risk phenotype. More studies need to utilize nutrigenomic tools, particularly proteomics and metabolomics, to focus on the cellular and metabolic consequences of an adverse nutritional environment *in utero* or during early infancy. One of the major challenges of applying these approaches, at least in human studies, will be to separate the effects of early life programming and the interaction of early life events with the genome from the effects of lifestyle factors in adult life.

## KEY READINGS

Barker, D.J.P. (1998). *Mothers, babies and health in later life*. Churchill Livingstone. London.

Gluckman, P.D. and Hanson, M.A. (2006). *Developmental origins of health and disease*. Cambridge University Press. Cambridge, U.K.

Langley-Evans, S.C. (2004). *Fetal Nutrition and Adult Disease: Programming of chronic disease through fetal exposure to undernutrition*. CABI. Wallingford, U.K.

## REFERENCES

Barker, D.J.P. (2004). The developmental origins of adult disease. *J Am Coll Nutr.* 23(6 Suppl.), 588S–595S.

Campbell, D.M., Hall, M.H., Barker, D.J., Cross, J., Shiell, A.W., and Godfrey, K.M. (1996). Diet in pregnancy and the offspring's blood pressure 40 years later. *Br J Obstet Gynaecol.* 103, 273–280.

Dennison, E.M., Syddall, H.E., Rodriguez, S., Voropanov, A., Day, I.N., and Cooper, C. (2004). Polymorphism in the growth hormone gene, weight in infancy, and adult bone mass. *J Clin Endocrinol Metab.* 89, 4898–4903.

Eriksson, J.G., Lindi, V., Uusitupa, M., Forsen, T.J., Laakso, M., Osmond, C., and Barker, D.J. (2002). The effects of the Pro12Ala polymorphism of the peroxisome proliferator-activated receptor-gamma2 gene on insulin sensitivity and insulin metabolism interact with size at birth. *Diabetes* 51, 2321–2324.

Eriksson, J.G., Forsen, T.J., Osmond, C., and Barker, D.J. (2003a) Pathways of infant and childhood growth that lead to type 2 diabetes. *Diabetes Care.* 26, 3006–3010.

Eriksson, J., Lindi, V., Uusitupa, M., Forsen, T., Laakso, M., Osmond, C., and Barker, D. (2003b). The effects of the Pro12Ala polymorphism of the PPARgamma-2 gene on lipid metabolism interact with body size at birth. *Clin Genet.* 64, 366–370.

Gillman, M.W., Rifas-Shiman, S.L., Kleinman, K.P., Rich-Edwards, J.W., and Lipshultz, S.E. (2004). Maternal calcium intake and offspring blood pressure. *Circulation* 110, 1990–1995.

Gluckman, P.D. and Hanson, M.A. (2004). Living with the past: evolution, development, and patterns of disease. *Science* 305, 1733–1736.

Godfrey, K.M., Forrester, T., Barker, D.J., Jackson, A.A., Landman, J.P., Hall, J.S., Cox, V., and Osmond, C. (1994). Maternal nutritional status in pregnancy and blood pressure in childhood. *Br J Obstet Gynaecol.* 101, 398–403.

Jordan, K.M., Syddall, H., Dennison, E.M., Cooper, C., and Arden, N.K. (2005). Birthweight, vitamin D receptor gene polymorphism, and risk of lumbar spine osteoarthritis. *J Rheumatol.* 32, 678–683.

Kajantie, E., Rautanen, A., Kere, J., Andersson, S., Yliharsila, H., Osmond, C., Barker, D.J., Forsen, T., and Eriksson, J. (2004). The effects of the ACE gene insertion/deletion polymorphism on glucose tolerance and insulin secretion in elderly people are modified by birth weight. *J Clin Endocrinol Metab.* 89, 5738–5741.

Keen, R.W., Egger, P., Fall, C., Major, P.J., Lanchbury, J.S., Spector, T.D., and Cooper, C. (1997). Polymorphisms of the vitamin D receptor, infant growth, and adult bone mass. *Calcif Tissue Int.* 60, 233–235.

Kubaszek, A., Markkanen, A., Eriksson, J.G., Forsen, T., Osmond, C., Barker, D.J., and Laakso, M. (2004). The association of the K121Q polymorphism of the plasma cell glycoprotein-1 gene with type 2 diabetes and hypertension depends on size at birth. *J Clin Endocrinol Metab.* 89, 2044–2047.

Langley-Evans, S.C., Welham, S.J.M., Sherman, R.C., and Jackson, A.A. (1996) Weanling rats exposed to maternal low protein diets during discrete periods of gestation exhibit differing severity of hypertension. *Clin Sci.* 91, 607–615.

Langley-Evans, S.C., Bellinger, L., and McMullen, S. (2005). Animal models of programming. *Maternal Child Nutr* 1, 142–148.

Langley-Evans, S.C. (2004). Fetal programming of adult disease: an overview. In *Fetal nutrition and adult disease: Programming of chronic disease through fetal exposure to undernutrition.* Ed. S.C. Langley-Evans. CABI, Wallingford, pp. 1–20.

Langley-Evans, S.C. (2006). Developmental programming of health and disease. *Proc Nutr Soc.* 65, 97–105.

Lillycrop, K.A., Phillips, E.S., Jackson, A.A., Hanson, M.A., and Burdge, G.C. (2005). Dietary protein restriction of pregnant rats induces and folic Acid supplementation prevents epigenetic modification of hepatic gene expression in the offspring. *J Nutr.* 135, 382–386.

McMillen, I.C. and Robinson, J.S. (2005). Developmental origins of the metabolic syndrome: prediction, plasticity, and programming. *Physiol Rev.* 85, 571–633.

Seckl, J.R. and Meaney, M.J. (2004). Glucocorticoid programming. *Ann NY Acad Sci.* 1032, 63–84.

Vickers, M.H., Breier, B.H., McCarthy, D., and Gluckman, P.D. (2003). Sedentary behavior during postnatal life is determined by the prenatal environment and exacerbated by postnatal hypercaloric nutrition. *Am J Physiol Regul Integr Comp Physiol.* 285, R271–273.

Walker-Bone, K., Walter, G., and Cooper, C. (2002). Recent developments in the epidemiology of osteoporosis. *Curr Opin Rheumatol.*14, 411–415.

Waterland, R.A. and Jirtle, R.L. (2003). Transposable elements: targets for early nutritional effects on epigenetic gene regulation. *Mol Cell Biol.* 23, 5293–300.

Weaver, I.C., Cervoni, N., Champagne, F.A., D'Alessio, A.C., Sharma, S., Seckl, J.R., Dymov, S., Szyf, M., and Meaney, M.J. (2004). Epigenetic programming by maternal behavior. *Nat Neurosci.* 7, 847–854.

Yliharsila, H., Eriksson, J.G., Forsen, T., Laakso, M., Uusitupa, M., Osmond, C., and Barker, D.J. (2004). Interactions between peroxisome proliferator-activated receptor-gamma 2 gene polymorphisms and size at birth on blood pressure and the use of antihypertensive medication. *J Hypertens.* 22, 1283–1287.

# 10 Taste as the Gatekeeper of Personalized Nutrition

*Toshiko Tanaka, Danielle R. Reed, and Jose M. Ordovas*

## CONTENTS



## 10.1 INTRODUCTION

Human food preferences and intake are determined by a complex mix of innate, acquired, and contemporary societal factors. Understanding the individual drivers that determine what food is consumed and in which quantities, how it is prepared, and when it is eaten should provide avenues for successful dietary advice and interventions aimed at decreasing disease risk and achieving healthier aging. This chapter reviews the current knowledge regarding the genetics of taste with a focus on bitter taste perception and discusses how genetic variation in taste may be linked to the consumption of foods associated with disease protection and increased well-being, as well as avoidance of habits associated with increased risk of disease. Better understanding of the role of taste in dietary behavior may lead to the identification of genetic markers that can be utilized for the development of personalized dietary recommendations based on individual taste preferences. Such personalized guidelines may improve adherence to dietary recommendations and provide better preventive strategies for chronic diseases.

In many countries, chronic diseases such as cardiovascular disease and cancer are the leading causes of mortality. Moreover, the prevalence of conditions such as metabolic syndrome and obesity are on the rise worldwide. Although these diseases have complex etiologies, diet is thought to be a major contributing factor. One of the greatest public health challenges is to alter eating behavior in populations as a means of preventing chronic diseases. Adherence to dietary recommendations such as increasing fruit and vegetable consumption proves to be difficult for many people. Although there are various environmental and physiological factors that determine individual food selection, taste has been suggested as an important factor in consumer food choice. There is a wide variety of taste preferences in the population, and part of this variability is genetically determined [1]. It is of interest to elucidate whether there are genetic markers of taste that predispose a person to consume a certain type of diet. Such information would be useful to identify people who are at risk for diseases based on their "taste" genotype. The genetic markers may provide the foundations for tailored recommendations based on their preferences.

## 10.2 BIOLOGY OF TASTE

There are five modalities of taste that can be detected by most mammals: sweet, salt, sour, bitter, and umami (the taste of monosodium glutamate) [2]. For our ancestors, the ability to taste was important to ensure acquisition of nutrients and for avoidance of noxious substances. In general sweet, salt, and to a certain extent, umami, drive food consumption, whereas bitter and sour elicit food rejection.

Taste perception begins at the tongue, where specific tastants in food interact with taste receptors found on taste cells (TCs) [2]. The TCs are specialized epithelial cells with neuron-like properties, including depolarization, release of neurotransmitters, and formation of synapse to afferent neurons. Approximately 50 to 150 TCs organize into an onion-like configuration to form a taste bud. Taste buds are found distributed throughout the tongue in three specialized structures called fungiform, foliate, and circumvallate papillae. Some taste buds are also located on the soft palate, uvula, pharynx, larynx, esophagus, and in the epiglottis. Upon binding of the tastants to its receptors, the TC depolarizes to create an action potential and communicates either directly or indirectly with afferent neurons. This ultimately leads to the transmission of signals to the brain.

### 10.2.1 Bitter Compounds in Foods and Beverages

Bitter compounds generally elicit food rejection, a behavior critical to avoid ingesting potentially toxic compounds. Humans can detect various bitter tastes at very low concentrations, a trait that is presumed to be favorable for survival. However, there are some naturally bitter compounds in foods that have been shown to have beneficial effects on health. Some of these compounds include phenols (found in tea, citrus fruits, wine, and soy), triterpenes (citrus fruits), and organosulfur compounds (cruciferous vegetables) [3]. These phytochemicals have been investigated for their putative anticarcinogenic and antioxidant properties. Various epidemiologic studies have shown that increased intake of fruit and vegetables is associated with decreased risk of chronic diseases such as heart disease and cancer. Public health efforts to increase fruits and vegetable intake have been challenging, and the resistance to increased consumption may be in part due to the bitter tastes of these foods [4]. Indeed, many of the "healthy" vegetables such as cruciferous vegetables are often disliked for their bitter taste, especially by children [3].

For this reason, it has been hypothesized that variability in bitter taste perception may influence diet-related health outcomes. Much information investigating the association between bitter-taste sensitivity and food preferences has centered on the ability to taste a thiourea compound, phenylthiocarbamide (PTC). The N-C=S group in PTC is responsible for its bitter taste [5]. Although PTC is not found in nature, there are chemically related compounds such as isothiocyanates in cruciferous vegetables [6]. These bitter compounds often play a protective role for the plants. For example, glucosinolates are natural pesticides found in cruciferous vegetable and, when the plant gets damaged, they are hydrolyzed to goitrin, an isothiocyanate [3]. The abundance of bitter compounds in our food supply makes PTC sensitivity an ideal marker for the study of taste, food preferences, and dietary behaviors.

### 10.2.2 Phenylthiocarbamide Taste Sensitivity

The focus on the bitter compound PTC came about when A.L Fox discovered that some people found crystallized PTC to be bitter, whereas others did not [6]. Subsequent studies confirmed this observation and showed that in most populations, there is a bimodal distribution of taste thresholds dividing people into tasters and nontasters. Early studies used simple methods to dichotomize subjects, using PTC crystals or PTC saturated paper [7]. Many modern studies utilize another thiourea, 6-*n*-propylthiouracil (PROP), because PTC has a slight sulfurous odor. There have also been advancements in the psychophysical methods, in which subjects are exposed to varying concentrations of PTC to determine the threshold at which they can taste the bitterness. Various studies indicate that the thresholds are around $1.0 \times 10^{-4}$ mol/L for tasters and $>2.0 \times 10^{-4}$ mol/L for nontasters [6]. Further, it was shown that there are two types of tasters. Supertasters are extremely sensitive to PROP and perceive this compound to be more intensely bitter than medium tasters [8]. PTC/PROP sensitivity is modified by sex and age; there is a greater proportion of tasters among women, and sensitivity declines with age [5]. Anatomically, the tongue of supertasters has higher densities of fungiform papillae and taste pores. It was shown that, in general, women have higher densities of fungiform papillae, consistent with the observed higher frequency of tasters [7]. In most populations, there are more tasters than nontasters. The frequency of nontasters ranges from about 3% in western African populations to greater than 40% in some populations in India [5,6]. In North American Caucasians, the frequency of nontasters is estimated to be around 30% [5,9].

### 10.2.3 PTC/PROP and Phenotype Associations

PTC/PROP taster status has been associated with heightened bitter sensitivity and dislike of bitter foods such as cruciferous vegetables, coffee/caffeine/tea, cheese, grapefruit juice, and soy products [10 to 18] (Table 10.1). However, PTC/PROP sensitivity has not shown a consistent pattern of preferences regarding bitter foods [16]. This may be due to the low acceptance of bitter foods in the general population, thus minimizing the variability necessary to detect a difference. In addition to bitter foods and beverages, tasters have been reported to be more sensitive to sweet and spicy stimuli such as sucrose, saccharin, and capsaicin [19]. There is evidence that PTC/PROP sensitivity is associated with preferences for macronutrients, namely, fat. However, the direction of the association has not been consistent. In some studies, tasters liked foods with higher fat content [17] and disliked these foods in others [20,21]. There are some reports of no significant difference in fat preferences by taster status [22,23]. In one study, tasters were able to distinguish between 10 and 40% fat in salad dressing, whereas nontasters could not [19]. However, the taster did not report preferences for either types of dressing, whereas the nontasters preferred the high-fat dressing. It has been suggested that tasters are more sensitive to fat content because of the texture rather than the flavor of fat [19]. Thus, it is unclear whether ability to taste bitter flavors *per se* has an effect on preferences for fat content or whether the greater number of fungiform papillae determines the perceived pleasantness. Overall, these studies suggest that tasters have a heightened sensitivity to various tastes and a tendency to perceive these foods as unpleasant.

The connection between taste status and frequency of food intake is not as well established as food preferences (Table 10.1). Studies showing associations between PROP/PTC sensitivity and intake of bitter vegetables have been sparse. In one study, nontasters consumed more cooked turnip and watercress, but no differences were observed for nine other cruciferous vegetables [24]. In other studies, taste status was associated with bitter food preferences, and food preferences in turn were associated with frequency of intake [10,14]. Taste status, however, does not seem to be directly associated with frequency of food intake [10,14,25,26]. The general low consumption and small variability in intake of bitter foods may negate the ability of small studies to detect a difference, because of insufficient power. There has been more convincing evidence of taster status in association with the consumption of macronutrients, specifically for percentage of fat intake [20,27,28]. Using food frequency questionnaires, taster female college students reported higher intakes of energy from fat and lower intakes from protein [28]. In another study of children, female tasters had a lower intake of discretionary fat [20]. A feeding study in which subjects were given either a high-fat, high-carbohydrate, or mixed meal showed that tasters ate more fat and less carbohydrates during the mixed meal, but not the others [27]. Further studies are needed to clarify whether taste status is linked with fat intake and to determine the direction of the associations.

There have been several studies showing an association between PTC/PROP taste status and alcoholism. Initial case control studies revealed greater frequencies of nontasters in children with alcoholic family members compared to controls [29]. Taster subjects have been shown to perceive alcohol such as beer to be more bitter

**TABLE 10.1**
**Review of Studies Investigating PTC/PROP Sensitivity and Food Preference/Intake**

| Subjects: Sex (Age) | Food Preference and Sensory Assessment | Type of Food | Taster Classification Method | Difference by PTC/PROP Sensitivity Sensory or Dietary Intake | Reference |
|---|---|---|---|---|---|
| 146F, 136M (17–22 yr) | Food preference and consumption questionnaire | Twenty-five items that inhibit thyroidal iodine uptake, and six bitter foods | Tasting of PTC saturated filter paper | No | Mattes 1989 [26] |
| 17F, 17M (5–7 yr) | Verbal food preference questionnaire and sensory perception | Eight tasted foods, order-by-choice and 60 food checklist | Forced choice threshold detection and suprathreshold method | Sensory: Tasters disliked cheese and liked whole milk | Anliker 1991 [17] |
| 53F (20–45 yr) | Sensory rating | Tasted soy products and different dilutions of green tea | Forced choice threshold detection and suprathreshold method | Sensory: Tasters perceived green tea to be more bitter and dislike plain tofu, preferred vanilla flavor soymilk | Gayathri 1997 [15] |
| 45F, 30M (18–51 yr) | Sensory rating | Fats (10 vs. 40% salad dressing) capsaicin | Suprathreshold method | Sensory: Tasters reported more oral burn from capsaicin and distinguished fat content | Tepper 1997 [19] |
| 123F (20–60 yr) | Food preference questionnaire<br>Sensory rating | Rated fruits and juices<br>Sensory testing of naringin solution | Suprathreshold method | Sensory: Tasters disliked naringin and grapefruit juice | Drewnowski 1997 [18] |
| 118F (20–40 yr) | Sensory and hedonic rating | Fifteen Fat/sugar mixtures | Forced choice detection threshold suprathreshold method | Sensory: No | Drewnowski 1998 [23] |
| 159F (20–60 yr) | Food preference checklist<br>3-d food record (86 subjects) | One hundred and seventy-one items from various food categories | Suprathreshold method | Sensory: Tasters had lower preference for brussels sprouts, cabbage, spinach, and coffee<br>Intake: No | Drewnowski 1999 [10] |

*(continued)*

**TABLE 10.1 (CONTINUED)**
**Review of Studies Investigating PTC/PROP Sensitivity and Food Preference/Intake**

| Subjects: Sex (Age) | Food Preference and Sensory Assessment | Type of Food | Taster Classification Method | Difference by PTC/PROP Sensitivity Sensory or Dietary Intake | Reference |
|---|---|---|---|---|---|
| 50F (20–40 yr) | Sensory rating<br>FFQ | Six bitter foods tasted<br>Twenty-two bitter food items questionnaire | Suprathreshold method<br>Tasting PROP saturated paper | Sensory: Taste perception is associated with bitterness of food<br>Intake: No | Kaminski 2000 [14] |
| 24F, 22M (18–40 yr) | Food preference survey | Eighty-three items | Forced choice threshold detection and suprathreshold method | Sensory: In women sweet and high-fat foods negatively correlated with bitter sensitivity: in men a positive correlation was found | Duffy 2000 [21] |
| 326F (mean 47.6–51.7) | Food preference checklist | One hundred and seventy-one food items | Suprathreshold method | Sensory: Tasters dislike cruciferous, green, raw vegetables | Drewnowski 2000 [16] |
| 54F (18–30 yr) | Sensory rating | Sucrose, caffeine, chocolate | Suprathreshold method<br>Tasting PROP saturated paper | Sensory: Tasters perceived caffeine as being more bitter and disliked | Ly 2001 [12] |
| 92F, 55M (17–36 yr) | Sensory rating | Fattiness, saltiness, sweetness of four foods | Suprathreshold method | Sensory: No | Yackinous 2001 [22] |
| 85F, 38M (19–59 yr) | Food questionnaire for flavor, cost, effect on health | Forty-three food items representative of Tunisian diet | Taste recognition threshold<br>Suprathreshold method | Sensory: Tasters rated foods higher than nontasters overall; no differences in bitter foods except green tea, which tasters disliked | Pasquet 2002 [13] |
| 33F, 34M (4–5 yr) | Sensory test<br>FFQ (child and parent) | Tasted ten common foods/drinks that are bitter or varying in fat 114 items (FFQ) | Single concentration of PROP (yes/no) | Sensory: Tasters disliked broccoli, full-fat milk, American cheese<br>Taster girls disliked full-fat milk<br>Intake: Girl tasters had lower intake of discretionary fat | Keller 2002 [20] |

| | | | | | |
|---|---|---|---|---|---|
| 114F, 69M (17–36 yr) | FFQ | Ninety-five items | Suprathreshold method | Intake: No difference in men<br>Women tasters obtained lower percentage of energy from protein and fruit servings, higher from fat<br>Supertasters consumed less green salad compared to T, MT* | Yachinous 2002 [28] |
| 22F,14M (mean age 31) | Food intake | *Ad libitum* intake of high-fat, high-carb, or mixed meal | Suprathreshold method | Intake: Taster had higher fat intake, lower CHO intake *ad libitum* of mixed meal No difference for high-fat or high-carb meal | Kamphuis 2003 [27] |
| 71F, 39M (18–60 yr) | FFQ, food sampling | Block 98.1 | Suprathreshold method | Sensory: Tasters rated sampled bitter vegetables as most bitter (brussels sprouts, asparagus, kale). No association with perceived sweetness of sweet foods or from vegetables.<br>Intake: PROP sensitivity is inversely associated with vegetable intake; when examining other variables, however, taste sensitivity was not directly associated with vegetable intake | Dinehart 2006 [25] |

*T = taster; MT = medium taster

and unpleasant [30]. Taste status has also been linked with smoking habits [31]. In these studies the proportion of nontasters was greater in smokers compared to nonsmokers. It has been hypothesized that nontasters have less aversion to the bitterness of cigarettes and are thus at greater risk to smoke. Together, these data suggest that PTC/PROP sensitivity may mitigate the development of addictive behaviors such as smoking and alcoholism.

### 10.2.4 PTC/PROP Sensitivity and Disease

One of the first diseases that was investigated was goiter, because of the role of PTC as a thyroid inhibitor [5]. The isothiocyanates found in cruciferous vegetables are also natural thyroid inhibitors that PTC tasters find bitter. Goiters can be caused by both over- and underactivity of the thyroid gland. Hypothyroidism can occur in areas of low iodine, as this mineral is required for the production of thyroid hormones. In this case, tasters have the advantage, as they would avoid the consumption of "bitter" cruciferous vegetables. Conversely, in the case of hyperthyroidism, nontasters would have the advantage. In accordance with these hypotheses, several studies have found higher prevalence of nontasters in nontoxic goiter patients, and no association has been observed with diffuse goiter.

Other diseases examined include diabetes, cancer, ulcers, depression, and psychiatric disorders (reviewed in Reference 5). The underlying hypotheses for the associations include differences in dietary behavior, neurological activity, or unknown mechanisms. However, after initial reports, subsequent studies failed to replicate the findings. Therefore, it is difficult to draw conclusions regarding these associations. Further, many of these studies are small case control studies and the generalizability of the results may be questionable. Further examination of the mechanisms underlying the hypothesized associations may provide better understanding of the link between PTC/PROP and these diseases.

## 10.3 THE PURSUIT OF THE PTC GENE

Sensitivity to PTC/PROP is a heritable trait originally proposed to be monogenic but currently thought to involve several loci. Early linkage studies had shown that PTC sensitivity is linked with the Kell blood group on chromosome 7 [5]. This was supported by a study of PROP sensitivity in which significant linkage was found on chromosome 5p, with a possible linkage on chromosome 7q31 near the KEL locus [32]. In a subsequent study using PTC sensitivity, there was significant linkage to chromosome 7q, consistent with the previous studies [33]. Utilizing the results from these linkage analyses, the genes for bitter taste receptors have been identified by mining the human genome database. Electrophysiological studies showed that bitter tastants are mediated through the activation of G-protein-coupled receptors (GPCR). To identify the bitter receptor genes, segments of the genome linked with bitter taste perception were screened for novel GPCRs [34,35]. These efforts led to the identification of a family of bitter taste receptor genes (TAS2R) on chromosomes 5, 7, and 12. This family of receptors were found to be expressed in taste cells and showed specific interactions with bitter compounds *in vitro* [36].

In genomewide linkage analysis, one member of the bitter gene receptor family, *TAS2R38*, was shown to be responsible for PTC/PROP sensitivity [37]. Three single-nucleotide polymorphisms (SNPs) in the gene (P49A, A262V, and V296I) gave rise to five common haplotypes, named in the order of the amino acids at each SNP. These haplotypes accounted for 55 to 85% of the variance in PTC sensitivity. Based on associations with taste phenotypes, the taster haplotype was identified as PAV (proline-alanine-valine) and nontaster haplotype as AVI (alanine-valine-isoleucine). Functional analysis of the *TAS2R38* haplotypes provided further support for the hypothesis that this gene is the PTC gene. HEK293 cells transfected with PAV allele receptor displayed elevation of cytosolic Ca2+ in a dose-dependent manner, starting at PTC concentrations as low as 0.1 $\mu M$ [38]. On the other hand, cells expressing the AVI allele receptor did not respond to PTC at concentrations as high as 1 m*M*. This result is consistent with the observation of PAV as the taster and AVI as the nontaster haplotype.

### 10.3.1 Evolution of the PTC Gene

The identification of bitter taste receptor genes and the putative role of bitter taste perception as a defense system against environmental toxins have drawn interest from evolutionary biologists. The human *TAS2R38* shows 98.2 and 65.5% amino acid identity with chimpanzee (*chTAS2R38*) and mouse (*Tas2r138*) genes. Phenotypically, mice do not display a bimodal distribution, and the sensitivity to PTC or PROP is not correlated as in humans [5]. Thus, in mice, it is speculated that the *Tas2r138* gene is not a receptor for PTC/PROP as in humans, but rather serves as a receptor for another bitter compound. On the other hand, chimpanzees demonstrate both taster and nontaster phenotypes. However, the molecular basis of the variation is different [39]. The polymorphisms that give rise to the human taster haplotypes are absent in the chimpanzee gene. Instead, a polymorphism in the second position of the start codon is responsible for the taster phenotypes. This variation results in a truncated polypeptide that is not responsive to PTC *in vitro*. These molecular and phenotypic differences in PTC sensitivity between organisms suggest that this trait has evolved independently and may be a reflection of the different environments of the species.

In humans, evidence supports the notion that the PTC/PROP taster phenotype has been maintained through natural selection rather than by genetic drift [40]. Geneticists have hypothesized that those who are sensitive to bitter tastes will have a selective advantage because of their ability to avoid toxic foods [5]. However, the persistence of nontasters in most populations suggests that there are advantages to being insensitive to bitter compounds [5,40]. This may be explained by the multiple functions of bitter foods in our environment. Although bitter compounds can be toxic, many bitter foods have beneficial effects on health. For our ancestors, insensitivity to bitter taste may have provided availability of additional plant-based nutrient sources when food was scarce. For modern humans, it has been proposed that nontasters may be less prone to reject healthy bitter foods and may choose a diet with more variety [4].

### 10.3.2 PTC Gene Polymorphisms: Genotype–Phenotype Associations

The identification of *TAS2R38* has provided the tools to examine whether genetic measures of PTC sensitivity are linked to dietary behavior and disease status in humans. In a study of 143 children and their mothers, the P49A polymorphism was associated with bitter taste sensitivity [41]. However, the variability explained by the genotype was greater in children than in their mothers, indicating that age may be a significant modifier. Taste sensitivity was associated with greater preferences for sweets in children but not adults. In the mothers, ethnicity was the strongest predictor of sweet preferences, suggesting that cultural influences can override genetic influences of taste in adults. In another study of 84 healthy adults, *TAS2R38* haplotypes were a significant predictor of alcohol consumption [42]. Subjects with the nontaster haplotype reported higher use of alcohol in comparison to subjects with the taster haplotype. In a regression analysis, *TAS2R38* haplotype and number of fungiform papillae were both independent determinants of PROP bitterness. When the bitterness of PROP solution was recorded by *TAS2R38* haplotype, the intensity function was not as distinct as the results using taster groups determined by psychophysical methods. Nevertheless, this study supports the role of *TAS2R38* as a predictor of alcohol consumption.

In a cross-sectional study of older British women, the *TAS2R38* haplotype was not associated with dietary intake as measured by a food frequency questionnaire [43]. Further, no association was found between this haplotype and CHD risk factors or CHD. There was marginally greater prevalence of diabetes among the taster haplotype; however, the significance is unclear, given that multiple associations were examined. The lack of association in this study may be due to the older age of the subjects, as PTC sensitivity declines with age. However, this study may also indicate that this locus is not associated with measurable dietary behaviors in humans. Further studies are necessary to clarify the association between *TAS2R38* haplotype and dietary intake in both men and women.

These first studies examining *TAS2R38* provide tantalizing results for the use of this gene as a marker for food preferences and, potentially, dietary intake. The lack of association in the first epidemiologic study may be due to various confounding factors that were not measured in the study, such as restrictive dietary practices. Moreover, various cooking methods that cannot be deconstructed by most food frequency questionnaires can significantly alter the taste qualities of foods. Therefore, examination of these factors will provide better understanding on the role of *TAS2R38* on dietary behavior. It would be interesting to investigate whether there are differences in adherence to dietary recommendations based on *TAS2R38* haplotype. Future studies will most likely provide insight into the applicability of this marker as a tool to develop targeted dietary recommendations.

### 10.3.3 Other Bitter Taste Receptors

The PTC gene is one of an estimated ~30 bitter taste receptor genes in humans [34,35]. There is evidence that other bitter taste receptors are biologically important and have been linked with alcohol dependence as well as disease risk. For instance, sequence analysis of *TAS2R16* shows that the K172N polymorphism in the gene is under positive selection based on the observation of high frequency of the evolutionary derived variants in populations worldwide [44]. This result suggests that this receptor has adapted according to unique human environments. The K172N polymorphism lies in the third extracellular loop and functional analysis shows that the ancestral K172 allele has weaker response to ligands such as salicin, arbitun, and amygdalin than the evolutionary derived N172 allele. Consumption of foods containing these cyanogenic glycosides has been hypothesized to be protective against malaria [44]. Consistent with this hypothesis, the K172 allele has been found at higher frequencies where malaria is endemic. In addition, the K172 has been associated with increased risk for alcohol dependence [45]. Because *TAS2R38* has also been associated with alcohol consumption and both *TAS2R16* and *TAS2R38* are located on neighboring regions on chromosome 7, it would be interesting to examine both of these genes in relation to alcohol intake.

In an effort to identify genes associated with myocardial infarction (MI), an association study examining 11,053 polymorphisms representing 6,891 genes was conducted [46]. To identify the variants significantly associated with MI, three case control studies were analyzed sequentially. In the final analysis, five genes were significantly associated with MI, one being *TAS2R50* with odds ratio of 1.58 for the susceptible allele. Interestingly, another gene identified in this study was one of the olfactory receptors, *OR13G1*. The authors hypothesized that the association observed for both *TAS2R50* and *OR13G1* may be through dietary choices. Further studies are needed to confirm this hypothesis.

With the exception of the known alleles of *TAS2R38* and the sensitivity to the bitterness of PTC and related compounds, there are no known phenotype–genotype relationships between alleles of the other bitter receptors and the taste perception of their bitter ligands. However, there are many examples of a wide range of perceptual sensitivity by human populations to other bitter stimuli. Although PTC and *TAS2R38* are the first example of the effect of genetics on taste perception, the complement of taste receptors and their many alleles will probably reveal numerous relationships with bitter taste perception and the motivation to consume bitter foods.

## 10.4 OTHER TASTE MODALITIES

The discussion thus far has focused on bitter taste; however, there are four other conventional taste modalities: salty, sour, sweet, and umami — and perhaps a fifth taste, that for fatty acids. We briefly review these other genetic influences on these taste qualities and how they might contribute to the taste of food. Incorporating all the taste modalities may improve our understanding of the role of genetic variation in taste on food consumption and health.

### 10.4.1 Sweet and Umami

One of the universal experiences in human perception is that sweetness is considered to be good and desirable, and sugar is well accepted and well tolerated by people in all human populations studied to date. The initial step in sweet perception is the binding of the sweetener to the receptor, which is composed of two subunits, TAS1R2 and TAS1R3 (for a review of the discovery and biology of this receptor, see Reference 36). A second subunit (TAS1R1) when paired with TAS1R3, the common partner, is responsible for the transduction of umami (savory) taste. Alleles of *TAS1R3* are strongly associated with sweet intake in the mouse, and it has been hypothesized that alleles of human T1Rs may explain part of the variability of the intake of sugars. These phenotype–genotype studies have yet to be conducted in humans, although there are many known alleles in these taste receptors, especially the subunit specialized to sweet ligands. The umami-specific subunit of the receptor, *TAS1R1*, also contains many polymorphisms, and might be related to the sensory blindness to the savory taste of MSG experienced by a subset of people [47].

### 10.4.2 Sour

Individual differences in the ability to perceive sourness exist, but the genetic basis of this taste quality is unknown. The recent discovery of a key protein in sour taste in mice provides the foundations to investigate the mechanisms of sour taste transduction and the role of this taste modality on human dietary behavior and health [48]. Unripe fruit, types of milk and cheese and some vegetables are sour, and people often confuse sour and bitter, which contributes to the perception of a sour food as undesirable. Because many nutritious foods are slightly sour, its perception is an aspect of food selection that is understudied relative to its importance to human health.

### 10.4.3 Salt

The perception of saltiness differs from the other taste qualities because differences among people in sodium threshold and intensity ratings of saltiness are marked, but are related to immediate food intake rather than to genotype. Although some aspects of sodium transduction are understood, the search for the full complement of proteins that participate in this process is still on. It is possible that genetic differences among people are important, but it could also be that salt perception is labile, and the genetic differences would only be apparent if all subjects were fed diets equivalent in saltiness.

### 10.4.4 Fat

In addition to the basic tastes and their receptor genes, examination of unconventional taste qualities will likely be important in understanding human diet and health. Because fat is important to the sensory experience of food, differences in fat taste perception may influence dietary behavior. Several lines of evidence suggest there might be genetic determinants of oral fat perception, the most convincing of which is the observation that fat intake in humans is heritable [1]. There is debate about whether animals and humans have a sensory system that is specifically tuned to oral fats, largely because the receptor and transduction mechanisms are not known. Chewing or tasting fatty foods without swallowing is sufficient to stimulate digestion, which is evidence that fats are sensed on the tongue [49]. Whether fat perception is mediated through sensory stimulation of fat texture or a chemosensory detection of fat "taste" is controversial. Recently, the glycoprotein CD36 was shown to be involved in the orosensory detection of dietary lipids in rats and mice [50]. This protein has been described as a putative receptor for fats, suggesting that taste of fat may be the sixth taste modality.

There is a human form of the CD36 receptor, but whether it has the same taste function as in rodents is not known. If this gene is involved in the perception of oral fats, alleles of this gene might explain individual variation in perception [51]. One intriguing observation is that the *CD36* gene and its alleles in humans have been studied by investigators who noticed its relationship with diet-induced disease such as diabetes [52]. It may be that *CD36* alleles might change fat perception and intake, thereby contributing to metabolic diseases. The human homologue of the mouse *CD36* gene is located in the middle of human chromosome 7, and during the last several years, many alleles of the human *CD36* gene have been discovered [51]. Because there is a range in the ability of people to detect fat in foods [53], efficiency of oral fat receptors may differ among people, therefore influencing preferences and intake of dietary fat.

## 10.5 GENETICS OF EATING BEHAVIOR

A principal challenge of studying taste and its relationship to nutrition and health is translating differences among people in sensory perception of food and drink to what they actually choose to eat. By introspection we can immediately identify cases in which a food that is not preferred has been eaten for reasons unrelated to taste, but rather to social or economic influences. Therefore, it is useful to examine not only the relationships between taste perception and genotype, but also between human nutrient selection and genotype. It is the goal that these two fields will eventually expand to bridge the gap between taste perception and food intake. The current knowledge on the genetic basis of dietary behavior is reviewed in the following text.

Family studies have been used to determine the genetic contribution to dietary behaviors in humans. The heritability estimates for carbohydrates, protein, and fat range from 30 to 66%, 20 to 70%, and 10 to 56%, respectively [54]. Because macronutrients are energy yielding, some of the genetic components may include energy regulation rather than proportion of macronutrients. Heritability estimates for energy intake in these studies ranged from 11 to 70%. The different data analyses methods and varied acquisition of dietary intake make the studies difficult to compare and may explain the wide variability in the heritability estimates. Nevertheless, these studies support the role of genetics in food consumption. Given the complexity of human dietary behaviors, with the exception of monogenetic conditions such as with leptin deficiency, no single gene is likely to have a great impact on food intake.

Although candidate gene association studies of dietary behavior have been sparse, there have been several positive reports. The majority of the genes reported to date are those involved in the central control of energy intake including neuropeptides and monoamine systems (reviewed in Reference 54). For example, serotonin is a neurotransmitter that is involved in various physiological processes including sleep, appetite, mood, thermoregulation, pain perception, hormone secretion, and sexual behavior. Central and peripheral administration of serotonin decreases food intake, increases energy expenditure, and drugs that promote serotonergic activity have an anorectic effect. Serotonin reuptake blockers also increase sweet and bitter taste perception in humans. These observations collectively make the genes in the serotonin pathway candidates for influencing dietary behaviors. A SNP in the promoter region of the serotonin receptor 2A (*5-HT2A*) was associated with total energy and fat intake in Caucasian populations [55,56]. The minor allele carriers of the −1438G/A SNP consumed fewer calories, and in adolescents the differences in the energy were driven by fat intake. The major allele homozygotes consumed as much as 10% more energy in comparison to the minor allele homozygotes. These findings are interesting in light of the observation of lower frequency of the A allele in anorexic patients.

In addition to the *5-HT2A* gene, polymorphisms in other genes, including the dopamine transporter, agouti-related protein, and uncoupling proteins, have been associated with macronutrient intake [54]. These candidate gene association studies together support the involvement of multiple gene loci on dietary behavior. With the exception of *5-HT2A*, there have been no published reports replicating the observations in other populations. Replication studies are particularly important for candidate gene association studies because of the propensity of false-positive results. Furthermore, examination of multiple polymorphisms (or haplotypes) rather than a single SNP may provide better understanding of the significance of these genes as a marker for dietary behavior. The studies published thus far highlight the complexity and the diversity of genes that may mediate food intake. Therefore, future studies investigating the genetics of dietary behavior that consider multitude of genes rather than focusing on one aspect of dietary behavior may prove to be more fruitful.

One of the drawbacks of the candidate gene approach is that these studies are limited to current knowledge of the control of feeding behaviors. An alternative approach for the discovery of genetic contribution of food consumption is to use the whole-genome scan approach. There have been two genomewide linkage analyses of macronutrient intake in Mexican Americans, Caucasians, and African Americans. The first study examined 816 Mexican American participants from the San Antonio Family Heart Study [57]. Using FFQ developed specifically for this population, total energy and macronutrient [total protein, total fat, saturated fat (SFA), monosaturated fat (MUFA), polyunsaturated fat (PUFA), total carbohydrates, and sucrose] intake were examined. Heritability estimates for these dietary parameters were modest, ranging from 9% for PUFA to 21% for MUFA. Suggestive linkage was found on chromosome 2p22 with LOD score of 2.62 for SFA, 2.09 for total fat, 2.22 for total protein, and 2.05 for MUFA. The proopiomelanocortin (*POMC*) gene that encodes for a protein that is the precursor of appetite-regulating hormones was identified as a candidate gene within this region. However, two polymorphisms on exon 3 were not associated with saturated fat intake, suggesting that *POMC* is not the gene underlying the observed linkage. In the second study, total energy and macronutrient (fat, carbohydrate, protein, and sucrose) was examined in 794 Caucasians and 198 African American participants of the HERITAGE study [58]. In Caucasians a region on chromosome 1 (1p22.1-1q22) was linked with total energy and fat intake, 1p22-1p32 and 20q13.3 for total energy intake, and 12q14.1 for total fat intake. In African Americans, suggestive linkage found at 1q43-44 for sucrose intake, and regions 1p22.3, 6q22.31, and 12q24.21 for fat intake. No specific candidate genes were examined in the study; therefore, the genes underlying the linkage are yet to be identified. It is noteworthy that the linkage observed in the studies were specific to each ethnic group. This may be due to the differences in the methodologies for dietary assessment or linkage analyses used by the two studies. Or it may be an indication of different genetic architecture of dietary behavior by ethnicity. These studies provide clues regarding the regions of the genome that may contribute to macronutrient intake and may be the initial steps toward identifying novel genes involved in dietary behavior.

## 10.6 FUTURE PERSPECTIVE ON PERSONALIZED NUTRITION

The current nutrigenetic paradigm places an emphasis on interindividual differences in physiological response to diet. However, one of the biggest challenges for nutrition practitioners is to change dietary behaviors. Therefore, incorporating genetic markers that determine predisposition to certain dietary habits may be an important factor in the development of successful dietary intervention strategies.

In humans, taste is a powerful determinant of food selection. In the specific case of the bitter taste sensitivity, this may have served in ancestral times as a primary defense against ingestion of toxic compounds in foods. For modern humans, the role of bitter taste perception for the avoidance of noxious food is less important. However, it is thought that individual differences in bitter taste sensitivity may influence health outcomes through its effect on dietary behaviors. Sensitivity to PTC and PROP has provided some insight into the role of bitter taste perception on preferences and consumption of bitter foods. The haplotypes of the *TAS2R38* gene accounts for most of the variability of PTC sensitivity, and several studies suggest that it may serve as a marker for lifestyle and dietary behavior. However, current evidence does not yet support a link between genetic variability at this taste candidate gene, habitual consumption of certain foods, and health-related outcomes. This is expected when considering the complexity of the large number of taste-related genes as well as other pathways that modulate eating habits (i.e., serotonin and dopamine). Therefore, advances in this promising area of translational research will be driven by a more comprehensive approach to the problem encompassing wide genome coverage as well as the inclusion of behavioral, cultural, and economic determinants. It is foreseeable that a better knowledge of the physiology of taste and its genetic variation in humans will result in an increased ability to carry out successful personalized dietary recommendations that will be both appealing and successful in terms of preventing chronic disorders.

## ACKNOWLEDGMENTS

We thank Dr. Carol Christensen and Dr. Marcia Levin Pelchat for their generous contributions in the preparation of this manuscript.

## KEY READINGS

Herness, M. S. and Gilbertson, T. A., Cellular mechanisms of taste transduction, *Annu Rev Physiol*, 61, 873–900, 1999.

Mennella, J. A. et al., Genetic and environmental determinants of bitter perception and sweet preferences, *Pediatrics*, 115, e216–22, 2005.

Rankinen, T. and Bouchard, C., Genetics of food intake and eating behavior phenotypes in humans, *Annu Rev Nutr*, 26, 413–34, 2006.

Reed, D. R. et al., Diverse tastes: Genetics of sweet and bitter perception, *Physiol Behav*, 88, 215–26, 2006.

Tepper, B. J., 6-n-Propylthiouracil: a genetic marker for taste, with implications for food preference and dietary habits, *Am J Hum Genet*, 63, 1271–6, 1998.

## REFERENCES

1. Reed, D. R. et al., Heritable variation in food preferences and their contribution to obesity, *Behav Genet*, 27, 373–87, 1997.
2. Herness, M. S. and Gilbertson, T. A., Cellular mechanisms of taste transduction, *Annu Rev Physiol*, 61, 873–900, 1999.
3. Drewnowski, A. and Gomez-Carneros, C., Bitter taste, phytonutrients, and the consumer: a review, *Am J Clin Nutr*, 72, 1424–35, 2000.
4. Drewnowski, A. and Rock, C. L., The influence of genetic taste markers on food acceptance, *Am J Clin Nutr*, 62, 506–11, 1995.
5. Guo, S. W. and Reed, D. R., The genetics of phenylthiocarbamide perception, *Ann Hum Biol*, 28, 111–42, 2001.
6. Tepper, B. J., 6-n-Propylthiouracil: a genetic marker for taste, with implications for food preference and dietary habits, *Am J Hum Genet*, 63, 1271–6, 1998.
7. Bartoshuk, L. M., Comparing sensory experiences across individuals: recent psychophysical advances illuminate genetic variation in taste perception, *Chem Senses*, 25, 447–60, 2000.
8. Reed, D. R. et al., Propylthiouracil tasting: determination of underlying threshold distributions using maximum likelihood, *Chem Senses*, 20, 529–33, 1995.
9. Fox, A. L., The relationship between chemical constitution and taste., *Proc Natl Acad Sci*, 18, 115–120, 1932.
10. Drewnowski, A. et al., Taste and food preferences as predictors of dietary practices in young women, *Public Health Nutr*, 2, 513–9, 1999.
11. Reed, D., *Behavioral modulation of the path from genotype to obesity phenotype*, John Libbey & Company, Paris, 1999, pp. 199–208.
12. Ly, A. and Drewnowski, A., PROP (6-n-Propylthiouracil) tasting and sensory responses to caffeine, sucrose, neohesperidin dihydrochalcone and chocolate, *Chem Senses*, 26, 41–7, 2001.
13. Pasquet, P. et al., Relationships between threshold-based PROP sensitivity and food preferences of Tunisians, *Appetite*, 39, 167–73, 2002.
14. Kaminski, L. C. et al., Young women's food preferences and taste responsiveness to 6-n-propylthiouracil (PROP), *Physiol Behav*, 68, 691–7, 2000.
15. Gayathri Devi, A. et al., Sensory acceptance of Japanese green tea and soy products is linked to genetic sensitivity to 6-n-propylthiouracil, *Nutr Cancer*, 29, 146–51, 1997.
16. Drewnowski, A. et al., Genetic taste markers and preferences for vegetables and fruit of female breast care patients, *J Am Diet Assoc*, 100, 191–7, 2000.

17. Anliker, J. A. et al., Children's food preferences and genetic sensitivity to the bitter taste of 6-n-propylthiouracil (PROP), *Am J Clin Nutr*, 54, 316–20, 1991.
18. Drewnowski, A. et al., Taste responses to naringin, a flavonoid, and the acceptance of grapefruit juice are related to genetic sensitivity to 6-n-propylthiouracil, *Am J Clin Nutr*, 66, 391–7, 1997.
19. Tepper, B. J. and Nurse, R. J., Fat perception is related to PROP taster status, *Physiol Behav*, 61, 949–54, 1997.
20. Keller, K. L. et al., Genetic taste sensitivity to 6-n-propylthiouracil influences food preference and reported intake in preschool children, *Appetite*, 38, 3–12, 2002.
21. Duffy, V. B. and Bartoshuk, L. M., Food acceptance and genetic variation in taste, *J Am Diet Assoc*, 100, 647–55, 2000.
22. Yackinous, C. and Guinard, J. X., Relation between PROP taster status and fat perception, touch, and olfaction, *Physiol Behav*, 72, 427–37, 2001.
23. Drewnowski, A. et al., Genetic sensitivity to 6-n-propylthiouracil and sensory responses to sugar and fat mixtures, *Physiol Behav*, 63, 771–7, 1998.
24. Jerzsa-Latta, M. et al., Use and perceived attributes of cruciferous vegetables in terms of genetically-mediated taste sensitivity, *Appetite*, 15, 127–34, 1990.
25. Dinehart, M. E. et al., Bitter taste markers explain variability in vegetable sweetness, bitterness, and intake, *Physiol Behav*, 87, 304–13, 2006.
26. Mattes, R. and Labov, J., Bitter taste responses to phenylthiocarbamide are not related to dietary goitrogen intake in human beings, *J Am Diet Assoc*, 89, 692–4, 1989.
27. Kamphuis, M. M. and Westerterp-Plantenga, M. S., PROP sensitivity affects macronutrient selection, *Physiol Behav*, 79, 167–72, 2003.
28. Yackinous, C. A. and Guinard, J. X., Relation between PROP (6-n-propylthiouracil) taster status, taste anatomy and dietary intake measures for young men and women, *Appetite*, 38, 201–9, 2002.
29. Pelchat, M. L. and Danowski, S., A possible genetic association between PROP-tasting and alcoholism, *Physiol Behav*, 51, 1261–6, 1992.
30. Intranuovo, L. R. and Powers, A. S., The perceived bitterness of beer and 6-n-propylthiouracil (PROP) taste sensitivity, *Ann NY Acad Sci*, 855, 813–5, 1998.
31. Enoch, M. A. et al., Does a reduced sensitivity to bitter taste increase the risk of becoming nicotine addicted?, *Addict Behav*, 26, 399–404, 2001.
32. Reed, D. R. et al., Localization of a gene for bitter-taste perception to human chromosome 5p15, *Am J Hum Genet*, 64, 1478–80, 1999.
33. Drayna, D. et al., Genetic analysis of a complex trait in the Utah Genetic Reference Project: a major locus for PTC taste ability on chromosome 7q and a secondary locus on chromosome 16p, *Hum Genet*, 112, 567–72, 2003.
34. Adler, E. et al., A novel family of mammalian taste receptors, *Cell*, 100, 693–702, 2000.
35. Matsunami, H. et al., A family of candidate taste receptors in human and mouse, *Nature*, 404, 601–4, 2000.
36. Reed, D. R. et al., Diverse tastes: Genetics of sweet and bitter perception, *Physiol Behav*, 88, 215–26, 2006.
37. Kim, U. K. et al., Positional cloning of the human quantitative trait locus underlying taste sensitivity to phenylthiocarbamide, *Science*, 299, 1221–5, 2003.
38. Bufe, B. et al., The molecular basis of individual differences in phenylthiocarbamide and propylthiouracil bitterness perception, *Curr Biol*, 15, 322–7, 2005.
39. Wooding, S. et al., Independent evolution of bitter-taste sensitivity in humans and chimpanzees, *Nature*, 440, 930–4, 2006.
40. Wooding, S. et al., Natural selection and molecular evolution in PTC, a bitter-taste receptor gene, *Am J Hum Genet*, 74, 637–46, 2004.

41. Mennella, J. A. et al., Genetic and environmental determinants of bitter perception and sweet preferences, *Pediatrics*, 115, e216–22, 2005.
42. Duffy, V. B. et al., Bitter receptor gene (TAS2R38), 6-n-propylthiouracil (PROP) bitterness and alcohol intake, *Alcohol Clin Exp Res*, 28, 1629–37, 2004.
43. Timpson, N. J. et al., TAS2R38 (phenylthiocarbamide) haplotypes, coronary heart disease traits, and eating behavior in the British Women's Heart and Health Study, *Am J Clin Nutr*, 81, 1005–11, 2005.
44. Soranzo, N. et al., Positive selection on a high-sensitivity allele of the human bitter-taste receptor TAS2R16, *Curr Biol*, 15, 1257–65, 2005.
45. Hinrichs, A. L. et al., Functional variant in a bitter-taste receptor (hTAS2R16) influences risk of alcohol dependence, *Am J Hum Genet*, 78, 103–11, 2006.
46. Shiffman, D. et al., Identification of four gene variants associated with myocardial infarction, *Am J Hum Genet*, 77, 596–605, 2005.
47. Lugaz, O. et al., A new specific ageusia: some humans cannot taste L-glutamate, *Chem. Senses*, 27, 105–15, 2002.
48. Huang, A. L. et al., The cells and logic for mammalian sour taste detection, *Nature*, 442, 934–8, 2006.
49. Mattes, R. D., Fat taste and lipid metabolism in humans, *Physiol Behav*, 86, 691–7, 2005.
50. Laugerette, F. et al., CD36 involvement in orosensory detection of dietary lipids, spontaneous fat preference, and digestive secretions, *J Clin Invest*, 115, 3177–84, 2005.
51. Ma, X. et al., A common haplotype at the CD36 locus is associated with high free fatty acid levels and increased cardiovascular risk in Caucasians, *Hum Mol Genet*, 13, 2197–205, 2004.
52. Corpeleijn, E. et al., Direct association of a promoter polymorphism in the CD36/FAT fatty acid transporter gene with Type 2 diabetes mellitus and insulin resistance, *Diabet Med*, 23, 907–11, 2006.
53. Reed, D. R. et al., *Sensory and metabolic influences on fat intake*, Elsevier Applied Science, London, New York, 1992, pp. 117–137.
54. Rankinen, T. and Bouchard, C., Genetics of food intake and eating behavior phenotypes in humans, *Annu Rev Nutr*, 26, 413–34, 2006.
55. Aubert, R. et al., 5-HT2A receptor gene polymorphism is associated with food and alcohol intake in obese people, *Int J Obes Relat Metab Disord*, 24, 920–4, 2000.
56. Herbeth, B. et al., Polymorphism of the 5-HT2A receptor gene and food intakes in children and adolescents: the Stanislas Family Study, *Am J Clin Nutr*, 82, 467–70, 2005.
57. Cai, G. et al., Quantitative trait locus determining dietary macronutrient intakes is located on human chromosome 2p22, *Am J Clin Nutr*, 80, 1410–4, 2004.
58. Collaku, A. et al., A genome-wide linkage scan for dietary energy and nutrient intakes: the Health, Risk Factors, Exercise Training, and Genetics (HERITAGE) Family Study, *Am J Clin Nutr*, 79, 881–6, 2004.

# 11 Personalized Nutrition and Public Health

*Pieter van't Veer, Edith J.M. Feskens, and Ellen Kampman*

## CONTENTS



## 11.1 INTRODUCTION

Personalized nutrition (PN) addresses the idea that optimal nutrition differs between individuals as a result of their genetic makeup. One hundred years after Mendel and 50 years after Watson and Crick, the current deciphering of the human genome holds the promise that knowledge of the genetic makeup and the omic technologies will enable us to provide highly specific dietary advice fitting the nutritional requirements of individuals.[1]

Nutritional requirements are traditionally based on physiological needs, e.g., for growth and development, to maintain nutritional status, to minimize disease risk, or to optimize life expectancy. Based on this biomedical approach, nutritional requirements and recommendations are provided for energy intake and nutrient needs for specific populations according to age, sex, physical activity, health status, life cycle, etc. Beyond these variations in requirements at the group level, variability in nutritional requirements has been denoted as "natural" biological variation, stemming from genetic variation, uncontrolled environmental factors, and measurement error. Thus, effects of dietary factors may — at least in part — depend on inherited individual susceptibility, allowing the strength of the diet–health equation to differ between subjects. In this framework, "biological variation" in classical risk factors such as blood pressure and blood lipids serve as phenotypical intermediates of diet–gene interactions.

When we apply this biomedical approach of PN to disease prevention and health promotion, it enters the domain of public health, defined as "the science and art of preventing disease, prolonging life and promoting health through organized efforts of society."[2] To enhance public health, nutritional requirements and recommendations are translated into food patterns, which, at least implicitly, incorporate national and local traditions and cultural issues, consumer acceptance, economic interests, and feasibility. These dietary guidelines complete the sequence from requirements to recommendations and, subsequently, to guidelines, and the process provides a basis for evidence-based nutritional policy.

In the context of public health, PN can fulfill a role in effective implementation of dietary guidelines at the individual level, i.e., in dietetics and health promotion. Here, the challenges are similar to those of clinical nutritionists and dieticians treating specific distortions in blood pressure, lipid metabolism, etc.; both in a clinical and in a public health context, population nutrition recommendations have to be translated to an individualized dietary optimum in everyday food choice matching the lifestyle of the individual.

Thus, although the biomedical concept of PN is scientifically challenging and may help to further uncover and define physiological requirements, it also has an independent meaning in the domain of public health, where existing and future nutritional requirements are applied to populations (public health) and individuals (PN) aiming at disease prevention and health care.

In this contribution, we will delineate the link between PN and public health. We will do this from the viewpoint of epidemiology. We will first address the role of diet (and lifestyle) in chronic disease epidemiology at the global level and then clarify the basic concept of diet–gene interaction. Subsequently, developments in the status quo on research in nutrient/diet–gene interactions will be summarized for colorectal carcinogenesis and diabetes, representing two pathological processes of major importance to population health. Then, the so-called prevention paradox and its implications for PN will be illustrated and knowledge gaps will be touched upon. Finally, elements for a discussion framework on PN are proposed, and future prospects are delineated.

## 11.2 CHRONIC DISEASE ETIOLOGY

### 11.2.1 Nutrition and Environment

During the past century, improvements in environmental factors such as water supply, sanitation, housing, immunization, and health care have resulted in a major increase in life expectancy, accompanied by successive replacement of infectious diseases by health outcomes such as trauma (because of increased use of private transportation), and age-related cardiovascular disease and malignancies, with overweight and diabetes as intermediary health states. This epidemiologic transition has accompanied a nutrition transition, first focusing on food security (energy needs), followed by food safety and food distribution resulting in increased workforce and economic development, culminating in attention to food quality and dietary advice (food and nutrition policy). This evolution has mainly taken place in the Western countries, and is still occurring in developing economies. These subsequent stages of development require increasingly higher levels of societal infrastructures, and they are clearly visible cross-sectionally at the global level.

What are the main avoidable risk factors? The World Health Report[3] quantified attributable risks of death for the most important exposures: high blood pressure and high serum cholesterol are leading, and known to have direct dietary determinants; next, overweight, physical inactivity, and low consumption of fruits and vegetables also indicate an unbalanced diet and lifestyle. Alcohol and tobacco are addictive lifestyle factors. These exposures are much more important in Western economies compared to developing countries, but undernutrition in regard to zinc, vitamin A, and iron is almost unique for the latter.

The young are especially vulnerable to undernutrition, as is apparent from survival curves of developing countries. But in developed economies the risks of a Western lifestyle are becoming visible only after prolonged, lifelong exposure (which also implies that the risks are intrinsically low). The dramatic improvements in life expectancy and physical well-being during the past century resulted from gradual changes in dietary and environmental factors. Still, about one third of age-related cardiovascular and malignant diseases in developed economies remain diet related. Thus, now that major environmental risk factors have been controlled and have resulted in higher life expectancy, genetic variability between individuals within a population will become a relatively more important factor in explaining the remaining variability in life expectancy. International frameworks and consortiums such as the European Nutrigenomics Organisation, NuGO, are now deciphering the human genome and developing omics technologies, leading to deeper understanding of diet–gene interactions, potentially prolonging healthy life span and preventing disease.

The opportunities provided by the genomics revolution must be viewed against their relevance for individuals and the societies they are living in. For a rational approach to PN and public health, an important question is, to what molecular level we can break down human health and physiology into highly specific molecular cellular nutrition-related processes in order to provide scientific proof, without arriving at infinitely small subpopulations that lack any predictive meaning for (groups of) individuals and in our societies.

### 11.2.2 Genetic Factors and Their Interplay with Diet

Monogenetic traits, with high attributable risks have long served as a model to understand gene–environment interactions. Phenylketonuria (PKU) is a classical example. Phenylalanine (Phe) is a necessary nutrient, but in the absence of a normal phenylalanine hydroxylase enzyme (PAH), Phe metabolites accumulate and eventually lead to mental retardation. The frequency of homozygous deficient subjects is on the order of 1/10,000, which resembles the disease risk because of the ubiquitous exposure to Phe via dietary protein. Because the adverse effect of the nutrient is limited to the population that harbors the genetic variant, all cases can be prevented by adapting the diet in this specific group.

In epidemiologic terms, the PKU example basically envisages gene–environment interactions as the effects resulting from the interplay between a combination of two factors: Phe and PAH, both either present (+) or absent (–), yielding four possible combinations (++,+–, –+, ––) in which only the combination Phe+ (applicable to whole population) with PAH– (applicable to 1/10,000) exhibits a large increased risk of disease. Because of the ubiquitous exposure to Phe and the rare PAH defect, PKU is perceived as an inborn single-gene disease, although the successes of dietary treatment illustrate that it is in fact a highly specific gene–environment interaction. Note that in this example of gene–environment interaction, the risk of disease in Phe+/PAH– subjects is extremely high, whereas the other three combinations carry no risk. Also note that there are many different PAH polymorphisms leading to a similar distortion in Phe metabolism and subsequent mental retardation.

In epidemiology, it was initially hoped that relatively small population-based case control or cohort studies could suffice to detect such strong interactions as in the PKU example. It was stipulated that the weak associations for certain dietary risk factors might be the average of strong associations in certain (relatively small) subgroups of the population, with no association being present in the remainder. To account for the low gene frequency, genetic epidemiologists also developed efficient study designs making use of the genetic relationships between family members and corresponding data analysis techniques. Apart from shared lifestyle factors, it appeared that some syndromes have a major genetic component. In the field of CVD, these are, for example, familial hypercholesterolemia, and the hereditary forms of arrhythmias such as the long QT syndrome, or Liddle's syndrome in hypertension. In the field of diabetes, they are for example, maturity-onset diabetes of the young (MODY), and in the field of cancer examples are Li–Fraumeni Syndrome and hereditary non-polyposis colorectal cancer (HNPCC). The genes involved in these familial syndromes are responsible for only a small percentage (say, 5 to 10% at most) of the total burden of these diseases. These groups have very high risks of developing the disease and, hence, they develop it at a young age. Nevertheless, about 10 to 20% of the population has some type of positive familial history for a specific chronic disease with relative risks on the order of 2 to 3, depending on definitions of familiar risk and the disease as such; thus, about 20% of the case load involves some familial background. The next section provides an overview of the status quo of both types of population-based and family-based studies in the etiology of colorectal cancer and diabetes.

## 11.3 EXAMPLES OF THE STATUS QUO: CARCINOGENESIS AND DIABETES

### 11.3.1 Diet, Genes, and Colorectal Cancer

Already in 1968, MacMahon suggested that environmental factors may influence cancer risk through the genetic mechanism of mutation, whereas genetic mechanisms may modify the impact of the environment.[4] More recently, genetic mutations have been described in the etiology of cancer, such as mutations in the BRCA1 and BRCA2 genes in hereditary breast cancer, and mutations in mismatch repair genes, e.g., MLH1 and MSH2, in the HNPCC syndrome. Mutations in these genes result in a 40 to 80% lifetime risk of developing disease. Such alterations are rare, however, and taken together account for a very small proportion of cancer cases, probably not more than 1 to 5%. Because highly penetrant cancer genes in frequently occurring types of cancer have not been identified thus far, it seems likely that cancer results from biological interaction of both genetic and environmental factors such as diet.

Lifestyle factors, such as dietary habits, smoking, and alcohol consumption are considered to explain more than 30% of cancer incidence worldwide.[5] A common cancer that is thought to be predominantly influenced by lifestyle factors is colorectal cancer (CRC). It is the second most common cancer in the Western world, although it is relatively uncommon in most African, Asian, and South American countries. The marked international variation in CRC incidence, the rapid increase in incidence in families moving from a low- to high-CRC incidence country (migrant studies) and the results from association studies imply that lifestyle factors contribute importantly to the etiology of this disease. It is estimated that more than 50% of CRC may be preventable by reducing alcohol intake, avoidance of weight gain, more physical activity, and decreasing (processed) meat consumption, while increasing the consumption of plant-derived foods.[5]

Relative risks (RRs) observed for dietary factors and CRC in association studies are, however, relatively small (RR < 2). Two decades ago, inherited susceptibility to diet-related carcinogens or specific intakes of nutrients, vitamins, and nutrients provided a promising explanation for these weak associations and inconsistent findings in association studies. Research began to focus on more common genetic alterations that by themselves may not substantially impact disease risk but that in concert with environmental exposures may lead to development of cancer.

Although human experimental studies do show interesting individual variation in response to specific foods and nutrients,[6] the results of most observational studies on inherited susceptibility to dietary factors in cancer risk appeared to be disappointing.[7] Observed diet–gene associations are weak and inconsistent. So far, many individual studies have been designed to examine the main effects of individual factors and do not have adequate power to examine interactions. Often, only one or two single SNPs are studied simultaneously, the functionalities of which are not known. Thus, these studies are not equipped to take complex diet–gene and gene–gene interactions into account. Also, the focus on SNPs as markers of inherited variation may be insufficient to capture the complexity of cancer, given that it ignores other genetic alterations (loss of heterozygosity, epigenetic silencing, somatic mutations, etc.).

### 11.3.2 Diet, Genes, and Diabetes

The incidence of type 2 diabetes (T2DM) has risen rapidly during the past decades together with its major risk factor, obesity. According to the CDC in Atlanta (U.S.), the age-adjusted prevalence of diagnosed diabetes increased, for example, 81% for men and 59% for women from 1980 to 2004. Nowadays, the U.S. prevalence rate amounts to 5.1%, and the lifetime risk for U.S. inhabitants is 33%. Similar trends occur in other Western countries. The WHO has estimated that because of both demographic changes and increases in obesity, about 230 billion people will suffer from diabetes in 2030. The increasing prevalence illustrates that genes cannot be the rate-limiting factor, because the genetic background of the population cannot change that much so quickly. However, T2DM remains a good example of diet–gene interaction: already in 1927, Elliott P. Joslin stated that "heredity loads the canon but obesity and other stresses pull the trigger."

The heritability of T2DM in twin studies has been estimated to range from 25% to up to 80%.[8] Having a sibling with T2DM increases the risk about threefold. Indeed, McCarthy and his group pointed out that this sets the upper limit for the combined effects of all susceptibility variants.[9] Linkage studies have revealed QTLs associated with either T2DM or related continuous traits such as glucose levels and insulin levels (higher in prediabetes, indicating insulin resistance). So far about 17 QTLs on 12 different chromosomes have been identified.[10] Next, metabolic studies gave rise to a long list of candidate genes, such as glucose transporters, insulin-receptor-related factors, sulfonurea receptors, glycogen synthase, PPAR-gamma and related cofactors, but also lipid-metabolism-related factors, beta-2 and beta3 adrenergic receptors, and many obesity related factors as well.[9] Interestingly, but perhaps not surprisingly, the products of some of these candidate genes are diabetes drug targets. For example, the SUR1/KIR6.2 gene locus (ABCD8/KCNJ11 on chromosome 11p) plays a role in the membrane potential of the beta cell. Before the genetics was even fully disclosed, the sulfonureas were designed to stimulate insulin secretion in T2DM. The antidiabetic thiazolidinediones (TZDs) are PPAR-gamma agonists and work as an insulin sensitizer. Again, PPAR-gamma is an important candidate gene, for which the scientific evidence is so compelling that the Pro12Ala variant is associated with T2DM. Calpain 10 (CAPN10) is an interesting candidate gene as it is one of the few susceptibility genes that has been found by genomewide screening of families.[11] Finally, very recently, a new surprising gene has been discovered, TCF7L2, transcription factor 7-like 2,[12] of which the mechanism and targets for treatment or prevention are now being investigated.

Few studies so far have investigated the topic of diet–gene interactions in T2DM. Researchers of the Finnish Diabetes Prevention Study have been active in this field and their findings have been summarized recently.[13] PPAR-gamma was one of the first genes studied. Carriers of the low-risk 12Ala allele did not develop diabetes when they were part of the lifestyle intervention group (diet and physical activity), whereas there was an increasing trend for T2DM with 12Ala in the control group. This difference was accompanied by differences in weight loss. However, these findings also demonstrate the premature state of this type of research, as the high diabetes risk for 12Ala is contrary to what is generally found. An English group, for example, noticed that when the dietary P:S ratio is low, BMI and fasting insulin levels in Ala carriers are higher than that in Pro/Pro homozygotes, but when the P:S ratio is high, the opposite is seen.[14] In fact, this would suggest that on a low dietary P:S ratio diabetes risk is larger in Ala carriers, and on a high P:S ratio diabetes risk is larger in Pro/Pro homozygotes. As fatty acids are natural ligands for PPAR-gamma, these findings await confirmation and further study; also, a lack of power and other methodological issues make interpretation difficult.

## 11.4 PREVENTION PARADOX: SICK INDIVIDUALS AND SICK POPULATIONS

### 11.4.1 Prevention Paradox

In 1985, Sir Geoffrey Rose pointed at the so-called "prevention paradox." He stressed the importance of distinguishing sick individuals and sick populations.[15] Essentially, the prevention paradox implies that individual benefits and population benefits do not necessarily coincide and that cost efficiency must be included in the equation to find an optimal prevention strategy. With respect to the role of genes and environmental factors such as nutrition, Rose indicated that in populations with homogeneous exposures, the classical epidemiologic studies will fail to detect the role of environmental factors and they will only identify markers of susceptibility. With respect to nutrition, the major differences are between populations on the world scale, as illustrated by the epidemiologic transition; apart from socioeconomic gradients, the variation in nutritional exposures within populations is limited and the (relative) risks of nutritional factors are modest or weak indeed. Thus, markers of susceptibility become relatively more prominent in terms of the (relative) risks. Furthermore, Rose argues, strategies in disease control are the "high-risk" approach, which seeks to protect susceptible individuals (e.g., by PN) and the population approach, which seeks to control the causes of incidence.

Population strategies aim to shift the distribution of exposure as a whole. For instance, industry-mediated approaches (with or without legislative incentives) that control the distribution of foods over the population have proved effective and cost-effective. Apart from the classical example of John Snow,[16] who controlled water supply and eliminated cholera in London, other examples include fluoridated drinking water, iodized salt, and elimination of trans fatty acids; these approaches benefit to public health, whereas the risk reduction in any individual subject is of minor importance. Mass-media approaches also aim at reaching the population as a whole and changing lifestyles and dietary patterns; this, however, has not been very effective and is suspected to reach the well-educated socioeconomic strata of society, who already have relatively good health and low disease risks.[17]

In line with medical tradition, nutritional advice is also provided to individuals at high risk. For instance, food industries are also targeting lifestyle and food choice and offer functional foods (with or without health claims) specifically formulated for high-risk groups of the population or those motivated to improve their quality of life. Along these lines, it has been suggested that "knowledge of differential risks resulting from predisposing metabolic genetic traits … can be useful in behavior modification programs and chemoprevention strategies that will have the maximum impact."[18] Even apart from cost-efficiency issues, it remains to be seen if such high-risk approaches followed by behavioral modification and personalized nutrition are as effective as the whole-population approach.

### 11.4.2 Gene–Environment Interactions: Individual and Population Health

Now that data from association studies on nutrients, genes, and their interaction have become available from epidemiologic studies, individual and population benefits can be used to derive the case load from each of the components. We express the strength of associations as the relative risk RR, and we use $RR_N$ for nutritional factors, $RR_G$ for the genetic factor, and $RR_{NG}$ for the effect of their joint exposure. The population attributable risk (PAR) describes the (relative) case load owing to the joint distribution of nutritional and genetic factors relevant to public health; the PAR depends on both the RRs mentioned and the proportion of the population $P_{ij}$ in each of the population segments. Rather than providing formulas, we prefer to visualize the case load as a function of the prevalence of the genetic factor and presence/absence of nutritional exposure.

As an example, RRs and prevalences of the genetic variants are taken from a case control study on aflatoxins, polymorphisms in aflatoxin-metabolizing genes, and the risk of liver cancer in Sudan.[19] In this study, consumption of aflatoxin-contaminated peanut butter was taken as a marker of exposure to aflatoxins. Genes considered were GSTM1, GSTT1, and EPHX. The RRs obtained from this study are summarized in Figure 11.1. The y-axis depicts the RRs and the x-axis the

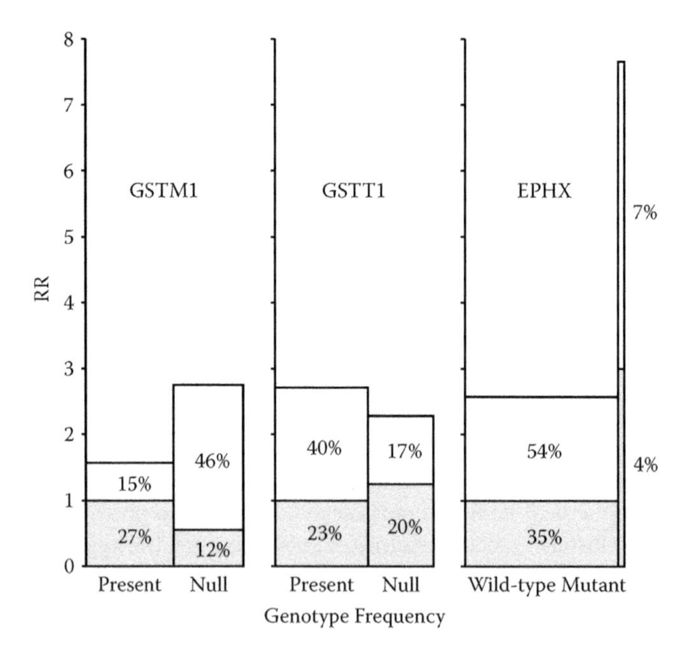


**FIGURE 11.1** Graphical representation of population attributable risk [PAR (%), surface area] as a function of relative risk (RR) and genotype frequency. Data were derived from a case control study on liver cancer as related to aflatoxin-contaminated peanut butter and genotypes of GSTM1, GSTT1, and EPHX, conducted in Sudan.

proportion of the population harboring the genotypes considered. Thus, for each genotype, the case load is graphically represented by the surface given by the product of the prevalence $P_{ij}$ and the RR of the nutritional exposure, here aflatoxin-contaminated peanut butter (this is the case because we have used a median split for aflatoxin exposure). For the three genes considered, aflatoxin reduction in the whole population would prevent about 60% of all cases, independent of genotype (we neglect the fact that the PARs for exposure to aflatoxin are not identical because of weak associations between genotype and exposure and rounding errors). For the highly prevalent GSTM1 and GSTT1 null polymorphisms, a substantial part of the case load derives from the exposed and genetically nonsusceptible subgroup. For the variant of the EPHX gene, only one tenth of all exposure-related cases are derived from the category of the genetically susceptible.

This example illustrates that any single screening test, even when the mutant genotype is highly prevalent (GSTs), tends to provide relatively small PARs for exposure, whereas major opportunities to prevent disease in large segments of the population are not seized. The RRs do not differ greatly according to genotype, and the rare frequency of the high-risk genotype renders the case load due to the interaction relatively small. As illustrated in the previous section, published diet–gene interactions in obesity, diabetes, and cardiovascular and malignant disease all suggest that this example of liver cancer reflects a general phenomenon.

### 11.4.3 Additive and Synergistic Effects

The way in which genetic and dietary factors act jointly is relevant to individual vs. population health and depends on the RRs and $P_{ij}$'s. This joint action may be additive or synergistic (or antagonistic).

When genes and diet work additively, the risks of exposure and genetic background tend to add, i.e., $RR_{NG} = 1 + (RR_N - 1) + (RR_G - 1)$. An additive model might apply when the etiological pathways in which the gene and the dietary factor are involved are completely disjoint. In fact, in such cases, diet–gene interaction is not really an issue: the nutritional factor adds the same risk independent of the genotype and, consequently, individuals with the mutant and those with the wild-type genes would reduce risk by the same extent by dietary modification.

In all other cases, nutritional and genetic risks act in a synergistic or antagonistic way. In synergistic interaction, the effect of genes and diet together exceeds their separate effects; in the case of antagonism, it is less. In synergism, individuals would benefit from screening, but the full potential of nutritional modification would not be met, because a large part of the case load will still derive from the exposed group with the low-risk genotype. In epidemiology, logistic regression models and Cox Proportional Hazards models tend to be used for estimating the independent risks of two or more factors, which implicitly assumes synergy of the form $RR_{NG} = RR_N * RR_G$. Of course, evaluation of this assumption by using statistical interaction terms may provide evidence for deviations from the multiplicative model, leading to additive or supramultiplicative effects.

When the prevalence of the high-risk genotype is small, $RR_{NG}$ must largely exceed $RR_N * RR_G$ to justify screening. When the risk of exposure is almost entirely restricted to the genetic variant (as in the PKU example), i.e., $RR_N = 1$, the case load resulting from exposure and the genetic factor coincide. In this specific and uncommon case of gene–environment interaction, dietary modification (if possible) can reduce the risk among the genetically susceptible. When $RR_N$ exceeds 1, the case load emerging from the relative large size of the "less susceptible" genetic subpopulation does not justify an individualized approach that only targets this subgroup, unless both the prevalence of the high-risk genotype is large and $RR_{NG}$ is large as well.

The foregoing observations become highly relevant if results on different genes are considered simultaneously. The study on liver cancer could provide a hypothetical example: One could speculate that — if the genes mentioned are independent and if the RRs are multiplicative — that the RR of liver cancer for exposure to aflatoxin contaminated peanut butter could rise to RR = 2.7 * 2.3 * 7.7 = 48, which would be applicable to a population segment of 0.44 * 0.41 * 0.04 = 0.007, resulting in a very low PAR. Thus, when several genes are addressed simultaneously, the RRs and individual benefits can be large. However, the higher the RR, the smaller the population segment it applies to. Finally, any of the data in this example should be used with caution, both because of uncertainties due to sampling and because of uncertainties with respect to independence of the polymorphisms and the biochemical pathways involved.

Thus, for combinations of specific diet–gene interactions, the biological interaction (synergism or antagonism) of genes and diet is superimposed on background risk. Joint effects can be quantified using theoretical models, but we still have to learn what type of model applies most commonly to gene–environment interactions. It is highly questionable whether elucidation of biochemical pathways can contribute to valid inference on additivity, multiplicativity, or other synergistic/antagonistic effects; at the same time, high-throughput mass approaches that simultaneously include a large number of gene variants and dietary factors in epidemiologic research are often incapable of yielding sufficient evidence for specific gene–nutrient interactions. Uncertainty on individual risks is a necessary consequence and will limit the possibilities for PN advice.

## 11.5 DISCUSSION FRAMEWORK FOR PN

### 11.5.1 CONTEXT

Discussions on possibilities and limitations of PN would benefit from a framework that distinguishes the context in which PN is applied (clinical, prevention), the research angle (genomics), and issues relevant to individual advice (tailoring).

For effective treatment of clinically sick and very-high-risk individuals, drug treatment is indicated. Genetic factors are gradually being incorporated in clinical settings to optimize treatment according to prognostic indicators. In the preventive domain, risks are much lower, metabolic aberrations are relatively mild and interventions in lifestyle are implemented via, e.g., dietetic advice, the basic form of PN. The objective is to successfully alter habitual dietary intake and thereby reduce risk factors of disease (blood lipids, blood pressure, overweight, etc.) within the individual's range of possibilities. Apart from compliance issues (also relevant to drug treatment), such individual advice can indeed lead to direct changes in dietary intake, but demonstrating effects on habitual diet, nutritional status, risk factors of disease, and long-term disease risk is increasingly difficult.

In contrast to effective individual treatment, an important issue in prevention is effective communication. Mass-media approaches to low-risk populations are known for poor efficacy, conceptually similar to poor compliance in drug treatment. Group approaches (e.g., at schools) to communicate dietary recommendations are considered more effective, and the idea is that tailored dietary advice based on individual genomics data would be even more effective. This notion is questionable, however. As we can see in the practice of clinical dietetics, dietary advice incorporates dietary assessment, provides options for dietary change, helps to set priorities, is practical, and monitors changes, provides feedback on dietary intake (and exposure/health markers). For the individual, the trade-off is between lowering a high risk at the expense of giving up a habitual diet. For PN the healthy individual will make a trade-off between (unsure) future risk reduction and rewards of (positive) feedback on the one hand and direct losses of well-being related to changing habitual patterns of food preparation, psychological aspects, taste, and social aspects of eating. Direct changes in "quality of life" must be balanced against uncertain future longevity. (See Chapter 13 and Chapter 14.)

### 11.5.2 Genomics

Research on diet–gene interactions and genomics research are in their infancy. So far, the results of diet–gene studies have not been equivocal. Several methodological issues may account for this, such as the need for large study samples, a consistent and well-measured phenotype, high-quality information on dietary exposures, etc. There certainly is an enormous growth potential for research, and we are beginning to see its potency in explaining variation of nutrient needs and risks between individuals.

In this chapter, we focused on genetic data; information on human disease risks as related to transcriptomics, proteomics, and metabolomics is not available nowadays. The genetic blueprint can be regarded as a somewhat static trait that tells us about the potential of our body, but differently so for different individuals and results are still scarce. Whole-genome scans employing thousands of SNPs will soon become available and indicate new relevant loci, with possibly surprising findings. This may enable the search for underlying pathways and study of the simultaneous effects of SNP-patterns and dietary modification. However, statistical methods and common scientific principles are still being developed. For instance, the etiological distance between SNPs and a clinical disease is long, and dilution occurs. Shortening this distance by reducing the phenotype from individual to organ, tissue, cellular, or molecular levels tends to increase the strength of scientific proof on specific interactions; at the same time, however, zooming in on molecular laboratory research excludes higher-level interactions and increases uncertainty due to other factors, thereby tempering the generalizability to individual subjects and populations. In addition to SNPs, future results of transcriptomics, proteomics, and metabolomics may provide powerful noninvasive techniques to screen populations and monitor the effect of dietary interventions. For instance, the role of folate in DNA methylation and other reversible epigenetic processes may be examined using these techniques on blood samples from a large number of individuals, taking inherited differences in folate metabolism into account. However, the current enthusiasm about scientific promises in genomics research should not result in overestimating the upper limit of gene–diet interactions on public health. For instance, for T2DM a relative risk of about 3 is provided by family history studies and similar figures apply to cancer etiology; as illustrated, extreme high-risk groups are clinically important, but they tend not to be of major public health importance.

An intrinsic scientific problem in genomics research is that genes and diets play their role in many biochemical pathways at the same time. Each gene may have many polymorphisms/SNPs relating to (slightly) different mRNAs, proteins, and metabolite patterns. Studying all functions under controlled conditions and assessing their associated risks is virtually impossible. Thus, there is a need for integrative markers, i.e., phenotypic markers reflecting pathophysiologically relevant distortions in metabolic pathways, attributable to key regulatory genes of that pathway or to genetic variation in the enzymes involved. This calls for identification of pathways starting from known classical risk factors of disease or of being healthy in old age and using the metabolites, proteins, transcriptome, and genetics as explanatory factors. In conclusion, even if the scientific hopes will be realized, it will take a long time, before the results are ready for use in individual advice and the benefits for population health remain limited.

### 11.5.3 Tailoring

As mentioned earlier, balancing direct gains in well-being against future risk is nowadays restricted to clinical settings with high and intermediate risks. However, ICT technologies can make tailored advice available to a larger proportion of the population in a cost-effective way. A personal balanced diet, however, should not be based on nutrient composition alone, but it should also include dietary assessment (as the starting point to identify options for change), energy balance (physical activity), lifestyle factors (e.g., smoking and drinking), and medical risk factors (BMI, blood lipids, blood pressure, etc.), whereas genomic markers might be added in the distant future. Nevertheless, PN targets the individual, and remains a high-risk-group approach, rather than the population-based approach advocated by Sir Geoffrey Rose.

The concept of PN also calls for defining health as "more than the absence of disease," also including personal well-being (as WHO does). If this is ignored, it may lead to adding "years to life" rather than "life to years." In a clinical high-risk context, risk reductions are paid for not only economically, but also personally by accepting side effects that adversely affect well-being in a physical (surgery), mental (pain, suffering), or social sense (hospitalization). The price individuals want to pay for reducing moderate or low risks are logically much less, but they are taken into account in tailored advice to individual patients. If well informed, individuals can decide their own personal balance of long-term risks (with attached values) and direct benefits in the domain of well-being (with their attached values). In this view, "personal" is based on individual values rather than genomic risks.

In practice, it appears that some people are willing to pay large amounts of money for genetic testing and tailored advice, even though the advice provided is quite similar to generic guidelines; however, individual risk cannot be addressed with reasonable accuracy and precision, leaving the predicted risks associated with high uncertainty. Thus, similar to the widespread use of supplements and the increasing use of functional foods, the PN approach may preferentially reach the worried, healthy, well-educated, and health-literate population segments that already have the highest life expectancy. This way, PN may contribute to widening the socioeconomic health gradient in populations. This calls for careful balancing of the population-targeted policies against the PN approach.

## 11.6 FUTURE PERSPECTIVES FOR PN

The idea that genomics research can lead to PN is theoretically sound, but has a very long way to go and is currently "a bridge too far." Data are available on a limited number of specific diet–gene interactions, but they are not promising for public health. Moreover, it is not clear what these data imply for polygenic and multifactorial interactions in disease etiology. Moreover, a theoretical framework is lacking that could help to reconstruct individual and population risks from the laboratory-based pieces of evidence of diet–gene interactions. And even when large-scale human data using genomic technology and systems biology become available, large uncertainties would remain when scientific data on risks among groups of subjects are applied to the individual.

Nevertheless, at some point in time, systems biology, individual, and population health might converge for some highly relevant gene–diet interactions. Requirements and technologies for PN may evolve parallel in time, probably starting from dietetic counseling practices. In the meantime, research on genomics and tailoring must be accounted for, as the idea and rough prototypes are already "on the market." This stresses the need to further explore the possibilities, limitations, and implications of full-scale implementation, simultaneously by scientists, stakeholders, and the public.

Nevertheless, if PN is realized, the prevention paradox remains, i.e., individual benefits and population benefits do not necessarily coincide, unless direct benefits in subjective well-being are included in the health concept. At least the time-scale of the risks, cost-efficiency, and personal well-being must be included into the equation to find the optimum balance. For now, the omics are not relevant to public health, as proteomics and metabolomics are expensive, and statistical techniques for interpretation are still in development. For the time being, family history probably remains the most useful tool as an easy and efficient summary measure of a large variety of highly specific genetic factors.

Applications of PN await convincing scientific evidence, and it is possible that such evidence may never materialize. This should be taken as a challenge for a serious debate between molecular sciences, social sciences, and public health professionals to balance the health and well-being of individuals and populations with respect to PN.

## ACKNOWLEDGMENT

The work underlying this chapter has been funded by a grant of the Wageningen University Board (VIVRE project "MyFood", 2004–2005).

## KEY READINGS

Brennan, P., Gene-environment interaction and aetiology of cancer: what does it mean and how can we measure it?, *Carcinogenesis* 23(3), 381–7, 2002.

Mutch, D.M., Wahli, W., and Williamson, G., Nutrigenomics and nutrigenetics: the emerging faces of nutrition, *FASEB J.* 19(12), 1602–16, 2005.

Ordovas, J.M. and Corella, D., Nutritional genomics, *Annu Rev Genomics Hum Genet,* 5, 71–118, 2004.

Perera, F. P., Environment and cancer: who are susceptible?, *Science* 278(5340), 1068–73, 1997.

Rose, G., Sick individuals and sick populations, *Int J Epidemiol* 14(1), 32–8, 1985.

## REFERENCES

1. Mutch, D.M., Wahli, W., and Williamson, G., Nutrigenomics and nutrigenetics: the emerging faces of nutrition, *FASEB J.* 19(12), 1602–16, 2005.
2. *Report of the committee of inquiry into the future development of the public health function and community medicine.* HMSO, London, 1988.
3. *The World Health Report 2002 — Reducing risks, promoting healthy lifestyle* WHO, 2002.
4. MacMahon, B., Gene-environment interactions in human disease, *J Psychiatr Res* 6, 393–242, 1968.
5. WCRF, *Food, nutrition and the prevention of cancer: a global perspective* WCRF/American Institute for Cancer Research, Washington, D.C., 1997.
6. Lampe, J. W. and Peterson, S., Brassica, biotransformation and cancer risk: genetic polymorphisms alter the preventive effects of cruciferous vegetables, *J Nutr* 132(10), 2991–4, 2002.
7. Brennan, P., Gene-environment interaction and aetiology of cancer: what does it mean and how can we measure it?, *Carcinogenesis* 23(3), 381–7, 2002.
8. Beck-Nielsen, H., Vaag, A., Poulsen, P., and Gaster, M., Metabolic and genetic influence on glucose metabolism in type 2 diabetic subjects — experiences from relatives and twin studies, *Best Pract Res Clin Endocrinol Metab* 17(3), 445–67, 2003.
9. McCarthy, M. I. and Zeggini, E., Genetics of type 2 diabetes, *Curr Diab Rep* 6(2), 147–54, 2006.
10. Florez, J. C., Hirschhorn, J., and Altshuler, D., The inherited basis of diabetes mellitus: implications for the genetic analysis of complex traits, *Annu Rev Genomics Hum Genet* 4, 257–91, 2003.
11. Sreenan, S. K., Zhou, Y. P., Otani, K., Hansen, P. A., Currie, K. P., Pan, C. Y., Lee, J. P., Ostrega, D. M., Pugh, W., Horikawa, Y., Cox, N. J., Hanis, C. L., Burant, C. F., Fox, A. P., Bell, G. I., and Polonsky, K. S., Calpains play a role in insulin secretion and action, *Diabetes* 50(9), 2013–20, 2001.
12. Grant, S. F., Thorleifsson, G., Reynisdottir, I., Benediktsson, R., Manolescu, A., Sainz, J., Helgason, A., Stefansson, H., Emilsson, V., Helgadottir, A., Styrkarsdottir, U., Magnusson, K. P., Walters, G. B., Palsdottir, E., Jonsdottir, T., Gudmundsdottir, T., Gylfason, A., Saemundsdottir, J., Wilensky, R. L., Reilly, M. P., Rader, D. J., Bagger, Y., Christiansen, C., Gudnason, V., Sigurdsson, G., Thorsteinsdottir, U., Gulcher, J. R., Kong, A., and Stefansson, K., Variant of transcription factor 7-like 2 (TCF7L2) gene confers risk of type 2 diabetes, *Nat Genet* 38(3), 320–3, 2006.

13. Uusitupa, M., Gene-diet interaction in relation to the prevention of obesity and type 2 diabetes: evidence from the Finnish Diabetes Prevention Study, *Nutr Metab Cardiovasc Dis* 15(3), 225–33, 2005.
14. Luan, J., Browne, P. O., Harding, A. H., Halsall, D. J., O'Rahilly, S., Chatterjee, V. K., and Wareham, N. J., Evidence for gene-nutrient interaction at the PPARgamma locus, *Diabetes* 50(3), 686–9, 2001.
15. Rose, G., Sick individuals and sick populations, *Int J Epidemiol* 14(1), 32–8, 1985.
16. Smith, G.D, Behind the broad street pump: aetiology, epidemiology and prevention of cholera in mid-19th century Britain, *Int J Epidemiol* 31(5), 920–932, 2002.
17. van der Pal-de Bruin, K.M., de Walle, H.E., de Rover, C.M., Jeeninga, W., Cornel, M.C., de Jong-van den Berg, L.T., Buitendijk, S.E., and Paulussen, T.G.. Influence of educational level on determinants of folic acid use, *Paediatr Perinat Epidemiol* 17(3), 256–63, 2003.
18. Perera, F. P., Environment and cancer: who are susceptible?, *Science* 278(5340), 1068–73, 1997.
19. Tiemersma, E. W., Omer, R. E., Bunschoten, A., van't Veer, P., Kok, F. J., Idris, M. O., Kadaru, A. M., Fedail, S. S., and Kampman, E., Role of genetic polymorphism of glutathione-S-transferase T1 and microsomal epoxide hydrolase in aflatoxin-associated hepatocellular carcinoma, *Cancer Epidemiol Biomarkers Prev* 10(7), 785–91, 2001.

# *Section II*

## *Personalized Nutrition and Stakeholders in Society*

# 12 Imminent Applications of Nutrigenomics: A Stakeholder Analysis

*J.T. Winkler*

## CONTENTS



## 12.1 INTRODUCTION

The promise of nutrigenomics is grand; the practicalities are daunting. Many scientists researching the frontiers of the field believe the complexities are such that useful applications are decades away. But, for better or for worse, scientists do not always determine what happens in the world. Other groups have interests in nutrigenomics. For them, benefits are in prospect — genetic understanding and personalized diets, better health and enhanced capacities, improved foods and targeted marketing, lower costs, and higher revenues. Rewards such as these may inspire a more optimistic interpretation of the scientific evidence. And provide incentives to immediate action. This chapter identifies probable actions of key interest groups whose interplay will shape the future of nutrigenomics. The intent is description, not prescription. The perspective is intentionally agnostic, to describe not what is desirable, but what is likely, for good or for ill. The method is stakeholder analysis. Five groups will be considered: scientists, food companies, consumers, competitive athletes, and health-care providers. Their behavior will raise issues on which policy decisions will have to be taken, sooner or later. For all these parties, the discovery of inherited susceptibilities and capabilities is a prerequisite for whatever actions they want to take. Hence, this chapter is as much about genetic testing as it is about nutritional interventions.

## 12.2 SCIENTISTS

Most people active in nutrigenomics at present are scientists, conducting research in genomics, transcriptomics, proteomics, metabolomics, and associated disciplines. In this field, as everywhere else, differing views coexist even among the cognoscenti.

Nonetheless, the view of numerous leaders is that, because of the multiple genes, multiple polymorphisms, and multiple metabolic pathways involved, unraveling genetic influences on diet-related diseases will take a long time. We are in the stage of basic science and likely to remain so for many years. With the present state of knowledge, speculation regarding practical applications of nutrigenomics would be premature.

Thus, for example, Ben van Ommen, Coordinator of the NuGO program: "I think it is way too early to give dietary advice based on your genes."[1] Similarly, Sian Astley, U.K. coordinator of NuGO, feels there is "no way that nutrigenomics is ready yet to give individual advice or help health policy."[2] "Not in our lifetimes," says "optimist" Bruce German.[3] "Never," feels Larry Parnell, because it is technically impossible to cover all possible gene–gene permutations.[4] Prudence is most vividly expressed by Jose Ordovas: "What we are seeing now is the very, very beginning. Nutrigenomics has established proof of concept, but that's it. To commercialize the science at this point is almost like throwing darts in the dark."[5]

Even within the scientific community, however, others urge immediate use. Most obvious are scientists in companies selling genetic tests, such as Sciona and Genelex. Among clinical geneticists, Aubrey Milunsky condenses the positive case into the title of his book, *Your Genetic Destiny: Know your Genes, Secure your Health, Save your Life*.[6] For others, moral as well as practical arguments encourage incremental application of nutrigenomic knowledge as soon as it emerges. Diet-related diseases are so widespread, responsible for so much mortality, morbidity and misery, that it would be "criminally negligent" to continue prescribing ineffective general diets when personalized nutrition is possible.[7]

## 12.3 TIMELESS ISSUES BEHIND CURRENT CONTROVERSIES

Between "Nutrigenomics Now!" and "Never!" lie issues in the philosophy of science. Among them is the classic: how much certainty is needed before initiating practical action? In translation: what percentage of the variance in disease rates needs to be explained by a set of genes before therapeutic interventions are justified?

That question has practical immediacy because nutrigenetic tests are not static, either useful or inadequate, once and for all. Rather, they are developed incrementally as evidence accumulates. Sciona's first test, for example, assessed 7 genes, then 19, with further expansions anticipated.

Another fundamental issue for nutrigenomics has surfaced in ironic form: should the use of tests be determined by the quality of available responses to the information they produce? Public health screening programs are sometimes postponed because no effective remedies exist or the cost of screening exceeds the population benefits of subsequent treatment.

In contrast, one criticism of nutrigenetic testing, following research by the U.S. Government Accountability Office, was that it only produced "commonsense" recommendations.[8] Many nutritionists would be flattered and surprised that contemporary dietary advice is now "common sense." The usual criticism of nutrition science is that some of its therapies are unproven, or only erratically effective, because the mechanisms of action are incompletely understood. To which the standard rebuttal has been: they may do good and probably will do no harm. Such benign insouciance will no longer suffice. With the advent of nutrigenetic testing, the standards of proof for nutritional therapies will rise. So too will the specificity of nutritional advice provided to the tested.

Indeed, one of the greatest promises of nutrigenomics is to identify the mechanisms of nutritional action, by monitoring genetic influences on metabolism, through genetic and other biomarkers along pathways. This provides an alternative to the orthodoxy of double-blinded randomized controlled trials, which are impossible with foods. Meanwhile, a prolonged debate is in prospect about the accuracy, acceptability, and advisability of nutrigenomic tests. It will include the scientist vs. scientist squabbles that enrage nonspecialists who want certainty. And exonerate those who would change nothing.

However, a related issue may hasten the introduction of tests. Expectations are rising for genetic controls on subjects in nutritional trials. For example, two issues in the relationship between salt and hypertension are the extent and strength of inherited "salt sensitivity." Those convinced that genetic influences on blood pressure are strong (including the salt and savory foods industries) feel the absence of genetic controls in earlier studies undermines the positive associations they produced. Researchers may henceforth feel it judicious to incorporate genetic controls, however imperfect, using whatever tests are available at the time.

Underlying all these issues is a common question: when is the science sufficient? The correlative question raised by stakeholder analysis is: who decides?

## 12.4 FOOD COMPANIES

That grand promise of nutrigenomics — to identify inherited susceptibilities to diet-related diseases, then provide personalized nutritional advice — creates commercial opportunities. There is a large prospective market for "targeted foods," products designed for genetically susceptible people. This is the nutritional analogue to pharmacogenetics, producing drugs tailored to patients' inherited characteristics. "Targeted foods" should be understood broadly. The category includes not just manufactured products, but also nutritional supplements, herbal remedies, and enhanced versions of fresh produce. Some fresh vegetables, fruits, eggs, meats, and fish containing higher levels of beneficial components may be produced by conventional breeding and feeding, others by genetic modification. Current examples of both approaches are provided by brassicas with higher levels of glucosinolates, offering a measure of protection against some cancers. Nutritionally modified plants (in which nutrient profiles are altered rather than agronomic properties) are not, at present, conceived as part of "nutrigenomics," although the concept could expand. The point, for present purposes, is simply that the commercial response to nutrigenomics will include a wide variety of targeted products.

Some will be niche products, such as glutenfree foods for celiacs. Some may become mass-market products, where the critical genetic variations are widespread in a population. Candidates, as nutrigenomics develops, might include genetic influences on insulin resistance, leading to new versions of traditional foods formulated with lower glycemic loads, relevant to obesity and diabetes. That topical example suggests targeted foods might also appeal to people suffering from the same problem without the inherited susceptibility, expanding the market. They are an advanced version of a 20th century industry development — functional foods, with added genetics. In fact, opportunities may be greater still. Nutrigenomics involves a two-way relationship. Nutrient intakes influence gene expression, and expressed or silenced genes influence nutrient metabolism.

Current practice is, by default, to adapt food intakes to inherited susceptibilities, through both reductions and additions. Those with familial hypercholesterolemia, for example, are urged to cut saturated fat intake and eat more "cardioprotective foods."[9] People inheriting galactosemia exclude milk products. Those suffering from cystic fibrosis supplement with fat-soluble vitamins.

As nutrigenomics develops, however, we may expect more targeted products designed to influence gene expression/silencing. Some of these genes may influence diseases that are not today considered "diet-related." "Targeted foods" could become a large category. If so, such products would arrive on the back of an already strong trend. To a degree unimaginable 30 years ago, foods are promoted for their nutritional strengths, on "health platforms." No longer just "less bad" (low-fat, reduced salt, sugar-free), high-tech fortified foods now promise positive benefits. Phytosterol-enriched margarines to lower cholesterol are the best-documented example.

At an abstract level, it is a form of progress that health is becoming a popular basis for choosing foods, alongside taste, price, and convenience. But assessing the nutrient profiles of products and linking them to personal genetic profiles is complex. Consumers will need help.

Dietary advice will become a routine part of genetic counseling. Conversely, dieticians will have to incorporate genetics into their repertoire. Nutrition education will be transformed, once one-size-fits-all recommendations are no longer plausible. Food companies will naturally offer pointed guidance, and they are much bigger nutrition educators than governments. Ahead lies a public contest for "share of mind."

### 12.4.1 Personalized Marketing

Genetic tests could also transform another trend in the food industry, toward "direct marketing." One cliché in advertising is that 50% of it is wasted, but we do not know which half. Much mass-market advertising is showered on people who will never be interested in the products being promoted.

Advertisers have long attempted to reduce this "wastage," to concentrate marketing on serious potential customers, a process also known as "targeting." Early efforts were primitive, based on media audience profiles, demographic characteristics, and attitudinal orientations. With widespread adoption of bar coding and supermarket loyalty cards, advertisers extract individual buying patterns from electronic-point-of-sale data, identifying established customers to encourage repeat purchases. Prospective buyers are now picked out from interests expressed though Internet search patterns. In contemporary marketing jargon, this is establishing a "personalized relationship with the customer."

In future, individuals' genetic test data could facilitate the ultimate personal relationship, "genetic marketing." When, eventually, nutrigenomics verifies individual susceptibilities and nutritional needs, it will simultaneously identify potential customers for targeted foods. In a sporting metaphor popular among marketers, this creates "the chance to go one-on-one with the customer in the kitchen."

Persuading consumers to share their genetic data, even bits of it, will probably provoke a larger and longer version of the competition between formula and baby food manufacturers to sign up new mothers for supplies while they are still in maternity wards. Inducements may be necessary, for institutions as well as individuals.

Economics enters the equation in another way. From a marketing perspective, targeted foods are archetypal "value-added" products. And the value they add beyond conventional foods is a particularly important one, health. In one version of market logic, better products justify higher prices.

In sum, nutrigenomics will stimulate new foods, new ways of selling them, and enlarged margins. These are powerful temptations to rapid applications of nutrigenomic research. So powerful that some food companies may force the pace, by making specific genetic tests directly accessible to consumers at subsidized rates, or indeed, free, a loss leader to recruit customers for new foods (see Chapter 14). Personalized nutrition will bring with it personalized marketing. Targeted foods will be promoted though targeted advertising. But, of course, this brave new commercial world will not be problem free.

### 12.4.2 The Counterpart to Promise

Those who buy targeted foods, as opposed to those who sell them, may view higher prices differently, as a levy tacked onto products that are alleged to do people good, a "health premium." Some economists will agree with them, because that pricing strategy creates economic problems.

Some people, made aware of their nutrigenetic susceptibilities, will become anxious about their future. In distress, some will feel they need to grasp whatever nutritional remedies are available, whatever the cost. In the language of economics, they become "price insensitive"; they have "inelastic demand" for those targeted foods that are relevant to their risks. This is the exploitation of anxiety. In many countries, commercial appeals to fear are prohibited by advertising regulations. But genetic susceptibility may be presented more subtly, fright disguised as fate (see Chapter 15).

Not only is individual psychology at issue, but macro health economics. Diet-related diseases are overwhelmingly diseases of poverty. With nutritional problems, as with much else, the poor suffer more. If targeted foods are permanently positioned at higher prices, then the people who need them most will be least able to acquire them. The public health promise of nutrigenomics would then not be realized (see Chapter 11).

But a different economic calculus leads to an intermediate position. Even for poor people, absolute price is not always the concern; sometimes they seek value for money. Targeted foods, if genuinely effective, would not only diminish disease risks and symptoms, but also associated costs. These include outgoings on care, but equally important, income foregone because of hindrances to employment. There may be net benefits, even if prices are high. Whether targeted foods really represent value for money, however, is conditional on another fundamental issue, namely, their efficacy. Will personalized nutrition be effective in coping with inherited, diet-related diseases? Even the most cautious researchers are optimistic on that point, or they would not be working in the field. But decades of nutrigenomic research may still not suffice, because this is as much a legal as a scientific issue.

### 12.4.3 Foods vs. Drugs, Science vs. Law

At present, the law says unequivocally that foods do not prevent, treat, or cure disease. In the U.S., foods cannot even ameliorate it. Or, more precisely, no one may claim that they do. Such "medicinal claims" are reserved for licensed drugs. That is one of the few points on which food laws around the world actually agree.

The prohibition has always been scientifically irrational. Modern nutritional science actually began with the demonstration that vitamins can prevent and cure "deficiency diseases." That, of course, is still true. For example, U.K. dietary recommendations state that the "essential and undisputed roles of vitamin C (ascorbic acid) are to prevent scurvy … [and] … 10 mg/d [is] also sufficient to cure clinical signs of scurvy … ."[10] So say scientists. But food manufacturers may not make the same statement about products containing vitamin C, no matter how enriched. These laws were, in fact, designed to staunch the gushing hyperbole of patent medicines. They did that job effectively. But foods were caught in the same net. Nutrients are treated the same as Victorian elixirs. Still, today, even the most nutrient-rich foods may not be presented as being prophylactic or therapeutic.

Meanwhile, most developed countries have resorted to fudge. A compromise emerged that, although companies may not claim that foods reduce disease, they may claim that foods reduce risk factors for disease. Companies may be required at some stage to present the scientific evidence behind their "health claims," a surrogate assessment of efficacy. The U.S. has adopted a particularly complex variant of this approach, with four grades of "qualified claims," depending on the quality of the evidence, with even "preliminary" and "unpersuasive" science allowed at the bottom rung.

Nutrigenomics has the potential to end this hotchpotch. When mechanisms of action are eventually proved, it will offer new and stronger forms of evidence, beyond normal nutritional arguments, about foods' beneficial actions against disease. That should, logically, undermine the legal distinction between foods and drugs.

However, doctors and most other health professionals receive little training in nutrition. They are often suspicious of dietary interventions, citing the absence of randomized controlled trials. This is part rationality, part protective mechanism against "alternative" therapies. Furthermore, interests have built up to defend the status quo, especially in pharmaceutical companies. Changing the law will be a lengthy, perhaps interminable, process. Legal pragmatism has already resisted science for more than a century and may continue to do so.

In the interim, possibly a long interim, nutrigenomic tests will be offered to people with varying degrees of completeness and certainty. Targeted foods will come wrapped in imprecise statements about what they do and how well. To paraphrase Eliot, this is the way nutrigenomics may begin, not with a bang but a whimper.[11] But food companies will strive for a more explosive beginning. They will actively promote both tests and products. Advertising may be as persuasive in implying the efficacy of targeted foods as it has been about many other goods. Consumers may respond more to these promises than to the scruples of scientists and lawyers.

## 12.5 CONSUMERS

Compared to the corporates, consumers have a more intense as well as a more personal interest in nutrigenomics. For some, their life depends on it. For others, only their quality of life hangs in the balance, but that is motivation enough for most. At present, relatively few consumers know about nutrigenomics, so they do not yet constitute a coherent "interest group." But targeted commercial promotions to the vulnerable will spread information quickly. And with it, hope.

Sick consumers sometimes employ a different rationality from scientists, defined by their context. In the early days of HIV/AIDS drugs, sufferers refused to wait for the conclusion of long randomized controlled trials. Their personal end might arrive before scientists had "proof." The rigor of three-stage clinical trials was seen, not as good scientific practice, but as delay, or worse, denial of treatment.

Seriously ill patients are increasingly demanding access to experimental, unapproved drugs.[12] The controversy over Herceptin for breast cancer is the latest example of consumer impatience with scientific method and regulatory due process. Sellers of remedies often encourage, support, and even finance, such demanding consumers. Elected politicians may respond to their appeals. They did in both the cases cited.

Diet-related diseases are usually chronic, lacking the life-and-death drama of these examples. But the popular perception of "genes-as-destiny" may lend nutrigenomics an urgency that nutrition has seldom acquired, outside famines. Consumers are already more accepting of nutritional remedies than doctors and regulators. Nutrigenomics will reinforce their preferences.

However, both the health and commercial benefits of targeted foods depend on consumers' willingness to share their nutrigenetic data with others, not just health professionals, but also food companies. Who will have access to genetic profiles?

### 12.5.1 To Regulate or Not to Regulate?

The initial public debate in many countries, led by consumer and patient organizations, suggests widespread reluctance, despite inducements. Attention has focused on possible misuses of data, especially by insurance companies and employers. The concern is potential discrimination against the genetically susceptible.

Advocates urge measures to protect privacy, forbidding compulsory testing and restricting access to the results of voluntary tests. Many call for more regulation — of tests, laboratories, biobanks, direct-to-consumer sales, promotional claims, products linked to test results, nutritional supplements, fortified foods, and more.

Historically, this is an unusual development. Normally, regulation trundles along belatedly after new technologies, like a rubbish van after a parade, sweeping up the mess. Those concerned about the new genetics are trying to preempt problems.

This strategy contrasts with another new technology that emerged around the same time, the Internet. For all its many virtues, the Internet is accused of facilitating numerous kinds of fraud, identity theft, mass disruptions through viruses, breaches of security and privacy through hackers, stimulating pornography and pedophilia, and not least for nutritionists, contributing to the surge in childhood obesity. Yet preventing regulation of the Internet is, for many, a point of principle. When Internet service providers accept some restrictions in China, this is interpreted as capitulation to power in pursuit of money.

"Preemptive regulation" is potentially a significant development in consumer protection. In part, it reflects the particular sensitivity many people feel about all things genetic, because of associations with eugenics and enduring battles with religion. Among its several purposes, this book is intended as a corrective to those apprehensions.

However, in many other areas of modern life, developed societies are in a deregulatory phase. Regulation is often presented as "red tape," a "burden" on enterprise. In some countries, deregulation is explicit policy. In the EU, all legislative proposals on foods must produce a "regulatory impact analysis."

At its grandest, we have here a conflict between two approaches to organizing modern society. Practically, we are in for a lengthy series of acrimonious regulatory battles about genetic testing and its unintended consequences.

### 12.5.2 Influences on Acceptability

But even within the field of genetic testing, nutrigenomics is different. Testing for diet-related susceptibilities is not like testing for Huntington's disease, the subject of much attitudinal research. For some inherited diseases, testing means disclosure of an unavoidable fate, even a death foretold.

Nutrigenomic testing has two distinct attributes that make it exceptional, and probably more acceptable. First, a positive response is always possible, changing diet. Second, that response is under the individual's control. These are intrinsic advantages of nutrigenomic testing, compared to other types of screening. Here, within economic constraints, knowledge empowers individual action.

But extrinsic factors will also influence the acceptability of these tests. Those who are not just at risk, but already ill with a diet-related disease, may be more insistent than resistant about testing. As with the aforementioned drugs, some will be more concerned about short-term relief from problems than long-term invasions of privacy. With nutrigenomics, as with other subjects, the views of consumer organizations are not always those of individual consumers.

The terms and conditions on which nutrigenomic tests are presented to the public will further shape uptake. Tests subsidized by industry would certainly be cheaper than those available individually from specialist testing companies. And perhaps more accessible, too, if distributed through local outlets, even unconventional ones such as pharmacies and supermarkets. Lower prices and easier availability would widen the customer base and help counter the allegation that nutrigenomics tests are merely a luxury for the worried well. They would become a resource for the demonstrably sick as well as those at risk.

Moreover, the agreement of consumers to share results with third parties, including food companies, might be a condition for providing subsidized tests. To those worried about privacy, such requirements will seem extortionate. But concerned consumers might be willing to share information with those they believe, rightly or wrongly, could help them, especially as initial tests are likely to be specific to genes for defined problems, rather than expensive whole-genome scans that could allow later fishing expeditions for other information.

Decisions on sharing personal data will not be taken by individuals in isolation, but within an evolving social context. Nutrigenomics is arriving at a time when skepticism toward conventional medicine is growing. Alternative or complementary therapies are increasingly popular, including dietary responses such as supplements, functional foods, and herbal remedies, as well as simply healthier eating. Nutrigenomics again reinforces an existing trend.

But it is already clear that nutrigenomics will be the focus of a public debate in its own right, amplified in popular media, about whether it is endangering or empowering.[13] The outcome is by no means certain. In Europe, the opponents of the "new genetics" in all its forms have had considerable success. Other parts of the world are more enthusiastic.

### 12.5.3 Familiarization with Genetic Testing

Underneath the fireworks of public polemic, however, a long-term process of cultural familiarization is under way, with both genetic testing and positive applications of its results. DNA tests add a new dimension to the already widespread interest in genealogy. DNA evidence, to identify murderers and rapists, often after years of conventional investigative failure, is already a staple of mainstream crime reporting and TV police dramas. A more compassionate use is to exonerate the victims of miscarriages of justice.[14]

Proceeding slowly and incrementally is preimplantation genetic diagnosis of embryos (PGD), to avoid disabling inherited diseases. At present, it is used only for couples attempting *in vitro* fertilization. In time, *in utero* testing may become possible, permissible, and popular.

Just entering public awareness is genetic testing for what is gently described as "paternity discrepancy," to determine whether the apparent father of a child is actually its biological father. The results, surprising to many, may foreshadow wider use of such tests.

The major instrument of familiarization, however, is likely to be pharmacogenetics. Genes influence the ability to metabolize pharmaceuticals, just as with nutrients. As a result, prescription drugs are in many cases, often in most cases, either ineffective or produce harmful side effects.[15] In theory, genetic testing could substantially reduce both waste and iatrogenesis. If such tests became routine, or indeed required, before the administration of drugs, the mass of the population would rapidly become accustomed to them in a helpful context.

Many practical obstacles lie ahead in this scenario. But considerable financial pressures are driving it forward. For health-care providers, pharmacogenetics promises to make treatments more effective, reduce drug bills, and cut the cost of treating side effects. For pharmaceutical companies, it should make their products more effective, preempt damage litigation and facilitate development of new drugs. Both sides have interests in applying pharmacogenetics widely and quickly.

None of these developments directly involves nutrigenomics. But increasing familiarity with genetic tests in various forms and perceptible benefits from their use may in time influence public acceptance of testing, including nutrigenomic testing.

In sum, it is possible that nutrigenomic tests, however imperfect, may actually be popular with consumers, whatever scientists may think and, hence, targeted foods too. The pull of demand reinforces the push of supply.

## 12.6 COMPETITIVE ATHLETES

Most of the discussion within nutrigenomics (and within this chapter, so far) has concentrated on identifying inherited susceptibility to disease, and then doing something about it. But, that is only half the potential. The other half is about promoting well-being as well as preventing disease, facilitating the good as well as preempting the bad.

That prospect is already subject to a complementary debate. In its strongest form, the issue is "human enhancement," the idea that human capabilities can be improved through a variety of means, including genetic and nutritional.[16] It is a large subject, beyond the broadest definition of nutrigenomics. For many, it seems a futuristic fantasy or nightmare, like Huxley's *Brave New World*, the fictional precursor of current concerns about "designer babies."

In fact, one form of human enhancement is an immediate prospect, possible "gene doping" of athletes at the 2008 Olympics in Beijing.

Gene doping is the thin but sharp end of a large wedge. It is introduced here to illustrate additional issues that nutrigenomics will face in future. Hence, among the stakeholders are elite athletes, as well as those who advise, coach, promote, and otherwise minister to them. More important for public health, this category also includes the much larger numbers who aspire to become leading, or at least improved, sportsmen and women, the millions who train for marathons, as well as the handful who win them. Hope is as vulnerable to exploitation as fear.

### 12.6.1 Gene Transfer: Therapy and "Doping"

Gene doping emerged as a public issue following announcement of experimental gene therapy to increase muscle bulk in elderly patients with muscular dystrophy. The researchers then reported receiving inquiries, not just from clinicians, but from coaches wanting a quick fix to build up players.[17] Gene doping is a dramatic pejorative but, as this anecdote indicates, it is really just one specific application of gene therapy and, hence, extendable; indeed, it already is being extended. Others are working on the same lines, identifying candidate genes that influence, for example, oxygen uptake, heart efficiency, fast muscle fiber responses, and blood flow. Different target tissues are appropriate for different sports. The goals include improving speed and stamina, as well as strength. The focus is "designer adults" rather than "designer babies."

In a parallel with nutrigenomics generally, many specialists feel gene transfer is at an early stage and much research is needed before it can be routinely applied. But it is widely recognized that "athletes are not so much interested in research, but outcomes. They will jump on a product or a technique or a strategy that they perceive to work, on the basis of no research at all."[18]

Prudence suggests gene doping is imminent. The World Anti-Doping Agency (WADA) has already convened two conferences on preventing it. They concluded the benefits are real and that it is feasible now. Initially, detection prospects seemed poor. Since then, at least eleven research projects have been commissioned, so WADA is now "optimistic" that it is "ahead" of potential sporting users.[19]

In practice, applications of genetics in sport, including nutrigenomics, will be introduced in stages. Initially, tests will identify individuals with the potential to become outstanding athletes. They have the capacity to improve, not only through high-tech interventions, but also with conventional training and sports diets, by "maximizing metabolic performance."

The first such test is already on the market, for variants of the ACTN3 gene, which allegedly separate sprinting sheep from long-distance goats.[20] Many more such tests will become available, with variable predictive value, but nonetheless appealing to the ambitious, and to their parents. Instead of identifying disease susceptibility, these tests indicate "performance predisposition." People are selected, not for treatment but enhancement.

Influencing gene expression is a more advanced stage. Expressing genes for IGF-I and silencing genes for myostatin are prime candidates for muscle enlargement. Pharmaceutical triggers are one route. Eventually, nutritional influences on gene expression/silencing might offer a truly invisible form of manipulation, becoming the cheating of choice: personalized nutrition for peak performance.

Simultaneously, using transcriptomics and proteomics to identify variations in gene expression is one of the most promising forms of detection for the full gene doping on the horizon.

### 12.6.2 Optimizing Nutrition

Introducing nutrigenomics into sport would extend another trend. Nutrition has long since moved beyond its original concerns with deficiency diseases and minimum daily requirements. Many now conceptualize the science as striving for "optimal nutrition," improving nutritional status in all phases of the life cycle; if not absolute well-being, at least better-being is the goal. Optimal nutrition has already been embraced by athletes: eat to compete. At a simple level, this logic is manifest in champions who foreswear fast food, dieticians advising at sports clubs, and health food shops selling the cornucopia of nutritional supplements that have become a routine part of competitive sport.

The most sophisticated example is the popular diet book, *The Zone*, which argues that human capabilities are optimized by maintaining nutrients within a narrow range, especially those influencing eicosanoids.[21] The approach was originally developed to improve the performance of a swimming team.

Adding nutrigenomics to the repertoire of sports nutrition will require new technical skills, but no leap in imagination. No imagination is needed either to envisage ethical issues that will erupt.

### 12.6.3 Ethics: Con and Pro

The heart of the matter is genetic manipulation of "human nature." This is not just about sporting prowess, but also other physical traits, including the cosmetic. Nor is it limited to the physical, but encompasses mental development, psychology, and behavior. Enhancement is not just for athletes; it could involve everyone. Improving health, the initial focus of nutrigenomics, is only part of the emerging agenda.

That prospect horrifies some, raising moral issues about life, about playing God. For others, it reopens the most notorious episode of the 20th century: "enhancement" as the acceptable face of eugenics. At its core is always some form of social selection, maybe not race, but something unpleasant. The alternative name for the process, *trans-humanism*, is even worse, with echoes of Frankenstein.

Current disputes over abortion, stem cells, and PGD prefigure the controversies ahead. These are some of the most passionately disputed social issues of the age. The debates over human enhancement will be of that intensity, and more, especially if they begin in the context of sporting nationalism.

Less familiar is the articulate affirmation of gene doping.[22] The new genetics introduces a new realism. Successful athletes have always had a genetic advantage. We used to call it "talent," now we can prove it is genes. Sports stars are "natural mutants." Manipulating genes of competitors is thus not cheating, it is actually fair play, leveling the genetic playing field. Further, if gene transfers are acceptable for the wasting elderly, why not for the promising young? If it is all right to manipulate physical capabilities, why not other talents? Why not, indeed, any traits people find desirable?

The future may include "premium enhancement" packages available to consumers to improve athletic performance. They would present parents with a moral/economic dilemma, whether to invest in their children's sporting futures. This is not scientific fantasy or commercial rip-off. It is actually one of the scenarios for 2025 being used now by the Department of Trade and Industry in the U.K. as the basis for public consultations on the ethics of science. If enhancement for sport arrives, purchasable "packages" for additional traits and talents will follow. They would put prices on the qualities people value most. They would create a market in superiority.

Ethicists will see gene transfer as raising fundamental questions about humanity. For the more worldly, it exacerbates eternal arguments about inequality. For others, this is just a new technical option for giving people what they have always wanted, but were previously unable to obtain.

Whatever the merits of arguments for and against, gene doping in popular sports would rapidly increase public familiarity with genetic testing and "beneficial" responses. In the long term, gene therapies for otherwise incurable diseases may be the more compassionate face of genetic modifications.

The point here is not to endorse any of these arguments, pro or con. It is merely to anticipate the imminent disputes, vicious but profound, about human enhancement in all its forms, including the nutrigenomic. Gene doping at the Olympics may fire the starting gun.

## 12.7 HEALTH-CARE PROVIDERS

Health-care providers everywhere, whether funded by taxation or insurance, are under financial pressure. Demand for health care is rising, and so are the costs of providing it, but budgets are not increasing proportionately. Providers respond variously, but basic strategies include cutting costs, restricting demand, and rationing provision.

One common component in cost control is transferring a proportion of bills to patients, in the form of charges, copayments, deductibles, or cost recovery schemes. A recurrent strategy for restricting demand involves limiting services to "essentials," excluding "nonessential" treatments. Dentistry is a frequent casualty. Demand is thereby transferred away from the normal provider. Patients must buy services from someone else, or go without.

### 12.7.1 Offloading Care

The radical solution, however, is to transfer treatment to the patient. It is never presented so bluntly, of course. Euphemisms abound. Patients are invited to assume more "responsibility" for their health, and to increase "engagement" in their own care. The U.K. government commissioned a banker to produce two reports on the "fully engaged patient," those who "monitor and treat their own conditions."[23,24] Programs followed to develop "self-managing patients," coping with minor illnesses and chronic conditions or, in complex cases, becoming "expert patients," and better yet "patient entrepreneurs."[25]

Patients' relationship with health-care providers is redefined as "partnership," increasing lay "involvement," to the point of "shared decision making"; shared care and costs, too. The role of the National Health Service is "empowerment, not nannying," said the British prime minister, a double-edged slash at his country's welfare state.[26]

In the market-oriented U.S., the language is different, but the goal is the same. The strategy is to "shift the incentives to people having ownership of their own health and therefore health care, as opposed to thinking some third party pays the bills."[27] In the misty past, when our proverbs were coined, sages spoke more plainly, "Patient, heal thyself." "Self-care" is the generic name for this approach. On balance, over time, it may or may not prove better for patients. But its sprouting in the 21st century has more to do with finance than therapeutics.

### 12.7.2 Personalized Nutrition as Self-Care

The relevance here is that personalized nutrition fits perfectly within the paradigm of self-care. It facilitates all three of the strategic transfers: costs, demand, and treatments. Genetic tests identify susceptibilities, for which the afflicted themselves take corrective action, changing their diets. To health-care providers, nutrigenomics offers help with both demand and supply. It can reduce demand in two ways. If effective, it prevents some diet-related diseases. If not, it deflects professional consultations into self-care.

Conventional screening programs are often viewed ambivalently by health ministers and managers. They identify formerly invisible problems, stimulating more treatments and additional costs. Nutrigenomic testing has opposite results. It shunts therapy onto patients, requiring fewer treatments and less expenditure.

Personalized nutrition also reduces costs in more fundamental ways. Appropriate remedies change from expensive drugs to cheaper foods. To reduce cholesterol, for example, take not statins, but phytosterol-fortified margarines. For hypertension, not ACE inhibitors, but weight loss. Statins and ACE inhibitors are, in many countries, two of the most commonly prescribed drugs. Even more importantly, although providers pay for much of the drugs, food is bought by consumers. This is not cost sharing, this is transferring the whole bill, passing the buck. For all these reasons, health-care providers will probably develop positive assessments of nutrigenomics.

### 12.7.3 Policy Options

This appreciation could manifest itself in different policies. Regulation, the priority for genetic skeptics, is but one of several options, and, for nutrigenomics, not the most likely. The easiest alternative is passive acceptance of commercial initiatives in testing and targeted foods, with no serious attempts at regulation. Why should the state or insurance companies control access to nutrigenomic tests? Why not "open access" for consumers? "Self-care" legitimizes laissez faire.

Alternatively, providers might actively engage with nutrigenomics, themselves offering selected tests for common or expensive diet-related diseases. Expanded clinical genetics services could cover some nutrigenomic testing and counseling. Savings could be large.

In between, benign facilitation would encourage cooperation among interested parties. For example, the U.S. Food and Drug Administration (FDA) recently reached an understanding with the pharmaceutical industry, whereby companies will share their pharmacogenetic test results with the government and in return receive "regulatory immunity." The FDA will not use the data in drug approval processes, but will gain valuable information.[28] This is co-optation rather than control.

This is an intimation of arrangements in nutrigenomics. In principle, even the limited genetic profiles produced by the initial testers would be useful for research, public health, and individual treatment. Health-care providers would value them for good diagnostic reasons as well as simple economics. Testers in turn would be keen to recover the costs of subsidized tests and to gain legitimacy amid controversy. All parties would favor an exchange, on terms and conditions to be negotiated.

### 12.7.4 Nutritional Compliance

The implications for individuals are mixed. One of the hopes of personalized nutrition is that it will increase people's motivation to eat healthily. Population dietary recommendations are widely disregarded, despite much claimed conformity. People may comply more readily with recommendations designed personally for them. So far, there is little evidence to support this scenario, but logic and anecdote make it plausible (see Chapter 13).

The policy question ahead is whether increased compliance will remain just an aspiration or become an enforceable obligation. What expectations will be placed on the individual to act on the results of nutrigenomic tests, to follow their personalized diet?

One template already exists. Parents of children with spina bifida or celiac disease are expected to control their diets strictly and, further, to train children to restrain their own intakes as they mature. Even optimists recognize that it requires "considerable effort" to enforce such regimes, which "leads to emotional stress in families," and which takes its "toll on the parents and the child."[29] However, failure to do so constitutes bad parenting, provoking interventions to protect children. These are extreme cases. But will analogous expectations gradually be applied, in some degree, to other genetically influenced dietary susceptibilities?

Already we see hints of social control. Increased insurance charges for some diet-related conditions are established, tolerated, and paid. Restrictive conditions on access to care is a further turn of the screw. For example, in the U.K., obesity drugs are reserved for the very overweight, who must also demonstrate a successful commitment to dieting.

A more sophisticated version of "conditional care" is being introduced in the U.S. "Personal responsibility" requirements are attached to publicly funded health programs for the poor.[30] Again, the logic is expressed in economic terms. It "gives people rewards and incentives to improve their health," and punishments if they do not.

Applicants must sign a pledge to attend health improvement programs, have routine screenings, keep appointments, and take medicines. If they do, they are entitled to enhanced benefits. If they refuse, or fail to keep their undertakings, they are reduced to basic services.

Such experiments are controversial and may not endure.[31,32] But the underlying logic is particularly applicable to diet-related diseases. Changing food consumption is essential for their cure, and nutrigenomic tests provide a technical basis for personalized rules about diet. Eating appropriately for your genes could become a prerequisite for care. Nutrigenomics will certainly create new norms. The issue then becomes: will compulsion be applied to ensure compliance? If so, how much?

In sum, health-care providers will probably embrace personalized nutrition. To others, pharmaceutical companies as well as patients, that may feel like a squeeze.

## 12.8 FUTURE PERSPECTIVES

There are many unresolved issues with personalized nutrition, concerning both tests and subsequent interventions. Much time and research will be needed to settle them. Scientists are right to be cautious, technically speaking. But they are lined up against other stakeholders with interests in rapid application of the developing nutrigenomics. Significantly, all have more resources to pursue their goals than scientists, and they all also have the prospect of increased revenues or substantial savings if they succeed. For them, nutrigenomics is an investment.

Food companies have the wherewithal to develop new products, to market targeted foods, to subsidize genetic tests, and to induce data sharing. Health-care providers have the purchasing power to conduct or buy in nutrigenomic testing, leading to substantial reductions in their drug bills and treatment costs. Most consumers are not rich, but their combined spending power could provide the economic base for both tests and products. These days, even elite athletes have more resources than scientists.

In the earlier sections on these four stakeholder groups, there have been two common themes. One is that their interests in nutrigenomics are all reinforcing existing trends — toward functional foods, alternative therapies, optimal nutrition, and self-care. They are swimming with the tide.

Nonetheless, second, nutrigenomics will be controversial, provoking public debates — about unproven science, exploiting the vulnerable, protecting consumers, and inadequate health services, with the grandest of them all, GM humans, just over the horizon.

Genetics has always been special — specially controversial. It began with polemics between Darwinism and religion that persist to this day, followed by the 19th century eugenics of criminality, the extensions to Social Darwinism, the 20th century eugenics of race, and the postwar emergence of sociobiology and ethology. Since the mapping of the human genome, the controversies have multiplied to include GM crops, intelligent design, genetic testing, *in vitro* fertilization, and genetic databanks, among others.

Nutrigenomics will not escape controversy. In the years ahead, there will be both scientific advance and mudslinging. It is potentially a major development, socially, economically, and politically, as well as scientifically, and for public as well as individual health. Understandably, people will feel strongly about it, one way or another.

At the end, this analysis returns where it began. It has been intentionally agnostic. It has not sought to decide who is right or what is better. It has drawn attention to policy issues that will arise, without predicting or prescribing how they might be resolved. The conclusion is not whether personalized nutrition is desirable or not, simply that it is likely to become a reality, and soon.

## KEY READINGS

Miller, P. and Wilsdon, J., *Better Humans? The politics of human enhancement and life extension*, Demos, London, 2006.

Milunsky, A., *Your Genetic Destiny: Know Your Genes, Secure Your Health, Save Your Life*, Perseus, Cambridge, 2001.

Sweeney, H.L., Gene doping, *Scientific American*, July 2004, p. 37.

U.S. Government Accountability Office, *Nutrigenetic Testing*, GA-06-977T, Washington, D.C., 2006.

Wanless, D., *Securing Our Future Health: Taking a Long-Term View*, HM Treasury, London, 2002.

## REFERENCES

1. Cited in, Pray, L.A., Dieting for the genome generation, *The Scientist*, 19, 14, 2005.
2. Astley, S., Nutrigenomics, presented at Demos Symposium, You eat what you are, London, April 20, 2005.
3. German, B., Nutritional phenotypes in the age of metabalomics, presented at NuGO Week Symposium, Pisa, September 10–13, 2005.
4. Parnell, L., The complexity of nutritional disorders presents a bioinformatic challenge to genotyping, presented at NuGo Week Symposium, Pisa, September 10–13, 2005.
5. Cited in Pray, L.A., op cit.
6. Milunsky, A., *Your Genetic Destiny: Know Your Genes, Secure Your Health, Save Your Life*, Perseus, Cambridge, 2001.
7. Gibney, M., Public communication at NuGO Week Symposium, Pisa, September 10–13, 2005.
8. Kutz, G., Nutrigenetic testing: tests purchased from four web sites mislead consumer, U.S. Government Accountability Office, GAO-06-977T, Washington, D.C. 2006.
9. Heart U.K., www.heartuk.org.uk.
10. Department of Health, *Dietary Reference Values for Food Energy and Nutrients for the United Kingdom*, HMSO, London 1991.
11. Eliot, T.S., The hollow men, in *Collected Poems 1909–1962*, Harcourt Brace Jovanovich, New York, 1991.
12. Groopman, J., The right to a trial, *The New Yorker*, December 18, 2006, p. 40.
13. Trivedi, B., Hungry genes?, *New Scientist*, 193, No. 2587, 34, 2006.
14. The true state of C.S.I. justice, *New York Times*, January 29, 2007.
15. Connor, S., Glaxo chief: our drugs do not work on most patients, *The Independent*, December 8, 2003.
16. Miller, P. and Wilsdon, J. (Eds.), *Better Humans? The politics of human enhancement and life extension*, Demos, London, 2006.
17. Sokolove, M., The lab animal, *New York Times Magazine*, January 18, 2004, p. 28.
18. Hamilton, B., Human enhancement technologies, uncorrected evidence, House of Commons Science and Technology Committee, October 25, 2006.
19. World Anti-Doping Agency, www.wada-ama.org.
20. Yang, N. et al., ACTN3 genotype is associated with human elite athletic performance, *Am J Hum Genet*, 73, 627, 2003.
21. Sears, B., *The Zone*, Regan Books, New York, 1995.
22. Miah, A., *Genetically Modified Athletes: Biomedical Ethics, Gene Doping and Sport*, Routledge, London, 2004.
23. Wanless, D. *Securing Our Future Health: Taking a Long Term View*, HM Treasury, London, 2002.
24. Wanless, D., *Securing Good Health for the Whole Population*, HM Treasury, London, 2004.
25. Cayton, H., Patients as entrepreneurs: who is in charge of change?, in Andersson, E., Tritter, J., and Wilson, R. (Eds.), *Healthy Democracy*, The National Centre for Involvement, London, 2006.

26. Donnelly, L., PM calls for empowerment instead of nannying, *Health Serv J*, 12, August 3, 2006.
27. McKinnell, H.A., cited in Berenson, A., An insider's critique of the health care system, *New York Times*, June 4, 2005.
28. Food and Drug Administration, Pharmacogenomic data submissions, final guidance, Issue 22, March 2005.
29. Milunsky, op cit.
30. Eckholm, E., Medicaid plan prods patients towards health, *New York Times*, December 1, 2006.
31. Steinbrook, R., Imposing personal responsibility for health, *New Eng J Med,* 355, 353, 2006.
32. Bishop, G. and Brodkey, A., Personal responsibility and physician responsibility: West Virginia's Medicaid plan, *New Eng J Med*, 355, 356.

# 13 The Personal Factor in Nutrition Communication

*Laura I. Bouwman, Maria A. Koelen, and Gerrit J. Hiddink*

**CONTENTS**



## 13.1 INTRODUCTION

Information that is personalized to take into account a targeted individual's characteristics and situation is more effective in influencing that person's health behavior than general information. The central factor for effectiveness is perceived personal relevance. In most theoretical models of behavior change, concepts relating to this personal factor are included, such as perceived personal risk, effectiveness of recommended actions, self-efficacy, and cost-benefit evaluation. In the field of nutrition, communication can be tailored to an individual's food-related needs, habits, preferences, and interests shaped by his or her physical and social circumstances. When the messages are also delivered in a location and at a time desired by the individual, we can speak of personalized nutrition communication. The innovative field of nutritional genomics (nutrigenomics) is expected to lead to more insights into the interaction between diet, genes, proteins and metabolites, and health. This will hopefully lead to evidence-based strategies for the development of stronger health messages that will influence both the perceived severity and effectiveness of the actions recommended in nutrition communication. Nutrigenomics aims to use genetic testing to assess "personal vulnerability" to the development of nutrition-related illnesses. Such a test could contribute to perceived personal vulnerability and to the perceived effectiveness of recommended actions, thereby influencing the perceived personal relevance of healthy eating. Next to a personalized assessment, the availability of a personalized "solution" by means of a diet, product, or nutrient that helps prevent nutrition-related diseases is a prerequisite for the concept of personalized nutrition to become integrated in health behavior change strategies.

Many causes of premature death and illness are preventable, or at least postponable, at the level of individual behavior. As individuals, if we did not smoke, exercised more, and ate less saturated fat and more fruits and vegetables, we would probably be healthier. In the last decades, a lot of effort has been put into improving dietary habits through nutrition communication. However, it has not been effective in changing the behavior of populations or individuals: in most European countries, actual consumption is not in line with basic recommendations for healthy nutrition. Although consumers know what they should be doing, diets still contain too much energy, saturated fat, sugar and salt, and insufficient vegetables, fruits, and fish. Dietary habits are important determinants of health because unhealthy eating, coupled with poor lifestyle choices, increases the risk of disease such as obesity, diabetes, cardiovascular disease, and cancer. The growing incidence of diet-related diseases accentuates the need for innovative approaches that motivate people to eat healthily [1–3]. A promising approach is personalization of nutrition communication. Reviews on health interventions [4,5] and research on the effect of personalization [6–8] have shown that information that is personalized to a targeted individual's characteristics and situation is more effective in influencing that person's health behavior than general information. Central to this chapter is perceived personal relevance, because personalized nutrition communication that is not perceived as being relevant to the individual will not induce motivation to eat healthily in the long term. We discuss how personal relevance is integrated in communication, fear arousing communication, and health behavior change theory. In most theoretical models, concepts relating to this personal factor are included, such as selective perception, perceived personal risk, effectiveness of recommended actions, and self-efficacy [9–14]. The innovative field of nutritional genomics is expected to lead to more insight into the interaction between diet, genes, protein, and metabolites, and health [15]. The possible influence of this innovation on perceived personal relevance of nutrition communication is discussed in Section 13.3. Finally, we discuss some of the issues surrounding the personalization of nutrition communication and topics for future research.

## 13.2 THE PERSONAL FACTOR IN THEORY: PERSONAL RELEVANCE

In communication, fear-arousing communication, and health behavior change theory, concepts include personal factors in several stages of the behavior change process: creating awareness, the threat appraisal, and the coping appraisal. Weinstein's *precaution adoption model* identifies a series of steps preceding the taking of preventive action, the first three of which relate to awareness [16]:

- Realize that a specific risk exists
- Acknowledge that the risk is significant and can affect people
- Recognize that one is personally vulnerable to the risk

### 13.2.1 Creating Awareness about Health Communication

Every day, we are confronted with an enormous number of messages. Nutrition information is provided through mass-media channels, on product labels, billboards, on the Internet and, in specific cases, through schools or by health professionals. It is impossible to pay attention to all of these messages: we have to be selective. People have a tendency to expose themselves to information that is consistent with their own attitudes and opinions [9]. This process is also known as *selective perception*. Attention is only given to information that is perceived as being somehow personally relevant; this means that exposure does not automatically elicit attention. However, what "personally relevant" means is not defined specifically in the literature. Batra and Ray [17] define relevant as "stronger" and providing topics that are "of interest" or "valued" by individuals. McGuire [18] describes relevant as "interesting." Personal relevance can be described as "consistent with personal attitudes and opinions." Sherif et al.'s *social judgment theory* [19] also states that people tend to accept ideas that agree with their own personal views. Messages that are not in line with their personal latitude (range) of acceptable options are ignored or dismissed. Another important factor relating to message content is the level of involvement. According to the *elaboration likelihood model* [10], the persuasive impact of a message can be central or peripheral. The key variable is involvement: the extent to which an individual is motivated and able to think about the position advocated in the message (issue-relevant thinking). When involvement is high, elaboration is also high. Elaboration involves cognitive processes such as evaluation, recall, critical judgment, and inference and occurs through the central persuasive route. Changes are stronger when induced through the central route. An issue that becomes more personally relevant to a recipient will increase his or her motivation to engage in thoughtful consideration and action [10]. Communication that contains information opposed to personal beliefs, attitudes, or opinions induces uncomfortable feelings. People tend to reduce those feelings by avoiding dissonant information. This process is known as "cognitive dissonance" [20]. A person who strongly believes that healthy food tastes bad will ignore information that aims to persuade him or her to eat healthily by saying that healthy food is tasty. Research has shown that many people have misperceptions about their personal food intake. They rate their food intake as "healthy" and therefore do not consider nutrition communication on healthy eating as being personally relevant [21–24].

### 13.2.2 Threat Appraisal in Health Communication

In between creating awareness and the behavior change process, feelings of personal risk will depend on the perceived severity of the consequences for an individual's health, and the effectiveness and costs of preventive behavior. Well-known models of preventive health behavior such as the *health belief model* [13], *theory of planned behavior* [25], and *protection motivation theory* [12] contain the concepts of perceived severity and vulnerability as influencing factors on motivation to change behavior. These models assume that people are able to adequately assess the risk to themselves associated with their behavior.

#### 13.2.2.1 Perceived Severity

In most communication about nutrition, the messages are about the consequences of unhealthy eating. The theory of planned behavior, protection motivation theory, and health belief model all rely on severity as the influencing factor for perceived personal relevance. Fear appeals are often made to spell out the severity of nutrition-related diseases such as diabetes and cardiovascular diseases, but the fact that these are outside the experience of most people may explain why the appeal is not effective. Gleicher and Petty [26] and Liberman and Chaiken [27] state that fear arousal can induce two different coping strategies: either acting as a motivator to induce intensive (and accurate) message processing or inducing defense motivation, both temporarily. Defense motivation is most likely to occur when a health threat is both severe and personally relevant because personal beliefs are being threatened. According to the *heuristic-systematic model* [27], the processing goal of defense-motivated people is to confirm the validity of a particular attitudinal position (I am eating healthily) and to disconfirm the validity of others (your eating choices place you at risk). Defense-motivated people will process information selectively in the way that best supports their own beliefs (see also: selective perception). Risk perception research has raised questions about the assumptions of most models in preventive health behavior, which is, as stated earlier, that people are able to adequately assess the risk to themselves associated with their behavior. Risk assessment is a complex process influenced by several factors that interfere with accurate assessment of personal risk. The catastrophic effect, controllability, reversibility, and whether the risk is taken on a voluntary basis or not influence risk perception and, thereby, fear arousal. For instance, perceived risks of unhealthy lifestyles (voluntary) are known to be lower than perceived risks of new technology (nonvoluntary) [28]. Thus, people tend to have misperceptions about their personal behavior, depending on the context in which the risk information is presented, the way the risk is being described, and their personal and cultural characteristics [11]. Furthermore, estimation of personal risks tends to be biased. Many people overestimate small probabilities (plane crashes) and underestimate large probabilities (heart disease). Risks that are cognitively available through personal experience or intense media coverage tend to be overestimated. This bias process is related to Tversky and Kahneman's [29] availability heuristic and refers to people's tendency to judge an event as more probable to the extent that it is more easily pictured or recalled. The lack of knowledge about the specific relationship between food intake and individual risk of disease may interfere with the perceived severity of nutrition communication and contribute to misperceptions of personal risk.

#### 13.2.2.2 Perceived Vulnerability

In protection motivation theory and the health belief model, perceived vulnerability or susceptibility refers to the subjective risk of acquiring an illness if no countermeasures are taken [30]. In combination with high perceived severity, perceived vulnerability is known to build fear and increase the personal relevance of messages. Research shows that people are quite aware of the relative risk of specific activities or behavior, but this tends to change when personal risk needs to be assessed. For instance, smokers accept the association between smoking cigarettes and disease but do not believe themselves to be personally at risk [31]. This is referred to as unrealistic optimism from Weinstein's [32] paper that focused on comparative risks in health risk perception. Van der Pligt [11] describes six causes of unrealistic optimism that can lead to perceived personal invulnerability, perceived control, egocentric bias, personal experience, stereotypical or prototypical judgment, self-esteem maintenance, and coping strategies. Risks judged to be under personal control tend to induce feelings of optimism [33]. People generally know more about their own protective behavior than about that of others, causing an egocentric bias that can generate optimism. They also tend to focus on their own risk-reducing behavior and are less aware of personal behavior that increases risk. Personal experience with a risk tends to be relatively vivid and can decrease unrealistic optimism. Stereotypical or prototypical judgment is a relatively extreme image people have of high-risk groups, which is unlikely to fit with their self-image, thereby increasing optimism. Generally, people tend to rate their own actions, lifestyle, and personality as better than that of others: this is known as self-esteem maintenance or enhancement. The last factor that influences unrealistic optimism relates to coping strategies. Conditions of high stress or threat can induce denial, thereby reducing emotional distress but also reducing the likelihood of preventive actions or their success. In general nutrition communication, vulnerability is addressed without reference to the personal factor. Recent research on the *stage model of processing of fear-arousing communications* developed by Das et al. [34] concluded that unless individuals can be persuaded of their vulnerability to health risk, they are unlikely to take protective action [35]. Through face-to-face consultation, vulnerability to nutrition-related disease can be made more personally relevant, based on assessment of the individual's lifestyle (e.g., calories), physical parameters (e.g., blood pressure), and environmental circumstances (e.g., sedentary work). As in relation to communication on severity, uncertainties about whether unhealthy eating will actually lead to illness, also known as probabilistic outcomes, interfere with the strength of the messages and, thereby, with perceived vulnerability [36].

### 13.2.3 Coping Appraisal in Health Communication

In the following section, personal factors in models of preventive health behavior that influence the coping appraisal, such as perceived effectiveness of the recommended action or response efficacy, perceived self-efficacy, and cost-benefit evaluation, are discussed.

#### 13.2.3.1 Perceived Effectiveness of the Recommended Action

The appraisal of recommended actions in terms of being effective in reducing or avoiding health risks is included in several theories. Having undertaken an extensive review, Sutton concludes that increasing communication on the efficacy of the recommended action strengthens the individual's intentions to adopt that action [37]. In protection motivation theory, motivation to engage in the recommended behavior is also codependent on the appraisal of both response efficacy and self-efficacy [12]. In the health belief model, the effectiveness of a recommended action is a function of the perceived extent to which preventive behavior will reduce the threat (perceived benefits) and the perceived negative aspects of a preventive behavior (perceived barriers) [13]. Recommendations in most nutrition messages are generic, or sometimes tailored to specific life stages such as childhood or pregnancy. Perceived effectiveness of the recommended action at the individual level can therefore be low. As during the threat appraisal, uncertainties about the effectiveness of recommended actions (or probabilistic outcomes) can interfere with perceived effectiveness of recommended actions. For instance, a healthy diet is not necessarily a safeguard against the development of cardiovascular disease [30].

#### 13.2.3.2 Perceived Self-Efficacy

In Bandura's [14] *social learning theory* (later called *cognitive learning theory*), the central concept relating to personal factors is "self-efficacy." It describes a cognitive state of taking control in which people believe they are capable of carrying out the specific behavior and can help create and control their environment in doing so. This concept of reciprocal determinism of behavior and environment is associated with concepts of self-management and self-control and is influenced by several processes, such as direct experience. It is also influenced by the storing and processing of complex information in cognitive operations that facilitate anticipation of the consequences of actions, represents goals, and weighs evidence from different sources to assess personal capabilities. This leads to a situation-specific self-appraisal that induces feelings of confidence or insecurity about behavior in new, unpredictable, or stressful situations. Self-efficacy is, then, the perception of one's own capacity to successfully organize and implement new behavior largely based on experience with similar actions and situations encountered or observed in the past, also called performance history [38]. Self-efficacy is also influenced by indirect or vicarious learning experience gained by observing others (modeling), such as a parent, teacher, or television personality who seems to enjoy a specific behavior. It is assumed that people learn more from models that are competent, attractive, likable, admired, and loved. Also, similarity to/empathy with the observer is known to influence learning [30]. Another influence on self-efficacy stemming from others is verbal persuasion. Strong persuasive messages from a respected, trusted person, such as a dietician, can have a positive influence on feelings of self-efficacy. Besides influencing behavior, self-efficacy affects thought patterns and emotional reactions, thereby inducing or reducing feelings of anxiety or coping ability. It is linked to specific skills and, by personalizing communication, attention can be paid to an individual's feelings of self-efficacy. Communication about what to eat can, for instance, be matched with an individual's level of cooking skills. Perceived behavioral control in the theory of planned behavior is closely related to self-efficacy and refers to the fact that people can have positive attitudes toward certain behavior but simply lack the resources to carry it out. In protection motivation theory, the coping appraisal will be positively influenced by response efficacy, the equivalent of effectiveness of recommended action and self-efficacy.

#### 13.2.3.3 Cost-Benefit Evaluation

The aforementioned theories on health behavior also include an evaluation of the material and immaterial costs and benefits of changing behavior in line with the recommended action. Those perceived benefits and costs are anticipated or expected, but not yet realized. The cost-benefit evaluation is integrated in both the threat appraisal (severity of health costs) and the coping appraisal (effectiveness/health benefits). At the same time, other consequences relating to physical, mental, social, and economic values will also be evaluated. Healthy meals that are not appreciated by certain members of the family can raise issues at meal times. These social "costs" of healthy eating can be perceived to be high and have a negative influence on the cost-benefit evaluation. In the theory of planned behavior, the behavioral beliefs reflect beliefs about the consequences of indulging in the behavior. Together with the evaluation of those consequences, attitudes toward certain behaviors are influenced. The perceived barriers in the health belief model refer to the perceived negative aspects of a particular recommended behavior, such as financial and social costs, and the efforts required to carry out the behavior. In protection motivation theory, these are referred to as response costs. If these costs are perceived to be too high, the personal relevance of the recommended action can be perceived as low [30]. Figure 13.1 represents important personal factors in the early stages of the behavior change process. In Table 13.1, an overview is presented of the discussed concepts. Table 13.2 provides an overview of the factors discussed relating to personal relevance and interfering concepts in stages of behavior change. Table 13.3 contains the personal factors in the discussed theory.

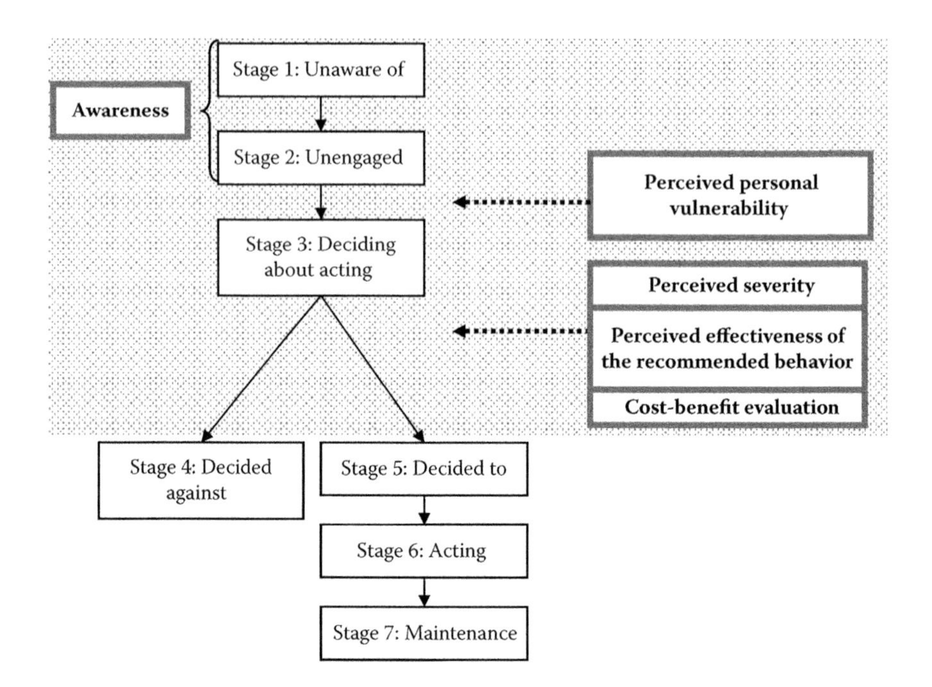


**FIGURE 13.1** Personal factors in different stages of behavior change. (From Weinstein, N.D., *Health Psychol.*, 7, 355, 1988. With permission.)

## 13.3 INFLUENCE OF INFORMATION ABOUT GENES, NUTRITION, AND HEALTH ON PERSONAL RELEVANCE

It has already been acknowledged that individual variability affects individual dietary and nutrient requirements, nutritional status, and, hence, health. Therefore, recommendations on nutrient intake vary according to age, sex, and ethnicity [39]. The relatively

**TABLE 13.1**
**Personal Factors Influencing Perceived Personal Relevance**

| Concepts | Reference |
|---|---|
| Optimistic bias/unrealistic optimism | Weinstein, 1980 |
| Selective perception | Sears and Freedman, 1971 |
| Defense motivation | Liberman and Chaiken, 1992 |
| Probabilistic outcomes | Zimbardo and Leippe, 1991 |
| Misperception/bias of personal risks | van der Pligt, 1996 |

## TABLE 13.2
## Factors Relating to Personal Relevance and Interfering Concepts in Stages of Behavior Change

| | Awareness | Threat Appraisal | Coping Appraisal |
|---|---|---|---|
| Personal relevance | Personal risk perception | Perceived severity<br>Perceived vulnerability | Perceived efficacy of the recommended action<br>Cost-benefit evaluation<br>Perceived self-efficacy |
| Interfering concepts | Selective perception<br>Cognitive dissonance<br>Optimistic bias | Defense motivation<br>Optimistic bias: unrealistic optimism | Probabilistic outcomes<br>Fatalism |

## TABLE 13.3
## Concepts Relating to Personal Factors in Discussed Theories

| Theories | Concept Related to Personal Factors | Reference |
|---|---|---|
| Heuristic-systematic model | Defense motivation | Liberman and Chaiken, 1992 |
| Social judgment/involvement theory | Involvement<br>Latitude of acceptance | Sherif, Sherif, and Nebergall, 1965 |
| Elaboration likelihood model | Involvement | Petty and Cacioppo, 1986 |
| Cognitive dissonance theory | Cognitive dissonance | Festinger, 1957 |
| Social learning theory/social cognitive theory | Self-efficacy | Bandura, 1982 |
| Theory of planned behavior | Behavioral beliefs<br>Outcome expectancy<br>Perceived behavioral control | Ajzen and Madden, 1986 |
| Protection motivation theory | Perceived severity<br>Perceived vulnerability<br>Intrinsic/extrinsic rewards<br>Response efficacy<br>Self-efficacy<br>Response costs | Rogers, 1983 |
| Health belief model | Perceived severity<br>Perceived susceptibility<br>Perceived benefits and barriers | Janz and Becker, 1984 |
| Precaution adoption model | Perceived awareness | Weinstein, 1988 |
| Stage model of processing fear-arousing communications | Perceived vulnerability<br>Perceived effectiveness of recommended actions | Das et al., 2003 |

new science of nutrigenomics examines the response of our genes, proteins, and metabolism to different foods. Nutrigenomics is expected to lead to evidence-based dietary intervention strategies for maintaining, and perhaps restoring, health and fitness and preventing diet-related disease. It is expected that, in the long term, nutrigenomic technologies will be used to determine how our body responds to foods that affect our long-term health [15]. Nutrigenomics is also targeting the assessment of personal vulnerability to the development of nutrition-related illnesses through genetic testing. Next to a personalized assessment, the availability of a personalized "solution" by means of a diet, product, or nutrient that helps to prevent nutrition-related diseases is a prerequisite for the concept of personalized nutrition to become integrated in health behavior change strategies. The assumption is that individuals will be able to use this information to reduce their risk of common diseases such as heart disease, diabetes, and obesity or to improve overall health and well-being. But not much is known yet about how individuals will actually use the information and whether it will contribute more to behavior change than the information currently supplied [40–43].

The most promising contribution to behavior change may lie in the reduction of uncertainties on a general and personal level, thereby reducing the influence of the interfering concept of probabilistic outcomes. The expected insights into the relationship between genes, nutrition, and health may provide a stronger base for designing clearer health messages about severity and effectiveness of the recommended actions. On a personal level, advice based on genetic testing can provide insight into individual vulnerability to nutrition-related illnesses and into the effectiveness of preventive strategies, thereby strengthening messages targeted at perceived personal vulnerability and perceived efficacy of recommended actions. Also, beliefs about the effectiveness of a treatment recommendation based on genotypic information could be strengthened. From research, it is known that tests offering great certainty of results (clinical validity), with available treatment and prevention options, are more readily undertaken [44]. Another potentially positive influence on perceived personal relevance is the avoidance of optimistic bias that leads to feelings of invulnerability. Uncertainties as to whether or not an individual is at risk of developing nutrition-related disease can be influenced by the results of genetic testing.

However, information on individual genetic makeup can also have undesired effects on motivation to change behavior. It is known that, when fear appeals become too strong, some people will react defensively; this leads to inaction. Also, higher susceptibility to developing nutrition-related disease can induce feelings of fatalism, thus decreasing motivation to change. Given the common perception that genetic risks are immutable, motivation to change behavior may be decreased by weakening beliefs that changing behavior will reduce risk. Perceived self-efficacy could also be negatively influenced by weakening the belief in the ability to change behavior: "It's in my genes so I can't change it."

Further research has to be undertaken to gain more insight into how people will include information on genetic makeup in the process of behavior change and whether it will either enhance or decrease motivation. In Table 13.4, an overview is presented of the possible contribution of innovations to perceived personal relevance of nutrition communication in respect of creating awareness, the threat appraisal, and the coping appraisal.

**TABLE 13.4**
**Possible Contribution of Information on Nutrition–Genes–Health to Perceived Personal Relevance of Nutrition Communication in Stages of the Behavior Process**

| | Awareness | Threat Appraisal | Coping Appraisal |
|---|---|---|---|
| Contribution of information on nutrition– genes–health | Reduce probabilistic outcomes | Strengthen severity messages<br>Strengthen effectiveness of recommended actions | |
| Contribution of genetic testing | | Increase accuracy of vulnerability assessment | Increase accuracy of recommended actions |

## 13.4 FUTURE PERSPECTIVES

The main conclusion to be drawn is that not enough is known yet about the impact of personalized nutrition interventions with respect to both reach and effect on behavior. The possible negative influence of information about the relationship between genes and health on perceived self-efficacy, as discussed in this chapter, is a point of concern. Current evidence does not suggest that providing people with DNA-derived information about risks to their health increases their motivation to change behavior beyond that achieved with nongenetic information [40,45]. In the authors' view, the question as to whether and how the inclusion of information on genes and health will influence perceived personal relevance of nutrition information, and thereby affect the motivation to eat healthily, needs to be the central focus in further research. Such insights could contribute to the development of more effective health communication. Figure 13.2 presents an amusing depiction of the dilemma faced.

The authors suggest that more effort needs to be put into understanding factors that influence personal eating style and are therefore perceived as personally relevant in nutrition communication. Eating style is an important, relatively constant characteristic that reflects individual beliefs and behavior concerning production, distribution, and consumption of food. It is often based on the notion that a certain diet offers specific individual benefits or causes harm and is constructed in the context of daily life. Research should start with exploring whether and how "genes" are currently represented in personal eating style.

A last point of discussion is the fact that personalized nutrition communication based on information from nutrigenomics will only contribute to health and well-being if end users are sufficiently motivated and enabled to follow up personalized recommendations on food intake. But the empowerment of individuals to improve their food intake depends not only on individual behavior but also on the interaction with the legal, physical, and social environment. Providing this stimulating environment in which the healthy choice is the easy choice is partly the responsibility of many: for instance, the government, for the right regulation; health professionals

I have the gene, so what can I do?
I have the gene, so I eat healthily

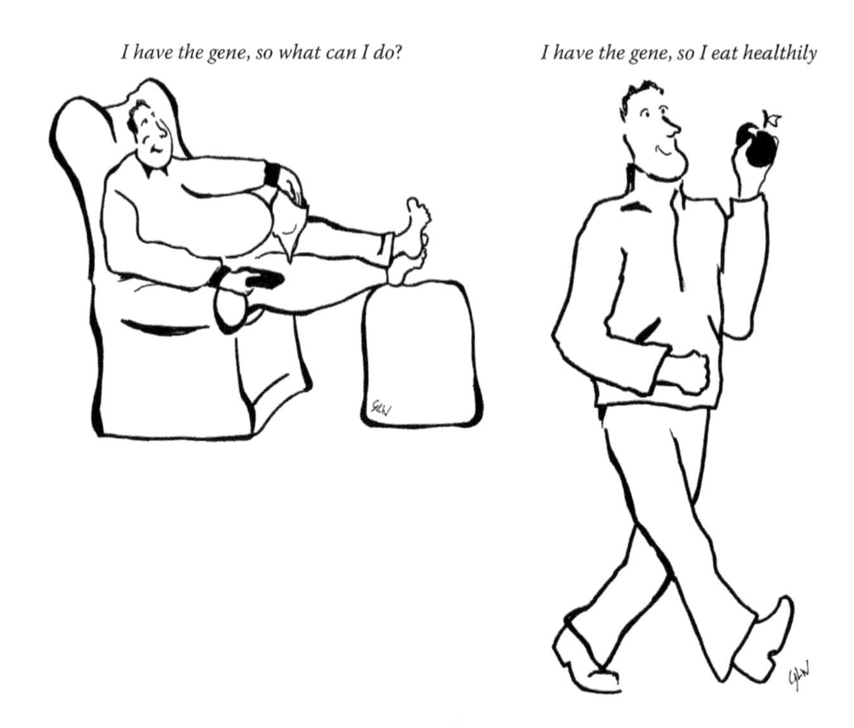

**FIGURE 13.2** What will be the effect of information on genes and health?

and education offices, for services, information, and social support; and industry, for products. Views on how nutrigenomics-based personalized nutrition communication will impact individuals and society need to be exchanged among all actors concerned to ensure its legitimate and successful introduction. As with other new technologies, personalized nutrition will entail benefits and risks and may change social structures, culture, norms, and values. These will best be addressed by the people that will be confronted with personalized nutrition in their daily life. Early involvement in the development and implementation process of innovations influences personal commitment to those innovations. The WHO also recently stated that capacity building through partnerships is an important strategy to promote health. Partnerships are important for bringing together diversity in expertise, skills, and resources for more effective health outcomes [46]. However, partnerships can only be successful if participants share visions about goals, leadership, and the necessary investment of each participant. Most often, this does not reflect reality.

A first step toward an open dialogue to create partnerships on personalized nutrition was taken at the round table discussion at the conference of the European Nutrigenomics Organisation in November 2005. The views of representatives from different scientific disciplines, industry, and government were collected about who should be involved in a dialogue and what topics should be on the agenda. Although the discussion was very lively, it was clear that its content remained scattered, leaving many topics touched upon unexplored in depth. The reactions of the participants were limited to their own specific interest, and the discussion did not elaborate further on specific topics. Further action is needed to facilitate extensive and fruitful dialogue about relevant topic such as dissemination of knowledge, practical relevance of scientific insights, and social-ethical issues such as expected high costs of applications.

## KEY READINGS

Frosch, D.L., Mello, P., and Lerman C., Behavioral consequences of testing for obesity risk, *Cancer Epidemiol. Biomarkers. Prev.*, 14(6), 1485.

Khoury, M.J., Genetics and genomics in practice: the continuum from genetic disease to genetic information in health and disease, *Genet. Med.*, 5, 261.

Lerman, C. et. al., Genetic testing: psychosocial aspects and implications, *J. Consult. Clin. Psychol.*, 70(3), 784, 2002.

WHO (2005) The Bangkok Charter for Health Promotion in a Globalized World. Available at http://www.who.int/healthpromotion.

## REFERENCES

1. Department of Health, Choosing Health: making healthy choices easier, Public Health White Paper; *Command paper CM 6374*, U.K., 2004.
2. Ministry of Health, Welfare and Sports, *Living longer in good health — also a question of a healthy lifestyle*. Dutch Ministry of Health, Welfare and Sports, The Hague, 2004.
3. World Health Organization, *The World Health Report 2002: reducing risks, promoting healthy life*, World Health Organization, Geneva, 2002.
4. Contento, I.R. et al., The effectiveness of nutrition education and implications for nutrition education policy, programs and research: a review of research, *J. Nutr. Educ.*, 27, 277, 1995.
5. Contento, I.R., Randell, J.S., and Basch, C.E., Review and analysis of evaluation measures used in nutrition education intervention research, *J. Nutr. Educ. Behav.*, 34, 2, 2002.
6. Curry, S.J. et. al., A Randomized trial of self-help materials, personalized feedback, and telephone counselling with non-volunteer smokers, *J. Consult. Clin. Psychol.*, 63(6), 1005, 2005.
7. Brug, J. et al., The impact of computer-tailored feedback on fat, fruit and vegetable intake, *Health Educ. Behav.*, 25, 517, 1998.
8. Kreuter, M.W. and Stretcher, V.J., Do tailored behaviour change messages enhance the effectiveness of health risk appraisals? Results from a randomized trial, *Health Educ. Res.*, 11, 97, 1996.
9. Sears, D.O. and Freedman J.L., Selective exposure to information: a critical review, in *The Process and Effects of Mass Communication*, Schramm, W. and Roberts, D.F., Eds., University of Illinois Press, Urbana, 1971, p. 209.
10. Petty, E.P. and Cacioppo, J.T., *Communication and Persuasion: Central and Peripheral Routes to Attitude Change*, Springer-Verlag, New York, 1986.
11. Van der Pligt, J., Risk perception and self-protective behaviour, *Eur. Psychol.*, 1(1), 34, 1996.
12. Rogers, R.W., Cognitive and psychological processes in fear appeals and attitude change: a revised theory of protection motivation, in *Social Psychology: A Source Book*, Cacioppo, J.T. and Petty, R.E., Eds., Guilford Press, New York, 1983, p. 153.

13. Janz, N. and Becker, M.H., The health belief model: a decade later, *Health Educ. Q.*, 11, 1, 1984.
14. Bandura, A., Self-efficacy mechanism in human agency, *Am. Psychol.,* 37,122, 1982.
15. Müller, M. and Kersten, S., Nutrigenomics: goals and strategies, *Nat. Rev.,* 4, 315, 2003.
16. Weinstein, N.D., The precaution adoption process, *Health Psychol.*, 7, 355, 1988.
17. Batra, R. and Ray, M.L., Advertising situations: the implications of differential involvement and accompanying affect responses, in *Information Processing Research in Advertising,* Harris, R.J., Ed., Lawrence Earlbaum Associates Publishers, London, 1983, p. 127.
18. McGuire, W.J., Attitudes and attitude change, in *Handbook of Social Psychology,* Lindzey, G. and Aronson, E., Eds., Random House, New York, 1985, p. 233.
19. Sherif, C.W., Sherif, M., and Nebergall, R.E., *Attitude and Attitude Change: The Social Judgement-Involvement Approach.* W.B. Saunders, Philadelphia, PA, 1965.
20. Festinger, L., *A Theory of Cognitive Dissonance.* Stanford University Press, Stanford, CA,1957.
21. Brug, J., Hospers, H., and Kok, G.J., Differences in psychosocial factors and fat consumption between stages of change for fat reduction, *Psychol. Health,* 12, 719, 1997.
22. Brug, J. et al., Self-rated dietary fat intake: association with objective assessment of fat, psychosocial factors and intention to change, *J. Nutr. Educ.,* 26, 218, 1994.
23. Glanz, K., Brug, J., and Van Assema, P., Are awareness of dietary fat intake and actual fat consumption associated? A Dutch-American comparison, *Eur. J. Clin. Nutr.*, 51, 542, 1997.
24. Lechner, L., Brug, J., and De Vries, H., Misconceptions of fruit and vegetable consumption: differences between objective and subjective estimation of intake, *J. Nutr. Educ.*, 29, 313, 1997.
25. Ajzen, I. and Madden, T.J., Prediction of goal directed behaviour: attitudes, intentions and perceived behavioural control, *J. Exp. Soc. Psychol.,* 22, 453, 1986.
26. Gleicher, F. and Petty, R.E., Expectations of reassurance influence the nature of fear-stimulated attitude change, *J. Exp. Soc. Psychol.*, 28, 86, 1992.
27. Liberman, A. and Chaiken, S., Defensive processing of personally relevant health messages, *Pers. Soc. Psychol. Bull.,* 18, 669, 1992.
28. Koelen, M.A. and Lyklema, S., (in Dutch) De consument en perceptie van voedselveiligheid, in *Ons Eten Gemeten.* van Kreijl, C.F. and Knaap, A.G.A.C., Eds., Bohn, Stafleu, Van Loghum, RIVM, Bilthoven, the Netherlands, 2004, chap. 8.
29. Tversky, A. and Kahneman, D., Judgement under uncertainty: heuristics and biases, *Science,* 185, 1127, 1974.
30. Koelen, M.A. and Van den Ban, A., *Health Education and Health Promotion,* Wageningen Academic Publishers, Wageningen, the Netherlands, 2004.
31. Pechacek, T. and Danaher, B., How and why people quit smoking: a cognitive-behavioural analyses, in *Cognitive Behavioural Intervention: Theory, Research and Procedures,* Kendall, P. and Hollon, S., Eds., Academic Press, New York, 1979, p. 389.
32. Weinstein, N.D., Unrealistic optimism about future life events, *J. Pers. Soc. Psychol.*, 39, 806, 1980.
33. Otten, W. and Van der Pligt, J., Risk and behaviour: the mediating role of risk appraisal, *Acta Psychol.,* 80, 325, 1992.
34. Das, E.H.H.J., de Wit, J.B.F., and Stroebe, W., Fear appeals motivate acceptance of action recommendations: evidence for a positive bias in the processing of persuasive messages, *PSPB*, 29, 650, 2003.
35. De Hoog, N., Stroebe, W., and de Wit, J.B.F., The impact of fear appeals on processing and acceptance of action recommendations, *PSPB*, 31(1), 24, 2005.

36. Zimbardo, P.G. and Leippe, M.R., *The Psychology of Attitude Change and Social Influence*, McGraw-Hill, Boston, MA, 1991.
37. Sutton, S.R., Fear arousing communications: a critical examination of theory and research, in *Social Psychology and Behavioural Medicine,* Eiser, J.R., Ed., John Wiley & Sons, Chichester, 1982, chap. 13.
38. Green, L.W. and Kreuter, M.W., *Health Program Planning: An Educational and Ecological Approach,* 4th ed., McGraw-Hill, New York, 2005.
39. Darnton-Hill, I.I., Margetts, B., and Deckelbaum, R., Public health nutrition and genetics: implications for nutrition policy and promotion, *Proc. Nutr. Soc.,* 63, 173, 2004.
40. Marteau, T.M. and Lerman C., Genetic risk and behavioural change, *BMJ*, 322, 1056, 2001.
41. Haga, S.B., Khoury, M.J., and Burke, W., Genomic profiling to promote a healthy lifestyle: not ready for prime time yet, Commentary, *Nat. Genet.*, 34(4), 347, 2003.
42. McCain, M. and Schmid, G., *From Nutrigenomics Science to Personalized Nutrition: the market in 2010.* Institute for the Future, Silicon Valley, California, 2003.
43. Massoud, M. et al., *The Future of Nutrition: Consumers Engage with Science,* Institute for the Future, Silicon Valley, California, 2001.
44. Marteau, T.M. and Croyle, R.T., The new genetics: psychological responses to genetic testing, *BMJ*, 316, 693, 1998.
45. Lerman, C. et. al., Genetic testing: psychosocial aspects and implications, *J. Consult. Clin. Psychol.*, 70(3), 784, 2002.
46. World Health Organisation, *The Bangkok Charter for Health Promotion in a Globalized World,* Available at http://www.who.int/healthpromotion, 2005, accessed June 2006.

# 14 A Marketing and Consumer Behavior Perspective on Personalized Nutrition

*Hans C.M. van Trijp and Amber Ronteltap*

## CONTENTS



## 14.1 INTRODUCTION

Adjusting marketing offerings to the identified needs and wants of consumers is at the heart of the marketing philosophy (e.g., Kotler and Keller, 2006). Essentially, marketing aims to achieve an exchange of values for the mutual benefit of both the customer and the supplier. What the customer receives in terms of need satisfaction from products or services and gives in terms of monetary and nonmonetary sacrifices to obtain the product is the mirror image of what the supply chain provides in terms of products and services, and receives in terms of money to satisfy its financial objectives of the value exchange. This process benefits both parties: the customer benefits from superior need satisfaction through consumption, whereas the supplier's benefits are financial means for growth and business continuity. When there are many customers and multiple suppliers, the processes of segmenting, targeting, and positioning become crucial. In other words, companies attempt to understand heterogeneity in consumer preferences, identify promising market segments, and position their marketing offerings (products and services) for maximum benefit. In strategic marketing, this is known as the STP process: segmenting, targeting, and positioning.

Historically, how this adjustment of marketing offerings to consumer needs has been achieved has depended largely on the market situation and the relative power of consumers and suppliers in the market economy. In the early days, many of the products were — literally — tailor-made. The industrial revolution changed the situation considerably. Economies of scale became a fact, and it became possible to produce products economically on a large scale. The key concerns were efficiency and the price of products, and the degree of personalization is probably best exemplified by Henry Ford, who in the 1920s stated that: "Any customer can have a car painted any color that he wants so long as it is black." Later, when markets became more abundant, supply more differentiated, and consumers exhibited greater purchasing power and more sophisticated articulation of their needs, market segmentation and product positioning became more crucial in the marketing process. Companies began to produce and market differentiated products targeted at identified market segments.

In the late 20th century this process reached a new level (Sheth, Sisodia, and Sharma, 2000; Wind and Rangaswamy, 2001; Pine and Gilmore, 1999). Companies now realize that the crucial objective of marketing strategy is customer value, that demand is heterogeneous and fragmented, that consumer segments are diminishing in size, and that the crucial element in competitiveness and marketing success has become the fit with the individual consumer. The variety of product and service is important, but as Pine, Peppers, and Rogers (1995: 103) state: "Customers, whether consumers or businesses, do not want more choices. They want exactly what they want — when, where and how they want it — and technology now makes it possible for companies to give it to them." A key concept in this trend is personalization. Personalization is about "building consumer loyalty by building a meaningful one-to-one relationship; by understanding the needs of each individual and helping satisfy a goal that efficiently and knowledgeably addresses each individual's needs in a given context" (Riecken, 2000: 27). So, personalization is about reducing the information gap between consumers and the supply chain (information asymmetry) beyond the level of traditional segmentation. It implies a degree of interactivity between supply chains and consumers, such that information about the consumer becomes available in an actionable format and that the fit of marketing offerings with those needs becomes more explicit. Personalization is central to the firm's customer relationship management (CRM) and to customer involvement, such as through consumer intimacy strategy (e.g., Treacy and Wiersema, 1993).

Personalization has pervaded many different fields, most prominently that of digital products and services, where it is relatively easy to obtain and analyze consumer input interactively and adjust the marketing offerings accordingly. The field of nutrition, too, is becoming increasingly affected by personalization, both in terms of information provision and in terms of products tailored on the basis of consumer information (e.g., Bouwman et al., 2005; Brug, Oenema, and Campbell, 2003; Brug, Campbell, and van Assema, 1999). The recent advances in nutrigenomics have given extra impetus to the field of personalized nutrition. The Institute of the Future defines personalized nutrition as "the application by individuals of their knowledge of nutrigenomics to their everyday decisions about nutrition" (Cain and Schmid, 2003: 2). However, we believe that personalization goes beyond the field of genetics and includes other information related to personal preferences as well, such as perceived state of health, tastes, values, and other relevant segmentation variables.

Personalization in the field of human nutrition provides great potential to all stakeholders, including the consumer, the firm, and those concerned with public health. The process of personalization provides consumers with the opportunity to find an offer that is better tailored to their specific needs. This might be in the form of nutritional information, personal advice, and even customized food products. In this way, personalization may also help consumers to reduce their search and evaluation costs in product choice behavior. For the firm, personalization may help to distinguish it from competitors, build customer relationships, and increase customer loyalty. If well executed and substantiated in nutritional science, personalized nutrition may contribute to the improvement of public health. However, there are benefits and costs associated with personalization — both to the individual consumer and to the company.

In this chapter we will address personalization from a consumer and marketing perspective. First, we will delineate the definition of personalization and distinguish it from customization. Then, we will review process models of the personalization process and use these models to identify and discuss the costs and benefits involved in personalization. Next, we will focus on consumer evaluation of personalization, before we turn to the operational dimensions of personalized nutrition. Lastly, we will discuss critical success factors from a marketing perspective, turn to conclusions, and look at the outlook for personalized nutrition.

## 14.2 PERSONALIZATION AND CUSTOMIZATION

Although personalization has quite a long history, particularly in the area of Information and Communication Technology (ICT), there is still a lack of consensus about its definition (Vesanen and Raulas, 2006). Also, personalization has been approached from many different perspectives (Riecken, 2000). Table 14.1 provides an overview of various definitions of personalization as they appear in literature. Some definitions focus on personalization as a capability of the company, whereas others (e.g., Peppers and Rogers at www.1to1.com; Riecken, 2000) define it in terms of its implementation in marketing execution. However, the majority of the definitions define personalization as the process of adjusting the marketing offerings (products, services, or information) to the identified needs of customers. Several key elements can be identified from the variety of definitions (Adomivicius and Tuzhilin, 2005).

Personalization involves the following:

1. Tailoring certain offerings, such as information (e.g., Web pages), services, personalized product and service recommendations (e.g., books, CDs, and vacations), and E-commerce interactions
2. Made available by a certain provider, such as E-commerce Web sites, or a food company

**TABLE 14.1**
**Definitions of Personalization**

| Reference | Definition |
|---|---|
| Peppers and Rogers (www.1to1.com) | One-to-one marketing based on the idea of an enterprise knowing its customer. Through interactions with a customer, the enterprise can learn how a customer wants to be treated and can then treat that customer differently from other customers. |
| Hagen (1999) | The ability to provide content and services tailored to individuals based on knowledge about their preferences and behavior. |
| Personalization consortium (2005) | The use of technology and consumer information to tailor electronic commerce interactions between a business and each individual customer. Using information either previously obtained or provided in real time about the customer, the exchange between the parties is altered to fit that customer's stated needs, as well as the need perceived by the business based on the available customer information. |
| Dyche (2002) | The capacity to customize customer communication based on knowledge preferences and behaviors at the time of interaction with the customer. |
| Peppers and Rogers (1997) | The process of using a customer's information to deliver a targeted solution to that consumer is known as personalization or one-to-one marketing. |
| Riecken (2000) | Personalization is about building customer loyalty by building a meaningful one-to-one relationship; by understanding the needs of each individual and helping satisfy a goal that efficiently and knowledgeably addresses each individual's needs in a given context. |
| Hanson (2000) | A specialized form of product differentiation in which a solution is tailored to a specific individual. |
| Peppers, Rogers, and Dorf (1999) | Customizing some feature of a product or service so that the customer enjoys more convenience, lower cost, and some other benefit. |
| Allen, et al. (2001) | Company-driven individualization of customer Web experience. |
| Imhoff, Loftis, and Geiger (2001) | Personalization is the ability of a company to recognize and treat its customers as individuals through personal messaging, targeted banner ads, special offers on bills, or other personal transactions. |
| Wind and Rangaswamy (2001) | Personalization can be initiated by the customer (i.e., customizing the look and contents of a Web site) or by the firm (i.e., individualized offering, greeting customer by name). |
| Coner (2003) | Personalization is performed by the company and is based on a match of categorized content to profiled users. |
| Roberts (2003) | The process of preparing and individualizing communication for a specific person based on stated or implied preferences. |
| Riemer and Totz (2003) | To match one object's nature to one subject's needs. More precisely: to customize products, services, content, communication, etc., to the needs of single consumers or customer groups. |
| Bonnett (2001) | Personalization involves a process of gathering user information during interaction with the user, which is then used to provide appropriate assistance or services, tailor-made to the user's needs. |

*Source:* Adapted from Vesanen, J. and Raulas, M., *Journal of Interactive Marketing*, 20(1), 5–20, 2006 and Adomavicius, G. and Tuzhilin, A., *Communications of the ACM*, 48(10), 83–90, 2005.

3. To the needs of their customers, such as consumers or Web site clientele
4. Based on knowledge about those customers, which may be explicit or implicit knowledge, preferences, or behaviors
5. Through an iterative process in which the customer often directly or indirectly acts as codesigner
6. With certain profit goals in mind, which can be simple (improving browsing and shopping experience, such as by presenting only content relevant to the consumer) to much more complex (e.g., building long-term relationships with the customer)

Personalization thus requires knowledge about the consumer and his or her specific needs, and adjusting offerings to fit those needs. Some offerings, such as services (which are by nature often developed in interaction with the consumer) and information can be adjusted to consumer needs relatively easily. However, adjusting physical products to individual consumer needs entails substantially increasing the complexity of the supply chain, with potential additional costs as a consequence. This is the field of customization.

Sometimes referred to as "product personalization" (Riemer and Totz, 2003), mass customization is the field of research that focuses on using flexible manufacturing processes to customize physical products to the needs and preferences of consumers with mass production (or near mass production) efficiency (Piller and Müller, 2004). Personalization and mass customization are different but closely related terms. Wind and Rangaswamy (2001) differentiate between the two terms, arguing that personalization is the process located on the consumer side of the marketing spectrum, whereas mass customization is the process on the operational product side. Much of the mass customization literature originates from the literature on flexible manufacturing. In customization, consumers can alter or even create products that contain precisely those attributes that the individual consumer specifies (Godek, 2002). In other words, the marketing offerings are being adjusted by, or for, the user very close to the moment of purchase or consumption. An example would be companies such as Dell and Gateway, which have adopted flexible and responsive manufacturing systems that create products to meet the needs of individual consumers upon their request (Pine, 1993). In contrast, personalization does not presuppose on-the-spot personalized production. Usually based on directly elicited or indirectly inferred consumer preferences, the firm recommends those products from an existing range that provides the best fit with those preferences (Godek, Yates, and Yoon, 2002). An example of personalization would be Amazon.com, which recommends alternatives on the basis of consumer-expressed preferences ("customers who bought this item also bought … "). In conclusion, customization goes one step beyond personalization, in that the customer is an active codesigner of the product (Bonnett, 2001). Mass customization in the context of nutrition involves a large number of complex supply chain issues that are beyond the scope of this chapter. We will only discuss its important implications for the marketing of personalized nutrition (see Section 14.7).

Personalization implies an interaction between the customer and the supply chain. Simonson (2005) discusses this interactive process and emphasizes that customer satisfaction is not only enhanced through delivering products with superior fit to the customer's individual preferences, but also that through self-assessment, the interactive process itself can help shape the customer preferences, particularly when customers do not yet have stable preferences. In this way, personalization may be a means to offer customers what they want, often even before they know that they want it (i.e., latent needs). Others (Fotheringham and Owen, 2000) have argued that although interaction is important, personalization is not restricted to synchronous interaction. Personalization may be based on previously collected consumer information. Also, personalization issues are dominant in — but not restricted to — online interactions (Murthi and Sarkar, 2004) but can be realized at all user interfaces (Riecken, 2000).

## 14.3 PROCESS MODELS FOR PERSONALIZATION

In the personalization literature (see Table 14.2), process models have been proposed that describe personalization as a number of consecutive and interlinked steps (Vesanen and Raulas, 2006). These models differ, depending on the specific fields they originate from, and tend to be biased toward the marketing side rather than the consumer evaluation side of the personalization process. Several authors

**TABLE 14.2**
**Several Proposed Process Models for Personalization**

| Adomavicius and Tuzhilin (2005) | Murthi and Sarkar (2003) | Pierrakos et al. (2003) | Vesanen and Raulas (2006) |
|---|---|---|---|
| Understanding the consumer<br>Collecting data<br>Creating consumer profiles | Learning about consumer preferences | Collecting data | Customer<br>*Interactions*<br>Customer data |
| Delivering personalized offering<br>Matching<br>Delivery and presentation | Matching offerings to customers | Preprocessing data<br>Discovering patterns<br>Postprocessing knowledge<br>Personalization | *Processing*<br>Consumer profile<br>*Customization*<br>Marketing output<br>*Delivery* |
| Measuring impact of personalization<br>Adjusting personalization strategy | Evaluating the learning and matching processes | | Customer<br>*Interaction* |
| | | Reports | Customer data<br>*Processing*<br>Customer profile |

*Source:* Summarized in Vesanen, J. and Raulas, M., *Journal of Interactive Marketing*, 20(1), 5–20, 2006. With permission.

(Steckel et al., 2005; Piller, 2005) have argued for more research on consumer evaluation, as successful personalization depends on an enduring learning relationship between the customer and the firm. Hence, the existing process models as included in Table 14.2 should be conceived of as cycles rather than linear processes, with their success depending on the ability to generate repeated interaction with the customer.

Process models by Murthi and Sarkar (2003) and Adomavivius and Tuzhilin (2005) separate the personalization process into three stages: (1) understanding and learning about customers' preferences, (2) delivering personalized offerings to customers, and (3) evaluating the learning and matching process. Pierrakos et al. (2003) describe the personalization process as having four basic features, namely: (1) the two-way nature of the communication system, (2) the level of response control that each party has in the communication process, (3) the personalization in the communication process, and (4) the use and involvement of database technology. However, the specific tasks they distinguish in the personalization process again relate to the understanding (data collection), personalization (data preprocessing, pattern discovery, knowledge postprocessing), and evaluation (reports) substages.

Vesanen and Raulas (2006) synthesize these process models by distinguishing between four *objects* (customer, customer data, customer profile, and marketing output) and four *operations* (interactions, processing of information, customization, and delivery) as the key variables that together define the marketing process with individual consumers.

The Vesanen and Raulas (2006) model defines the personalization process as a loop, with the customer as the starting point. Through interactions with a customer, relevant data are collected, such as expressed preferences (e.g., through questionnaires), Web site/purchasing behavior, or other more objective measurements such as blood parameters and genetic typing. This customer information is processed into relevant customer profiles that serve as a basis for the differentiation and segmentation of customers. Sophisticated techniques such as data mining and neural networks are increasingly being used for this purpose. The customer profiles are used to generate personalized marketing output, such as tailored communication material, personal advice, or personalized products. The delivery stage describes how (e.g., through which channel) the personalized marketing offerings reach the customer and will bring about a response from the customer as a new interaction, resulting in new customer data. This closes the loop in the Vesanen and Raulas (2006) model, as this new customer information will be processed into customer profiles as a new input into the customization process.

At a more general level, the proposed stages can be classified in terms of three responsibility domains: (1) consumer, (2) consumer–firm interaction, and (3) firm. The consumer domain refers to those stages that involve consumer actions, whereas the consumer–firm interaction domain comprises the processes by which the supply chain and the consumer interact through various interfaces. Finally, the firm domain includes the value-creation process undertaken by the supply chain on the basis of the consumer's personal information.

Ronteltap et al. (2006) have developed a process model specifically for the area of personalized nutrition, which defines specific stages in each of the three responsibility domains within the personalization process: the consumer, the interaction,

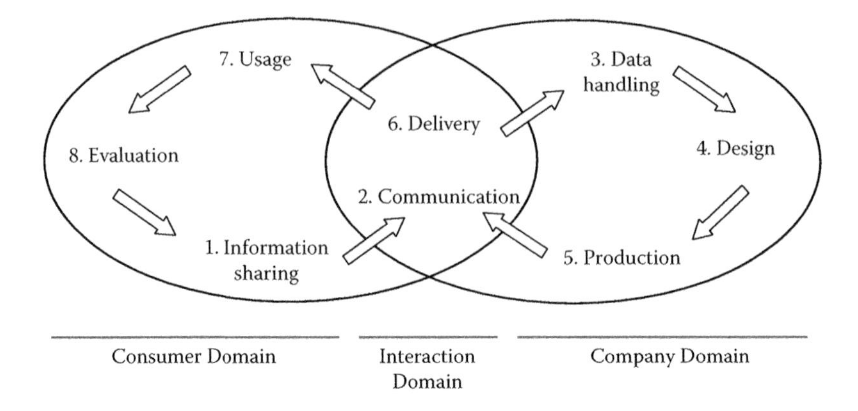


**FIGURE 14.1** The structure of a personalized recommendation system.

and the firm. The model (see Figure 14.1) describes the personalization process in eight different stages (see also Steckel et al., 2005; Wendel et al., 2006). During the first stage of the exchange process, consumers make available certain personal, and possibly sensitive, information (e.g., current health condition) to the supply chain (*stage one: information sharing*). In the next stage, this information passes through a physical interface (e.g., service desk), a digital interface (e.g., electronic questionnaires), or a combination (*stage two: communication*). *Stage three* of the exchange process (*data handling*) pertains to the receiver of the information (i.e., the supply chain) that will transform the personal information into a personalized solution on the basis of a decision model (*stage four: design*). Subsequently, the supply chain will create or select personalized recommendations (information or lifestyle or product advice) that address the needs of a particular client (*stage five: production*). In *stage six* (*delivery*), this personalized advice, involving different types of information possibly combined with products or services, is communicated and distributed via a user interface (e.g., e-mail) and received by the consumer. After acting upon the recommendation (*stage seven: usage*), the consumer may evaluate the added value of the recommendations and assess any personal benefit obtained from the interaction (*stage eight: evaluation*). This evaluation will then serve as input to the next cycle and the decision about whether or not to repeat the interaction.

By emphasizing the three domains, the model illustrates the joint responsibility of the consumer and the firm in establishing the personalized interaction. Whether such interactions occur depends largely on the perceived costs and benefits from the personalization process, which we will review next. In Section 14.5 and Section 14.6 we will specifically focus on the consumer evaluation of personalized nutrition.

## 14.4 COSTS AND BENEFITS INVOLVED IN PERSONALIZATION

To assess the marketing feasibility of personalization requires an analysis of the perceived costs and benefits for the actors in the personalization process. Some authors (e.g., Piller and Müller, 2004) argue that from a marketing perspective, the consumer decision to engage in the personalized advice process (on nutrition or another matter) is basically the result of a simple equation: "if the (expected) returns exceed the (expected) costs, the likelihood that customers will engage in this option will increase." The decision of suppliers to provide personalized advice follows the same logic: only if the expected returns exceed the expected cost will the firm offer personalized advice. The costs to the company are the costs of collecting personalized consumer information and differentiation (e.g., delivering personalized advice and the costs of resources required to do so). The returns are the price premium that can be charged for individualized options, the relationship and customer loyalty that individualization may build, and the enhancement of corporate or brand image. The key question is how to define the costs and returns at the consumer level. Although the firm's costs and benefits can be expressed in monetary units, the consumer value is more complex and involves psychological and ethical factors, too (Karat et al., 2003). At the consumer level, costs and benefits are usually (e.g., Piller and Müller, 2004; Simonson, 2005; Karat et al., 2003) differentiated into those emerging from the outcomes of the personalization process and those emerging from the interactive process itself.

### 14.4.1 Consumer Costs and Benefits at the Outcome Level

Consumer benefits of personalized offerings arise from the increased utility of products and services that better fit personal needs compared to the best standard option attainable. In terms of personalized nutrition, the benefits would be represented by the added contribution to personal health and the simplification of the choice process. Provided that the information is simple and trustworthy, personalized advice can reduce confusion and the costs of sifting through the amount of nutrition information available.

The costs factor would constitute the costs of what the consumer would have to compromise in terms of taste and convenience value and the price premium the consumer would have to pay for personalized offerings compared to standard offerings (Piller and Muller, 2004).

### 14.4.2 Consumer Costs and Benefits at the Interactive Process Level

Consumer costs and benefits at the interactive process level are much more diverse and are often psychological rather than economic in nature. Consumers may derive value from codesigning the marketing offerings (Piller and Muller, 2004), i.e., being totally immersed in the interaction process itself (Csikszentmihalyi, 1990), successfully fulfilling the codesign task (Dellaert and Stremersch, 2005; Franke and Piller, 2004), and appreciating the presentation format or context (Simonson, 2005). Consumers may also experience symbolic benefits from the process of codesign, such as pride of authorship, sheer enjoyment, and a sense of creativity in task accomplishment (Piller, 2005). The interactive process itself can help consumers construct their preferences, adding to a sense of self-knowledge (Simonson, 2005). Further, personalization in nutritional advice can facilitate the empowerment of the individual consumer (e.g., Bouwman et al., 2005) in terms of access to information, improved decision making, and ultimately to "exercise control over genetic destiny" (Chadwick, 2004).

However, the interactive process also involves perceived costs on the part of the consumer. These costs primarily constitute the cost of disclosing personal information (Karat et al., 2003); here, privacy issues become pertinent. This is particularly problematic in the case of genetic information, as the information is hard-wired and stable over time, may be relevant to many different parties (e.g., insurance companies), and it is uncertain what applications the information may yield in the future (Chadwick, 2004). As a result, consumers may be reluctant to accede to their genetic information being stored, as in future it may be used against them (Chadwick, 2004; Economist, 2005). As a psychological cost, consumers may experience a lack of freedom and may feel that marketers are trespassing on their personal preferences; or they may interpret personalization as attempts to persuade and manipulate (Simonson, 2005). Also, the active involvement in the codesign task may result in the consumer feeling psychologically at a disadvantage, because the manufacturer possesses much more information. The consumer has few options available, other than trusting that the manufacturer will propose the best personalized option.

### 14.4.3 Value to the Company

Value to the company can be expressed in terms of the costs and benefits associated with the gathering of personal information from customers and the costs and benefits obtained from marketing personal solutions (Karat et al., 2003). Piller and Müller (2004) distinguish between the differentiation, cost, and relationship aspects of personalization. Offering products and services tailored exactly to the customer's needs gives the firm a competitive advantage, takes the offerings out of the commodity offerings, and, if recognized by customers, may generate consumer preference for these differentiated offerings. The cost aspect of personalization depends on the extra costs the firm incurs in the production and marketing of personalized solutions in relation to the price premium that can be charged for the personalized offerings. The relationship aspect of personalization and customization arises from a customer bonding with the company and the increase in customer loyalty arising from that (Simonson, 2005). Importantly also, this enduring learning relationship with the customer may result in specific information that is often hard to capture by conventional methods of market research. Building on this "difficult to obtain" information may in turn deter competitors.

Riemer and Totz (2003) elaborate on the company's economic motivation of personalization in relation to customer retention, which may be the result of the consumer's technological (e.g., incompatibility of technological systems), contractual (contract periods), or psychological obligations (e.g., brand preferences caused by satisfaction) to the company. Each of these obligations constitutes a so-called "lock-in" effect, caused by switching costs, which — from a customer perspective — are defined as any cost associated with the migration to a new supplier, vendor, or service provider. The costs of switching customer relationships can be subdivided into direct switching costs, opportunity costs, and sunk costs. Consumers experience direct switching costs because they find it more difficult to compare personalized products from rival companies and because personalized products increase their emotional obligations to the firm. Once a customer has entered into a relationship on the basis of personalized information, he or she is confronted with direct switching costs, and with opportunity costs associated with the probability of losing the advantageous effects of the current relationships. Finally, sunk costs (although economically irrelevant) associated with consumers' irreversible prior investments in establishing the current relationship are likely to reduce consumers' willingness to invest in a new relationship (Riemer and Totz, 2003). As a result, successful personalized relationships based on trust in the supplier "might drive customer satisfaction, trust and investment and increase switching costs — preventing customers from defecting" (Riemer and Totz, 2003: 38–39).

## 14.5 CONSUMER EVALUATION OF PERSONALIZATION

As identified earlier, an area less well understood (Steckel et al., 2005; Piller, 2005; Piller and Müller, 2004) is how consumers evaluate and choose consumer–firm interaction mechanisms as complex as those in personalized nutrition. Two fields of research that may be informative here are the technology acceptance model (e.g., Davis, Bagozzi, and Warshaw, 1989) and the self-service technology acceptance model (e.g., Dabholkar and Bagozzi, 2002), both building on Rogers' seminal work on the adoption and diffusion of technological innovations. Rogers' (2003) diffusion of innovations theory states that the speed of adoption of innovations can be partly explained by consumer characteristics (such as innovativeness) and the perceived characteristics of the innovation: (1) relative advantage to the user, (2) compatibility with existing habits and values, (3) perceived complexity of the innovation, (4) ability to try out the innovation on a small scale, and (5) the visibility of results of applying the innovation. Rogers' theory has enjoyed wide application in the marketing and innovation literature. In a meta-analysis of applications, Tornatzky and Klein (1982) show that three of the perceived innovation characteristics (relative advantage, complexity, and compatibility) are indeed consistently related to adoption (see also Meuter et al., 2005). The research tradition on consumer adoption of information technology in the working place has subsequently emphasized the so-called Technology Acceptance Model (Davis, 1989; Venkatesh, Morris, Davis, and Davis, 2003), which posits that ease of use and perceived usefulness are the key determinants of adoption of information technology. The model has also been applied in consumer adoption of self-services in the supermarket environment (e.g., Dabholkar and Bagozzi, 2002), where it has been shown that perceived enjoyment in using the system adds to predictive validity of the adoption models over and above ease of use and usefulness.

In a first systematic study on consumer evaluation of personalized nutrition systems, Wendel et al. (2006) extended the Technology Acceptance Model with consumer perceptions of privacy or safety (see Figure 14.1). They showed that usefulness, enjoyment, and privacy protection are the key perceived benefits on which consumers base their evaluation of personalized recommendation systems, together accounting for 80% of the variance in consumer preferences. They also show that these perceptions of benefits almost completely mediate the effects of personalized nutrition features on consumer preferences. It thus seems that variants of the Technology Acceptance Model are useful for understanding consumer evaluations of personalized nutrition, with usefulness, enjoyment, and privacy protection as key benefits.

## 14.6 OPERATIONAL DIMENSIONS OF PERSONALIZED NUTRITION

To our knowledge, no studies to date have elicited consumer responses to different operationalizations of the personalized nutrition process. In this section we will summarize the results from two working papers (Wendel et al., 2006; Ronteltap and Van Trijp, 2007) on this issue. Both studies are empirical tests of the model shown in Figure 14.1. In both studies, each stage of the model was operationalized at three levels (see Table 14.3). Based on these levels, systematically varied scenarios were

**TABLE 14.3**
**Factors and Factor Levels Applied in the Scenario-Rating Tasks**

| Factors and Factor Levels |
|---|
| 1. Information sharing |
| a. Blood composition |
| b. DNA/genetic makeup |
| c. Food consumption habits |
| 2. Communication |
| a. Through fitness club |
| b. Through hospital |
| c. Through family practitioner |
| 3. Data handling |
| a. Fully anonymous |
| b. Patient and family practitioner |
| c. Available to commercial food company |
| 4. Design |
| a. Commercial company |
| b. Insurance company |
| c. Government nutrition center |
| 5. Production |
| a. At ingredient level |
| b. Food product groups |
| c. Special branded products |
| 6. Delivery |
| a. Through e-mail |
| b. Through fitness club |
| c. Through family practitioner |
| 7. Usage |
| a. Within existing meal patterns |
| b. Add special products to diet |
| c. Prepare own adjusted meals |
| 8. Evaluation |
| a. No feedback for verification |
| b. Feedback for verification optional |
| c. Feedback for verification mandatory |

**Box 14.1 Consumers' Evaluation of Alternative Operationalizations of Personalized Nutrition**

You go to your *family practitioner* [fitness club] to deliver *information on your food habits* [DNA information].

The personal information you provide will be to *known only to you and your family practitioner* [shared with commercial companies].

On the basis of your personal information, the *Nutrition Center* [an insurance company] will compile personalized nutritional advice, which you will receive *through your family practitioner* [fitness club].

The personalized nutritional advice is in the form of *product groups* [branded food products] that you should eat more often or avoid. It is put together in such a way that *you can easily implement it in your regular diet* [you have to prepare separate meals, with special products].

After 3 months, you will probably already feel better, and this system *gives you the opportunity to verify* the improvements in your health status [does not provide feedback].

*Note:* The most *(italics)* and least [in brackets] preferred scenarios are shown.

developed as different combinations of levels of each of the eight stages (see Figure 14.1). These scenarios (see Box 14.1 for an example) were then evaluated by consumers in a conjoint task (Ronteltap and Van Trijp, 2007) and a scenario-rating task (Wendel et al., 2006). Consumer evaluation measures included overall preference and intended use (Ronteltap and Van Trijp, 2006), and the perceived benefits ease of use, usefulness, privacy protection, and enjoyment (Wendel et al., 2006). As both of these studies have been reported elsewhere in detail, only the main results will be discussed here.

Together, the two studies confirm that:

- The personalization process can indeed be conceived of as consisting of three domains: a consumer domain, an interactive domain, and a firm domain.
- Efforts in each of these domains contribute to overall consumer evaluation.
- Each of the eight stages of the personalization process (see Figure 14.1) contributes to the overall evaluation of personalized nutrition offerings, lending support to the personalization process model.
- What consumers are most suspicious of are commercial applications in terms of the type of offerings (i.e., branded food products), the ownership of the database technology (to translate the consumer profile into a personalized diet), the sharing of personal information with commercial companies, and the route to interaction (e.g., through fitness clubs).
- Consumers prefer to receive personalized nutritional advice through established health institutions, particularly the family practitioner.

- Consumers prefer to be able to choose the specificity of nutritional advice (preferring advice at the level of ingredients and product groups, rather than about specific brands and products) and optional (rather than mandatory or no) feedback.
- Consumers prefer solutions that they can easily incorporate into their daily lives.
- The effects of design features on consumer attitude and intentions appear fully mediated by the perceptual dimensions of ease of use, usefulness, enjoyment, and privacy (Wendel et al., 2006).

As an illustration of the conjoint task results, in Box 14.1 we show the two scenarios from the Ronteltap and Van Trijp (2006) study that consumers thought were the most (italics) and least (between brackets) desirable scenarios for personalized nutritional advice.

Overall, the results as presented in Box 14.1 show that there are still a number of hurdles to be overcome before personalized nutrition can be applied commercially in marketing. In the next section, we will discuss the critical success factors from a marketing point of view.

## 14.7 CRITICAL SUCCESS FACTORS FROM A MARKETING POINT OF VIEW

From a marketing point of view, personalized gene-based nutrition implies that food companies would focus on smaller and smaller consumer segments that are homogeneous in terms of genetic profiles and associated nutritional needs (e.g., Jiang, 2000). To be justifiable as a strategic marketing tool, any segmentation needs to conform to a set of specific criteria: (1) measurability, (2) substantiality, (3) accessibility, (4) responsiveness, and (5) actionability (Kotler and Keller, 2006). In this section we assess the feasibility of personalized gene-based nutrition in terms of these criteria. Segments need to be *measurable* to the extent that individual consumers can accurately and consistently be assigned to segments at justifiable cost. In the case of genetics-based segmentation, this would mean that it should be relatively easy to accurately identify which consumers belong to which genetic segment. Also, segments should be *substantive*, in the sense that the segments identified should be large enough to justify separate marketing programs. Segments should be *accessible*, in the sense that targeted marketing programs could be developed that effectively reach the segment of consumers. Segments should be *responsive*, in the sense that different segments respond differently to the differentiated marketing mixes, as otherwise it would not be profitable to develop these separate marketing programs. Finally, the segments should be *actionable*, in the sense that it is both possible and advantageous to target different segments with different marketing programs. Much of the marketing potential of personalized nutrition will depend on further and as yet unknown scientific progress in the areas of nutrigenetics and nutrigenomics. However, the five criteria for effective segmentation provide a useful tool for reflecting on the marketing potential of personalized nutrition.

In terms of *measurability*, genetics-based personalized nutrition has the advantage that genotype is a segmentation variable that is stable over time. However, the measures are not easily obtained, because of consumer resistance to divulging personal genetic information to third parties, particularly when these are not in the public health domain. Uncertainties exist about how this information will be used now and in the future. For food companies, it is unclear how they can obtain this information with sufficient accuracy and in large enough quantity. In terms of *substantiveness* of the segments, the key question is whether homogenous consumer groups of sufficient size can be identified to justify targeted marketing. In other words, if these are very small groups of consumers, it will not be feasible for the mainstream food industry to develop targeted marketing programs, although it may be a relevant niche market with marketing opportunity for entrepreneurial small- and medium-sized companies. However, such small segments are probably catered to more efficiently and effectively through the medical segment than through the commercial segment of food companies. In terms of *accessibility*, given that genetic constitution is highly idiosyncratic and not overtly visible, it will be necessary for food companies to reach the segment members through an individualized approach. Consumer reluctance to share this sensitive genetic information directly with commercial food companies complicates such one-to-one marketing interactions with the individual consumer.

The greatest opportunity for marketing personalized nutrition — assuming that once consumers experience the health benefits of personalized nutrition they are likely to actively seek the personalized foods that fit their specific preferences — is *responsiveness* to personalized offerings. However, most of the health benefits are long term and not easily discernible by the consumer. Hence, it is crucial for personalized nutrition to have demonstrable short-term effectiveness: for example, inducing a change in consumer-relevant biomarkers (such as lowering cholesterol level), or an improved feeling of well-being. *Actionability* touches on the distinction between personalization and mass customization. There is great potential for giving personalized advice to consumers about which *existing* products to choose or to avoid. However, the situation becomes much more complex when the challenge is to develop and market *personalized food products*. This would require customizing product offerings to match smaller and smaller segments of consumers, which in turn requires substantial adjustments to the existing food supply chains that are currently based on large-scale production. One possibility would be to develop specialized foods for particular genotype segments; whether this is feasible depends largely on the willingness of this segment to pay a premium price that will cover the extra costs involved in production, distribution, and marketing. Another option would be to add specific nutrients and ingredients to products in the very last step in the production chain, rather like a coffee-vending machine, which allows the consumer to add certain ingredients to the basic product in-store to make it fit with his or her personal nutritional needs. However, this would bring the application of personalized nutrition very close to that of supplements and medicine, and a key challenge would be to meaningfully differentiate the personalized food option from supplements and medicine. Further complicating the marketing of personalized nutrition are the regulations regarding nutrition and health claims (note that in the European Union, such regulations have recently come into force). It is expected that genetics-based products will focus either on maintaining health or on reducing risk of disease (or maybe even curing disease). Although claims to this effect are now permitted under the new European Union regulations, they are strictly regulated on the basis of scientific substantiation. The high costs of this scientific substantiation will be borne by a relatively small market segment, because the alternative is to make genomics knowledge publicly available, which would substantially reduce the competitive advantage of the institutions that create knowledge.

Overall, we believe that current developments in nutrigenomics augur well for improving our understanding of the relation between food, health, and disease, and individual differences therein. There is potential for personalized nutrition advice for those segments of consumers willing to make their genetic information available in order to obtain such advice. Some commercial companies such as Sciona (www.mycellf.com) are already practicing this particular application of nutrigenomics. Provided that these applications are scientifically sound and consumers are willing to share their genetic information, this may be one route for personalized nutrition to explore. But note that the Sciona business model relies heavily on the marketing of diagnostic kits, not on customized food products. Also, we believe that further advances in the science of nutrigenomics may be helpful in the marketing of food products whose selling point is the absence of certain ingredients and possibly nutrients ("guaranteed free from") as is currently already the case in "allergen-free" foods. If nutrigenetics provides evidence for sufficiently large consumer segments, this may be an opportunity for the mainstream food industry; otherwise, gene-based personalized nutrition may be a niche market relevant for smaller food companies. However, at present there are too many factors that hinder the commercial application of nutrigenetics-based practices for marketing food products on the basis of their content of specific combinations of ingredients and nutrients. It is unlikely that in the near future the benefits arising from customer loyalty and willingness to pay will outweigh the costs associated with personalized nutrition. The consumer segments are likely to be small and the additional production, distribution, and marketing costs high. For most larger food companies, this will deviate too much from their current business models to justify the effort. There may be potential for small specialist companies, provided that they can get the distribution channel right. However, such applications are more likely to be closer to the medical and supplement businesses than to the food business. In the short term, the added value of nutrigenomics is more likely to emerge from the better insight into the fundamental processes underlying health and disease than in the application of marketing for personalized diets. From consumers' great confidence in and reliance on their family practitioner, we further see that it is this "communication" channel that has most potential. We therefore believe that genetics-based insights can be best implemented through the existing health systems, with a central role being played by the family practitioner. Our consumer research suggests that commercial applications through fitness and health centers are still a step too far for most consumers.

Much of the existing segmentation and targeting in the food industry is being conducted on the basis of phenotype information rather than genotype information. Market potential should therefore be assessed by examining the added value of genotype segmentation over and above existing phenotype segmentation. For example, it is possible to identify a relevant segment of consumers at risk based on their current blood cholesterol level, on specific lifestyle features (age, lifestyle, job stress, etc.), or based on their genotype information. Blood cholesterol levels are relatively easy to measure and specific psychographic and lifestyle factors are an accessible feature to which communication to the target audience can be tailored. This raises the question of what added value genotype information related to blood cholesterol levels will have for marketing purposes. Clearly, genotype information has the potential for identifying individuals at risk much earlier in their lives, before the phenotype with the high cholesterol level has developed, and this may be important for preventive purposes. However, the crucial factor is the reliability of genotype information for predicting later development of high cholesterol levels, and the extent to which the effect of the genotype can be attenuated by environmental factors such as nutrition. Currently, the predictive accuracy seems to be low, especially for diseases such as diabetes and obesity that involve multiple genes. Finally, regarding actionability in terms of the development of specific dietary advice and tailored products, the question arises as to whether the additional genotype information would lead to relevant adjustments in the current dietary recommendations about the consumption of macro- and micronutrients.

## 14.8 CONCLUSION

Personalized nutrition based on insights from nutrigenomics is a relatively new concept. Building on marketing literature about personalization and effective market segmentation, in this chapter we have reviewed the marketing potential of personalized nutrition. Although personalization has revolutionized the marketing approach in many fields (see Wind, 2001; Wind and Rangaswamy, 2001 and Riemer and Totz, 2003 for more details), we have specifically focused on the potential of personalization in the food domain. We have argued that personalized nutrition based on nutrigenetics may provide potential for personalized nutritional advice with the purpose of assisting consumers to make better choices from the existing product supply. In terms of personalized food products, we have argued that currently there is limited marketing potential for the mainstream food industry, because the consumer segments are likely to be small and the additional costs involved in production, distribution, and marketing are large. However, niche markets of sufficient size and purchasing power might develop that can profitably be catered to by smaller and specialized food companies. Another potentially successful application of nutrigenomics knowledge in the short term may be foods personalized on the basis of the *absence* of certain ingredients and nutrients.

## 14.9 FUTURE PERSPECTIVES ON PERSONALIZED NUTRITION

Despite these constraints to personalized nutrition becoming a large-scale marketing opportunity, we believe that it has potential to add to public health in the more medically oriented domain. Again, this depends on the advances in the science of nutrigenomics, as complex states of health and disease cannot currently be predicted from genetics. Health-care professionals such as the family practitioner, a highly trusted source of health information, could be important gatekeepers in this process of advising consumers about personalized nutrition.

This chapter has highlighted that only a limited amount of scientific marketing and consumer research has been done on personalization in the food domain. There is clearly a need for more research in this area, not just from a marketing and consumer behavior perspective, but also more broadly at the interface between biochemical and nutrition science on the one hand and social sciences such as communication, ethics and marketing, and consumer behavior on the other. Only such a multidisciplinary approach will ensure that consumer triggers and reservations can be identified up front and serve as input to the further development of nutrigenomics practice to make it a substantive success both commercially and in terms of public health.

## KEY READINGS

Adomavicius, G. and Tuzhilin, A., Personalisation technologies: a process-oriented perspective, *Communications of the ACM*, 48(10), 83–90, 2005.

Murthi, B.P.S. and Sarkar, S., The role of the management sciences in research on personalization. *Management Science*, 49(10), 1344–1362, 2003.

Piller, F.T., Mass customization: reflections on the state of the concept. The *International Journal of Flexible Manufacturing Systems* 16: 313–334, 2005.

Vesanen, J. and Raulas, M., Building bridges for personalization: a process model for marketing. *Journal of Interactive Marketing*, 20(1), 5–20, 2006.

Wind, J. and Rangaswamy, A., Customerization: the next revolution in mass customization. *Journal of Interactive Marketing*, 15(1), 13–32, 2001.

## REFERENCES

Adomavicius, G. and Tuzhilin, A., Personalisation technologies: a process-oriented perspective, *Communications of the ACM*, 48(10), 83–90, 2005.

Bonnett, M., Personalization of Web services: opportunities and challenges. *Ariadne* 28 (June), www.ariadne.ac.uk, 2001.

Bouwman, L.I., Hiddink, G.J., Koelen, M.A., Korthals, M., Van't Veer, P., and Van Woerkum, D., Personalized nutrition communication through ICT application: how to overcome the gap between potential effectiveness and reality. *European Journal of Clinical Nutrition* 59(Suppl. 1), S108–S116, 2005.

Brug, J., Campbell, M., and Van Assema, P., The application and impact of computer-generated personalized nutrition education: a review of the literature. *Patient Education and Counseling* 36, 145–156, 1999.

Brug, J., Oenema, A., and Campbell, M., Past, present and future of computer-tailored nutrition education. *American Journal of Clinical Nutrition* 77(Suppl.), 1028S–1034S, 2003.

Cain, M. and Schmid, G. *From nutrigenomic science to personalize nutrition. The market in 2010.* Palo Alto (CA): Institute for the Future. New Consumer New Genetics Program, report SR–793 (www.ifth.org), 2003.

Chadwick, R., Nutrigenomics, individualism and public health. *Proceedings of the Nutritional Society* 6, 161–166, 2004.

Csikszentmilhalyi, M., *Flow: The Psychology of Optimal Experience.* New York: Harper and Row, 1990.

Dabholkar, P.A. and Bagozzi, R.P., An attitudinal model of technology-based self-service: moderating effects of consumer traits and situational factors. *Journal of the Academy of Marketing Science*, 30(3), 184–201, 2002.

Davis, F.D., Perceived usefulness, perceived ease of use and user acceptance of information technology. *MIS Quarterly* 13(3), 145–158, 1989.

Davis, F.D., Bagozzi, R.P., and Warshaw, P.R., User acceptance of computer technology: a comparison of two theoretical models. *Management Science* 35(8), 982–1002, 1989.

Dellaert, B.G.C. and Stremersch, S., Marketing mass-customized products: striking a balance between utility and complexity. *Journal of Marketing Research* 42(May), 219–227, 2005.

Fotheringham, M.J. and Owen, N., Introduction — Interactive health communication in preventive medicine. *American Journal of Preventive Medicine* 19(2), 111–112, 2000.

Franke, N. and Piller, F.T., Value creation by toolkits for user innovation and design: the case of the watch market. *Journal of Product Innovation Management*, 21: 405–415, 2004.

Godek, J., Personalization and customization: implications for consumer decision making and behavior. *Advances in Consumer Research* 29, 155–157, 2002.

Godek, J, Yates, J.G., and Yoon, Y., Customization and personalization: the influence of perceived control and perceived capability on product evaluations. *Advances in Consumer Research* 29, 155–157, 2002.

Jiang, P., Segment-based mass customization: an exploration of a new conceptual marketing framework. *Internet Research: Electronic Networking Applications and Policy*, 10(3), 215–226, 2000.

Karat, C.M., Brodie, C., Karat, J., Vergo, J., and Alpert, S.R., Personalizing the user experience on ibm.com. *IBM Systems Journal*, 42(4), 686–701, 2003.

Kotler, P. and Keller, K.L., *Marketing Management: analysis, planning, implementation and control*, 12th ed. Englewood Cliffs, NJ: Prentice Hall, 2006.

Meuter, M.L., Bitner, M.J., Ostrom, A.L., and Brown, S.W., Choosing among alternative service delivery modes: an investigation of customer trial of self-service technologies. *Journal of Marketing* 69(April), 61–83, 2005.

Murthi, B.P.S. and Sarkar, S., The role of the management sciences in research on personalization. *Management Science*, 49(10), 1344–1362, 2003.

Pierrakos, D., Paliouras, G., Papatheodorou, C., and Spyropoulos, C.D., Web usage mining as a tool for personalization: a survey. *User modeling and User-adapted interaction*, 13: 311–372, 2003.

Piller, F.T., Mass customization: reflections on the state of the concept. *The International Journal of Flexible Manufacturing Systems* 16: 313–334, 2005.

Piller, F.T. and Müller, M., A new marketing approach to mass customisation. *International Journal of Computer Integrated Manufacturing*, 17(7), 583–593, 2004.

Pine, B.J., Customizing for the new consumer. *Fortune* 128(December 16), 45, 1993.

Pine, B.J. and Gilmore, J.H., *The Experience Economy*. Boston, MA: Harvard Business School Press, 1999.

Pine, B.J., Peppers, D., and Rogers, M., Do you want to keep your customers forever? *Harvard Business Review* 73(March–April), 103–114, 1995.

Riecken, D., Personalized views of personalization. *Communications of the ACM* 43(8), 27–28, 2000.

Riemer, K. and Totz, C., The many faces of personalization: an integrative economic overview of mass customization and personalization. In Tseng, M.M. and Piller, F.T. (Eds.), *The customer centric enterprise: advances in mass customization and personalization*. Berlin: Springer, 2003, pp. 35–50.

Rogers, E.M., *Diffusion of innovations*, 5th ed. New York: Free Press, 2003.

Ronteltap, A. and Van Trijp, H.C.M. (2007). Consumer preferences for personalised nutritional advice: a conjoint analysis study. Wageningen University; Marketing and Consumer Behaviour Group. Working Paper (in preparation).

Ronteltap, A., Wendel, B.S., Van Trijp, H.C.M., and Dellaert, B.G.C., Marketing van producten die passen bij de genetische structuur van het individu [Marketing of products that fit the genetic predisposition of the individual]. *Jaarboek van de Nederlandse Vereniging van Marketing Onderzoekers*, 2006, pp. 127–141.

Simonson, I., Determinants of customers' responses to customized offers: conceptual framework and research propositions. *Journal of Marketing* 69(January), 32–45, 2005.

Sheth, J., Sisodia, R., and Sharma, A., The antecedents and consequences of customer-centric marketing, *Journal of the Academy of Marketing Sciences*, 28(1), 55–66, 2000.

Steckel, J.H., Winer, R.S., Bucklin, R., Delleart, B.G.C., Dreze, X., Haubl, G., Jap, S.D., Little, J.D.C., Meyvis, T., Montgomery, A.L., and Rangaswamy, A., Choice in interactive environments. *Marketing Letters* 16(3/4), 309–320, 2005.

Tornatzky, L.G. and Klein, K.J., Innovation characteristics and innovation-adoption implementation: a meta-analysis of findings. *IEEE Transactions on Engineering Management* 29(1), 28–45, 1982.

Treacy, M. and Wiersema, F. (1993), Customer intimacy and other value disciplines. *Harvard Business Review* 71(1), 84–93.

Venkatesh, V., Morris, M.G., Davis, G.B., and Davis, F.D., User acceptance of information technology: toward a unified view. *MIS Quarterly* 27(3), 425–478, 2003.

Vesanen, J. and Raulas, M., Building bridges for personalization: a process model for marketing. *Journal of Interactive Marketing*, 20(1), 5–20, 2006.

Wendel, S., Ronteltap, A., Dellaert, B.G.C., and Van Trijp, H.C.M., Customer–Firm Interaction in the creation and delivery of personalized recommendations. Working paper, 2006.

Wind, J., The challenge of customerization in financial services. *Communications of the ACM*, 44(6), 39–44, 2001.

Wind, J. and Rangaswamy, A., Customerization: the next revolution in mass customization. *Journal of Interactive Marketing*, 15(1), 13–32, 2001.

# 15 U.S. Consumer Attitudes toward Personalized Nutrition

*David B. Schmidt, Christy White, Wendy Reinhardt Kapsak, Josh Conway, and Elizabeth Baily*

**CONTENTS**



## 15.1 METHODS

Since 2004, the *Cogent Syndicated Genomics Attitudes and Trends* (CGAT) survey has been annually taking the public's pulse regarding the issue of genomics. CGAT explores public awareness, understanding, favorability, and interest in genomics and its applications, including nutrigenomics and pharmacogenomics. This chapter describes data from the CGAT survey, collected in January 2006, via a Web-based 205-question survey of more than 1000 Americans. Using both balancing and weighting techniques, the sample was designed to reflect the U.S. population in terms of key demographics, including education, age, income, and gender.

Data in this chapter are also from the International Food Information Council (IFIC) survey, *Consumer Attitudes toward Functional Foods/Foods for Health*. This survey measures consumer awareness of, and interest in, functional foods/foods for health as well as the application of genomics to nutrition and personal health, a science otherwise known as nutrigenomics or "personalized nutrition." This trending survey was first commissioned in 1998, with subsequent surveys conducted in 2000 and 2002; some survey questions gauge trends in consumer attitudes toward nutrition and health. Questions regarding consumer perceptions of "personalized nutrition" were added in 2005. The quantitative Web-based survey was fielded in May 2005 with more than 1000 randomly selected U.S. adults, aged 18 years and older. The findings were weighted by education, age, and ethnicity, reflecting the 2003 U.S. population census estimate, to allow the findings to be representative of the American public as a whole.

The findings from both surveys rely primarily on univariate analyses and cross-tabulations. The data were analyzed according to the demographic profile of the population, including primary characteristics (e.g., age, income and gender), health-based characteristics (e.g., health history, and current health status), and in some cases, attitudinal characteristics (e.g., receptivity to medical advances).

## 15.2 RESULTS

### 15.2.1 Genomics: General Attitudes and Perceptions

#### 15.2.1.1 Awareness and Interest Regarding Genomics

Although three fourths (76%) of the American public say they have heard or read something about genomics (defined as "using individual genetic information to understand and optimize health"), a closer analysis indicates that this broad awareness is quite limited in depth. First, only a very small number (6%) of Americans say they have heard "a lot" about genomics, whereas half (49%) say they have heard only "a little bit." Further, when those who say they have heard something about genomics were asked to describe what they have heard, about one fourth (27%) were unable to recall any details, and another one third (36%) mention having heard only about the basic connection between genes and health (Chart 15.1).

Still, there is a small group of Americans who understand the concept of genomics and some of its practical implications. Specifically, of the approximately 75% of Americans who have heard something about genomics, only about 15% say they have heard that genes can be altered for health benefits and about 5% have heard that genomics can aid in early detection of disease or that genomics can be used to help customize health-related treatments.

Although knowledge is limited, more than half (52%) say they favor the idea of using individual genetic information to understand and optimize health. Similarly, nearly half (46%) of Americans say they are interested in using their personal genetic information to understand and optimize their health. This includes using their personal

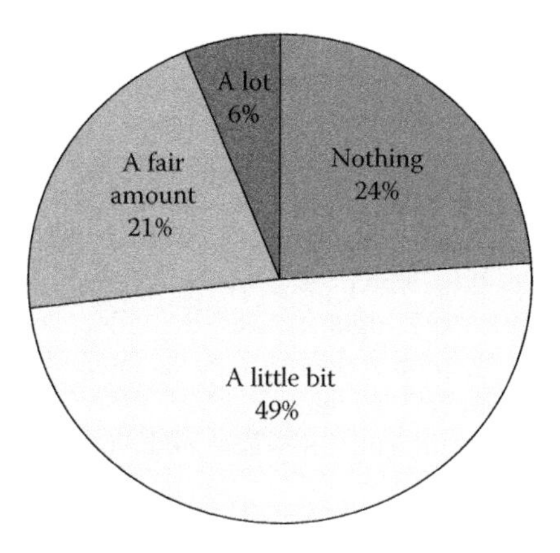


**CHART 15.1** U.S. consumers' genomics awareness. $n = 1015$.

genetic information to provide nutrition and diet-related recommendations (i.e., nutrigenomics or personalized nutrition). Findings specific to personalized nutrition will be explored later in this chapter.

Consumer interest in using genomics is highest when it can be connected to identifiable health benefits. For example, three fourths (72%) of the public are interested in using genomics to reduce risk of specific diseases. Furthermore, less than half (46%) of Americans say they would be even more interested if the test results could indicate they were certain to get the disease. In contrast, about one fourth (27%) of Americans would be more interested in using genomics if the test results were able to tell them that they carry the relevant gene but not whether they will develop a disease. The public is particularly interested in using genomics to target diseases that are treatable.

**Privacy.** Among the most interesting findings is the number of people who are concerned about privacy issues. Two thirds (66%) of the American public is concerned about how personal genetic information would be stored and who would have access to that information. One third (33%) of the public say their concern about privacy would actually prevent them from having a genetic test. A potential reason for this may lie in the fact that 36% of the public sees genetic tests as being more sensitive, and thus more personal, than other kinds of medical tests.

Regarding information misuse specifically, about half of Americans say they are concerned that their "DNA sample may be used for tests other than ones [they] have authorized." More generally, the public is worried about "misuse" by insurance companies, government, and employers (51%).

*Insurance discrimination.* Almost two thirds (64%) of the public agree with statements regarding insurance discrimination, including: "insurance companies will do everything possible to use genetic information to deny health coverage" and "insurance companies will use information to deny coverage for drugs people need if their genetic profile indicates a low chance of responding." This may be why more than half (56%) of the American public say they would be less interested in using genomic services if their test results would become "part of their medical record and therefore be obtainable by insurance companies." Conversely, the public does want insurance companies to pay for genetic tests. Almost half (48%) indicated they would be less interested if their "health insurance company would not cover the cost of genetic testing."

*Government discrimination.* A similar dynamic exists with regard to the government and its role in genomics. First, about two thirds (65%) say they are concerned that the government might obtain unauthorized access to their personal genetic information, and only 2% say they would want the government to receive a copy of the results of any genetic test they might choose to conduct. However, Americans are looking to the government to protect their privacy, as three fourths (72%) of the public believe the federal government "should establish specific laws and regulations to protect the privacy of genetic information." That said, 70% of Americans do not know whether laws to protect the privacy of their genetic information currently exist, and of those who are aware of existing laws, 60% believe the public needs more protection. Clear and strict protections could alleviate concerns, given that about 60% of Americans say they would be more interested in genomics if they were "assured by law that no one could access [their] DNA information without [their] consent."

*Employer discrimination.* Lastly, Americans are concerned about employers accessing their genetic information. More than half (54%) of Americans say they are concerned that their "employer would gain unauthorized access to their personal genetic information." Furthermore, only 1% say they would want their employer to receive a copy of the results of any genetic test they might choose to receive.

**Moral issues**. Another challenge facing genomics is public concern about moral issues. According to the research, there is a segment of the population that holds deep moral reservations about genomics. In this case, this group is a minority. One fourth (25%) of the public agree that "the recent advances surrounding the use of genetic testing make me uncomfortable from a moral standpoint." Slightly less (21%) agree that "meddling with our genes and DNA is trying to play God [and that] scientists, researchers, and doctors should stay out of it altogether."

The CGAT survey shows two trends that have emerged that may be important to consider. First, although the number of Americans who have moral reservations is low, this cohort has grown slightly over the past year (see Chart 15.2).

Second, about one third (33%) of the American public has not yet developed a firm moral stand on these issues; that is, they neither agree nor disagree with these

| | 2006 | 2005 | 2006 | 2005 |
|---|---|---|---|---|
| | Top 2 Box (Agree) | Top 2 Box (Agree) | Bot. 2 Box (Disagree) | Bot. 2 Box (Disagree) |
| We shouldn't meddle with our genes | 21% | 16% | 46% | 50% |
| Genetic testing should be stopped | 19% | 15% | 47% | 55% |
| Genetic testing makes me morally uncomfortable | 25% | 23% | 42% | 46% |

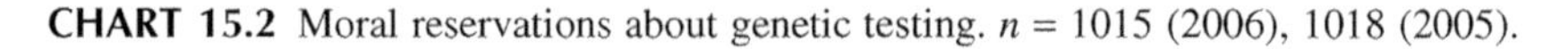

**CHART 15.2** Moral reservations about genetic testing. $n$ = 1015 (2006), 1018 (2005).

statements noted in Chart 15.2. Perhaps speaking to both moral and privacy concerns, we see that almost half (46%) of all Americans agree with the statement, "I am torn on the use of genetics. The potential benefits are incredible, but the potential for misuse is considerable."

**Emotional uncertainty**. The third challenge facing genomics is the emotional burden that genetic test results can bring. For example, about one fourth (26%) of the public agree that knowing their genetic profile "is too great a responsibility because it impacts [them], [their] spouse, and ultimately [their] children." Similarly, one third (32%) agree that it would be "too depressing to know [they were] going to get a disease, particularly if there is nothing [they] can do about it." This finding reinforces the consumer appeal of genomics when it addresses treatable diseases and actionable preemptive choices.

## 15.3 THE OPPORTUNITY FOR PERSONALIZED NUTRITION

### 15.3.1 Key Findings on Consumers' Perceptions regarding Health and Nutrition

Survey findings indicate that most Americans (94%) believe that they have some control over their own health. In addition, the majority of consumers (69%) believe food and nutrition play "a great role" in maintaining or improving overall health. Interestingly, more consumers (90%) said in 2005 that family health history plays a "moderate" to "great" role in maintaining and improving health than in previous years (82% in 2002, 80% in 2000, and 85% in 1998). This finding likely indicates consumers' increasing awareness of how their unique genetic makeup, inherited from their parents, may affect their future health status.

The majority (88%) of American consumers agree that certain foods have health benefits that go beyond basic nutrition and may reduce the risk of disease or other health concerns. Consumer interest in learning more about foods for better health remains high. Specifically, more than eight out of 10 (83%) Americans are interested in learning more about foods that have health benefits that go beyond basic nutrition and may reduce the risk of disease or promote better health. Those who are "very interested" in learning more about healthful foods are those who feel that food and nutrition play a "great role" in overall health (45% vs. 40% of those who say it plays a "moderate role," and 22% of those who stated "no role"); are more likely to be vitamin/supplement users (49% vs. 27% of nonusers); consumers with a college degree or higher (49 percent vs. 38 percent of those with some college or less); and consumers aged 35 to 54 (48% vs. 41% of those aged 18 to 34 and 35% of those who are 55 years and older).

#### 15.3.1.1 Interest in and Favorability toward Personalized Nutrition

More Americans have heard or read about using individual genetic information in the context of nutrition and diet-related recommendations (42%) than in any other context, including prescription drugs (36%), over-the-counter medications (29%), and beauty and cosmetic products (19%). In fact, nearly half (47%) of all Americans say they have heard or read something about personalized nutrition (defined as using genetic information to make informed dietary choices).

When asked what they thought about various terms to describe the practice of using genetic information to develop nutrition and diet-related recommendations, Americans overwhelmingly preferred either "personalized nutrition" (70% like "a lot" or "a little") or "individualized nutrition" (68% like "a lot" or "a little") over terms such as "nutrigenomics" (19% like "a lot" or "a little").

As with genomics in general, slightly more than half (51%) of the American public hold a highly favorable view of personalized nutrition. Among the 48% of Americans who hold an unfavorable opinion of personalized nutrition, most indicate that their favorability is low due to a lack of knowledge about the science. Whereas 20% cite lack of knowledge directly, most do so indirectly, saying they are "not sure how they could benefit" from personalized nutrition (17%) or "don't see a need for the science" (14%). Others say they fail to see how genomics would be superior to their doctor's opinion or to "good-old" common sense. A small number (14%) say they are not favorable at this point in time because "the unknown consequences" of personalized nutrition may be harmful, whereas others have more immediate concerns such as the perceived high cost of this technology (4%).

Interestingly, given Americans' fears of discrimination when it comes to genomics in general, only about 10% say their lack of favorability toward personalized nutrition is attributable to concerns regarding misuse of genetic testing information. When the topic turns away from general favorability toward using this technology for a personal benefit, just less than half (42%) of the American public express a strong level of interest in using genetic information to receive personalized, diet-related recommendations. Only one fourth (27%) of the American public characterizes their interest in personalized nutrition as low.

#### 15.3.1.2 Applications for Personalized Nutrition

*Desired benefits of nutrigenomics.* Although Americans find numerous potential benefits of personalized nutrition to be appealing, distinct preferences for specific applications are apparent. Specifically, more holistic, preventive health benefits rank highest, with 63% of consumers interested in disease prevention and 61% interested in overall wellness. Singular, less general health benefits, such as mental alertness (58%), stamina (53%), weight loss (52%), and vitamin/mineral optimization (48%) fall into a second tier, but are still appealing to a large number of people — about half of all Americans. Using personalized nutrition for appearance benefits ranks lowest of all the areas tested (40% interested). An overwhelming percentage (86%) of Americans favor receiving personal nutrition recommendations that provide guidance on both additions to and subtractions from their diet.

*Products of interest.* As shown in Chart 15.3, when it comes to the specific types of products Americans would be most interested in having tailored to their specific dietary needs, vitamins and supplements top the list. Interest in fortified foods and "natural" foods appeals to 50% of the American public, whereas only about 25 to 38% are interested in specific food products, including beverages and meal replacement bars.

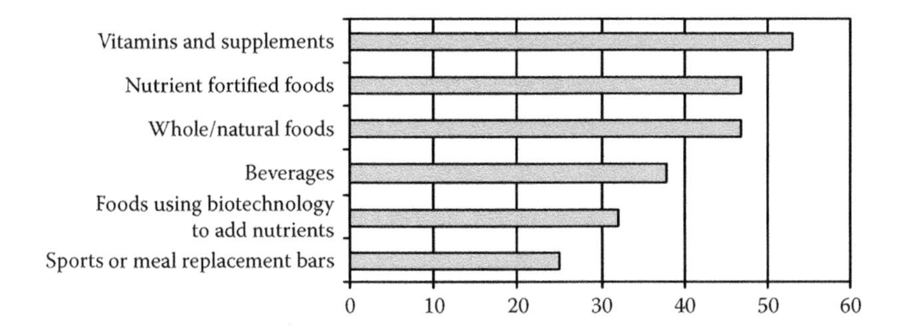


**CHART 15.3** Interest in genetically tailored products. $n = 1015$.

*The power of the physician as guide and gatekeeper.* Nearly 90% of Americans say they would consult their doctor when deciding to pursue a genomics test to facilitate personalized nutrition and diet-related recommendations, and almost a third (31%) of all Americans would only pursue testing after receiving a doctor's specific recommendation.

The role of the doctor goes beyond deciding whether or not to have a test. Once Americans have decided to take a genetic test for the purpose of receiving personalized nutrition recommendations, 67% cite the doctor's office as the most desirable location for administering such a test. The majority of Americans (70%) are also most likely to indicate that they would want to receive their test results in a face-to-face consultation — similar to how many patients receive their medical test information today.

*The power of the individual and other sources in decision making.* Although the doctor's opinion is undeniably important, more than half (57%) of Americans say they will "make their own decision" after consulting their doctor, and an additional 10% say they will not consult their doctor at all. This means that a majority of Americans have some measure of confidence in their own ability to decide whether or not to pursue genetic testing.

Although secondary to physicians (70%), significant numbers of consumers rated nurses and physician assistants (58%), and dietitians (57%) as highly credible sources for information on using genetic information for personalized nutrition information. Genetic counselors (48%) were also considered among the highly credible sources. The inclusion of health associations as a credible source (52%) demonstrates that consumers may not necessarily need a face-to-face, intimate history for a high level of trust. Pharmacists (43%) were considered only slightly less credible than genetic counselors. Moderately credible resources also included university or other health newsletters (42%) and government agencies (37%). Other sources, ranging from news media to product labels and insurers, received relatively low ratings when it came to being a credible source on personalized nutrition (see Chart 15.4 for the remaining figures).

*Testing locations and results delivery.* This research has shown the doctor's office as Americans' most desirable testing location. However, a sizeable number of Americans

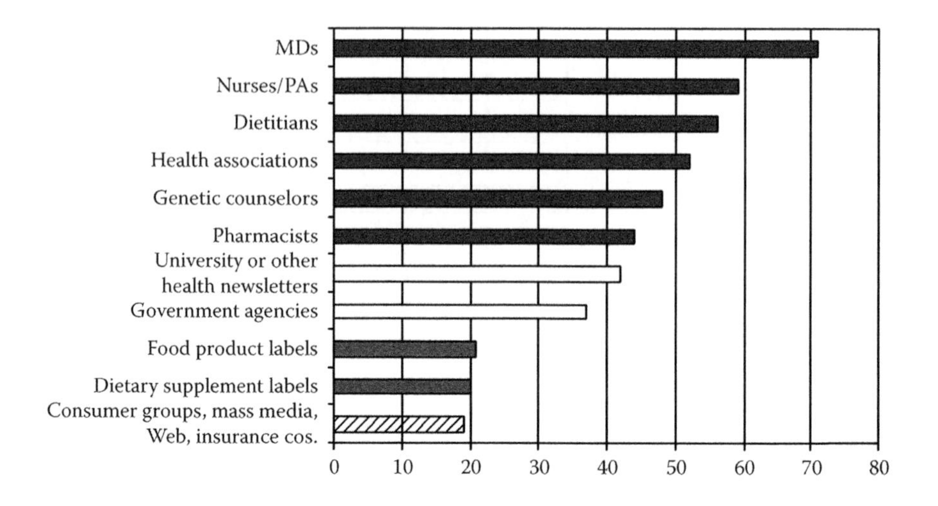


**CHART 15.4** Personalized nutrition resource credibility. $n = 1015$.

say they would be interested in testing at home (40%), perhaps because of the privacy it provides. In fact, at-home testing slightly edged out the offices of two other medical professionals — genetic counselors (39%) and dietitians/nutritionists (31%). Testing locations that are largely unacceptable to consumers include health spas, fitness centers, personal trainer's office, and health food stores (each with 8%).

Furthermore, although face-to-face delivery of test results tops the list (70%), not far behind are paper results (60%), which suggest that, given the right approach, home testing could be widely accepted. Americans were less interested in their willingness to receive their results through electronic media — 35% were willing to receive results via a secured Web site, 32% by e-mail, and 28% by disk. A phone call with a consultant was the least preferred means of receiving test results (26%).

## 15.4 DISCUSSION

### 15.4.1 Awareness, Interest, and Barriers regarding Genomics

Research results show that consumers' ideal scenario for genomics-related applications is one in which the genetic marker (or test) provides a high level of certainty that one would actually experience a specific disease for which there are known remedies. Given these high expectations, additional consumer education will likely need to address the many factors that can impact disease risk, including genetics as well as the environment (see Figure 15.1).

*Barriers to adoption.* Despite broad awareness, a positive perception, and general interest in genomics and its applications, there are some formidable challenges facing genomics. If left unchecked, the challenges have the potential of limiting widespread usage of genomics, or even becoming the flashpoint for a negative shift in public

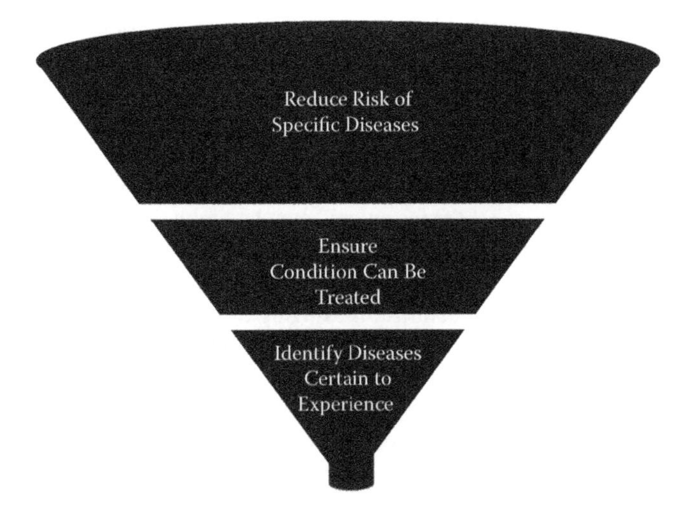


**FIGURE 15.1** Consumers are most interested in certain knowledge of treatable diseases.

opinion. The research showed there are three barriers of specific concern for genomic testing. These concerns include: privacy, moral issues, and perceived emotional drawbacks.

Almost two thirds of the American public were concerned about issues related to privacy, which included insurance, government, and employer discrimination. Given this finding, it is likely that a regulatory and statutory framework that takes these concerns into account will be debated before widespread adoption of genomics testing occurs. In the U.S., governing bodies are already beginning to look at genetic testing and some of the challenges to come. In the scientific and academic community, the Institute of Medicine held its first-ever meeting on nutrigenomics, sponsored by the National Institutes of Health's Office of Dietary Supplements, the National Cancer Institute, and the U.S. Department of Agriculture's Agriculture Research Service, which looked at the role of various stakeholders and their impact on this emerging area of science.[1] Additionally, in the U.S., the Department of Health and Human Services has formed the Secretary's Advisory Committee on Genetics, Health, and Society (SACGHS) to provide a forum for experts to discuss ethical, social, legal, and medical issues related to innovations and applications in genetic technology. The SACGHS also helps inform other government agencies about specific questions related to genetics and makes recommendations to the secretary on such issues.[2] For more than a decade, members of Congress have also been working to pass the Genetic Information Nondiscrimination Act (GINA) to address the growing concern surrounding the misuse of genetic information in insurance and employment decisions.

Around the globe similar discussions have also begun. In Canada, Genome Canada commissioned a project to compare different ethical approaches to public involvement in governing genomics.[3] The U.K. also has a commission in place that provides the government with advice about genomics. This commission has a particular focus on ethical, legal, and social issues related to human genetics.[4]

Genomics is entering a crucial phase in which scientific advances are blossoming, while simultaneously a sizable minority of the public is struggling to understand how these advances relate to their deeply held convictions. Given that about one third of the American public have not yet developed a firm moral stand on issues related to genetic testing, these "fence sitters" may be highly influenced by messaging regarding genomics — either pro or con. If a substantial number of these individuals are persuaded and join the concerned minority, the total group holding moral objections would form a near majority. In contrast, messaging that promotes the responsible use of genetic information as well as the implications for public (and personal) health may swing the balance more heavily toward positive viewpoints (see Figure 15.2).

Emotional concerns held by Americans may, in part, signal recognition of the significance —or even value — of genomics. However, there is also evidence that the emotional burden for some may be "too" great, enough to preclude interest for a sizable minority. Providers of genomic testing and products may be able to pursue strategies to lessen this burden, especially through professionals who provide testing coupled with consultation.

More research has been conducted to assess consumer acceptance and reactions to genetic testing than in the area of personalized nutrition. One area, which this research did not assess, was the behavioral consequences that could be associated with receiving a genetic test. One study, involving healthy individuals, asked participants to imagine that they were at increased risk for obesity based on the results of a genetic test. This preliminary study found that a positive test (i.e., showing that they were at increased risk of becoming obese) was a motivator for more healthful

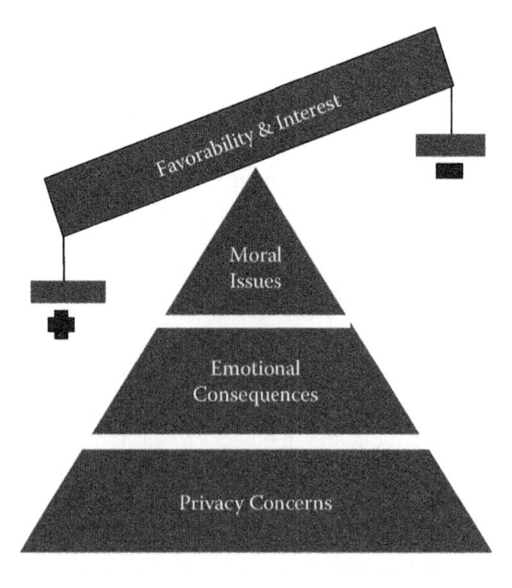


**FIGURE 15.2** Favorability and interest in genomics outweigh concerns.

dietary behavior.[5] This finding calls attention to the importance of providing motivational or behavioral information along with a genetic test to help consumers implement dietary or lifestyle changes.

### 15.4.2 Awareness, Interest, and Applications for Personalized Nutrition

Of the various genomic applications, the public is most aware of personalized nutrition. In addition, the public considers personalized nutrition to be aimed at general health, or as a more tailored diagnostic tool. Opportunities present themselves as the concept of using genetic information to provide personalized diet recommendations was favorably received by the majority of Americans, who are interested in learning more.

*Terminology related to personalized nutrition.* Research findings show that the majority of Americans preferred the terms "personalized nutrition" and "individualized nutrition" to other terms such as "nutrigenomics." Consumer insights from previous IFIC focus groups indicated that whereas the former terms are seen as focusing on one person ("speaking to me" or "about me"), consumers found the latter term too technical and difficult to understand. Even more worrying, many found this term to be "scary." Consumer communications that take into account such terminology preferences may be more effective in building acceptance of this emerging field.

*Applications of personalized nutrition.* In the case of pharmacogenomics, the CGAT survey showed that the public is most interested in identifying specific medical issues, as well as providing directional means to treat or prevent those issues. In contrast, personalized nutrition is held to a different set of success standards, according to which individuals are less concerned with specific treatments and more interested in general health and wellness outcomes. This difference in expectations may illustrate the public's belief in the functional limits of food and nutrition with regard to health. It also may be that the public is unaware of how specific genetic conditions or predispositions can be influenced by altering lifestyle choices, including the consumption of nutrients or food components over time (as opposed to taking prescription medications). In either event, it is again made clear that the public would benefit greatly from having a better general understanding of the interplay between genes and dietary choices in determining one's present and future health. Given the breadth of nutrition and lifestyle modifications that these tests may encompass, dietetic professionals are particularly poised to play a primary role in helping to meet this need.[6]

*Relaying genetic information to consumers.* At present, though awareness is high for personalized nutrition, the lack of familiarity with potential benefits, specific products, and the testing process would likely drive consumers to consult their trusted medical professionals for guidance regarding this emerging approach to personal health. Genetic testing, and by extension personalized nutrition, appear to be heavily rooted in the medical realm, and Americans are approaching them as they would any other medical need or concern.

It is not surprising, then, that for many, the doctor's office would be a preliminary step to pursuing any kind of genetic-based dietary approach. Thus, although efforts to communicate the general benefits and practical knowledge of personalized nutrition to the consumer are critical, so too is providing the latest developments and research in the field of genomics and its nutrition applications to the primary care physicians whose advice and knowledge would be sought by most individuals. This might, in part, help to alleviate the emotional burden that a lay reading of the genetic test results might produce. Such an unfamiliar medical test could potentially suggest a multitude of recommendations and changes. Creating an interdisciplinary partnership among health professionals could help mitigate the responsibility of one health professional being responsible for administering a genetic test, analyzing the results, explaining the results to a client, making recommendations on how to implement behavioral changes based on the results of the test, and following up with the client to determine how his or her life has been affected by the test results.

Considering the high levels of credibility and influence assigned to health-care professionals beside physicians, face-to-face result consultations may well provide an acceptable level of trust, particularly if performed by a dietitian/nutritionist or a pharmacist. In studies completed with consumers and genetic testing, it appears there are a multitude of factors that may influence an individual's decision to undergo genetic testing. Research has shown a decrease in genetic testing for women at risk of developing breast cancer after they spoke with a genetic counselor. However, in situations where a genetic test was offered without genetic counseling, people were more likely to undergo the genetic testing.[7] Partnerships and information sharing will be necessary to ensure that all those who work with genetic tests are providing the most accurate information to consumers and are equipped to answer any questions or concerns related to the genetic test being offered.

As public knowledge of and familiarity with the field grows, so too might consumers' willingness to test and use the information in the privacy of one's own home. One option could be to deliver paper results with an official seal of a trusted health association. However, business case studies have already shown that even with the best intentions of maximizing the benefits and minimizing the risks of a new science and technology, not all innovations will prove socially acceptable. Ideally, science, ethics, and the law working in concert could lay the foundation needed to ensure optimal social outcomes and public acceptance of this new technology.[8]

## 15.5 CONCLUSION AND PRINCIPLES FOR EFFECTIVE COMMUNICATION RELATED TO PERSONALIZED NUTRITION

Communicating the promise of personalized nutrition can be exciting and almost intoxicating for professionals working in the field. However, it is important to temper this enthusiasm with the reality of the pace of scientific discovery. Other chapters highlight some of the foremost international experts on nutrigenomics, and their research has uncovered fascinating implications for diet and gene expression. Yet, the scientific community would be the first to emphasize that there is more to discover about which genes are most important to our health and which may be impacted by nutrition. It is important to continue to communicate what we know about the promise of personalized nutrition, while at the same time communicating the limitations of that knowledge. Reports of scientific advances in this field should be accompanied by enough context to communicate the pieces of the puzzle that are still missing. Although the science continues to emerge, effective communication can help us move further down that road and avoid the obstacles that misinformation can create.

There are both challenges and opportunities in communicating the potential health benefits of foods and food components and how they ultimately may be associated with the practice of personalized nutrition. Overall, awareness of genomics is broad and interest is high, especially in regard to definitive tests for treatable medical conditions. At the same time, few adults have sufficient knowledge regarding genomics, leaving many unaware of the potential benefits to personal health or worse, vulnerable to misinformation. Moreover, the American public has a number of latent concerns that could quiet enthusiasm or even turn the tide against the entire field of genomics. According to the CGAT survey conducted by Cogent Research as well as the IFIC survey, *Consumer Attitudes toward Functional Foods/Foods for Health*, much of the American public is interested in using their personal genetic information to optimize their overall health through personalized nutrition. Communications about personalized nutrition should focus on balancing consumers' expectations with the reality of the science by not overpromising on potential outcomes. As applications of personalized nutrition become more widespread, it will be important to communicate both consumer benefits as well as address concerns. To build support, stakeholders, such as government, industry, health professionals, and others, need to work together to communicate effectively with each other and the public to increase knowledge of the benefits associated with personalized nutrition.

Consumers are primed for personalized messages about foods that provide benefits beyond basic nutrition and how to incorporate these foods into their diet. Because of this research finding and the fact that most Americans feel hopeful and curious about emerging science, a door is open for communicators to deliver more information that increases the understanding of personalized nutrition and helps consumers enjoy health-promoting foods as part of an overall healthful lifestyle. Keeping the consumer in mind, and adherence to the following communication principles, will be vital to consumer acceptance and success of personalized nutrition.

## 15.6 FUTURE PERSPECTIVES

The line of communication is not always a straight path. Americans acquire health and nutrition information from numerous sources. It is important for everyone in the communication chain to provide consistent and scientifically accurate information to consumers as they begin to apply this new technology.

To aid in this process, the IFIC Foundation partnered with the Institute of Food Technologists (IFT) to develop the *Guidelines for Communicating the Emerging Science of Dietary Components for Health*. These guidelines provide communicators with a checklist to help enhance the public's understanding of emerging science and the role it plays in overall health.[9] Communicators, ranging from health professionals, educators, scientists, scientific journal editors, government officials, and journalists, should consider these points when translating how the latest research about food and nutrition, including personalized nutrition, could change what is on the public's plate:

- Serve up plain talk about food and health.
- State that scientific research is evolutionary, not revolutionary.
- Carefully craft communications.
- Make messages meaningful.
- Cite study specifics.
- Point out the peer-review process as a key measure of a study's objectivity.
- Consider the full facts when assessing a study's objectivity.

One of the best ways to improve the public's understanding of personalized nutrition is to put partnerships in place that provide clear and consistent communication messages. Multiple communicators conveying the same messages increase the likelihood that those messages will resonate with consumers. It is particularly important that these partnerships be created while the science is still developing and less information has been imparted to consumers. These partnerships can help to ensure that the first information consumers receive, related to the applications and benefits of personalized nutrition, is the most accurate information.

## KEY READINGS

Borra, S., Kelly, L., Tuttle, M., and Neville, K. Developing actionable dietary guidance messages: dietary fat as a case study. *J Am Diet Assoc.* 2001; 101: 678–684.

International Food Information Council. 2005 Functional Foods/Foods for Health Executive Summary. July 2006. http://www.ific.org/research/funcfoodsres05.cfm. Accessed on January 22, 2007.

International Food Information Council Foundation. Tools for Effective Communication: Beginning a New Conversation with Consumers. http://www.ific.org/tools/intro.cfm. Accessed on January 22, 2007.

Kaput, J. et al. The case for strategic international alliances to harness nutritional genomics for public and personal health. *Br J Nutr.* 2005; 94: 623–632.

Sanderson, S.C., Wardle, J., Jarvis, M., and Humphries, S. Public interest in genetic testing for susceptibility to heart disease and cancer: a population-based survey in the U.K. *Prev Med.* 2004; 39: 458–464.

U.S. Department of Health and Human Services, National Institutes of Health, National Cancer Institute, *Making Health Communication Programs Work*, Bethesda, MD, 2001.

## REFERENCES

1. Institute of Medicine. Nutrigenomics and Beyond: Informing the Future. Nutrigenomics Workshop Presentations July 1–2, 2006. www.iom.edu/CMS/3788/31286/33150/35223.aspx. Accessed on December 18, 2006.
2. Department of Health and Human Services. Secretary's Advisory Committee on Genetics, Health, and Society. http://www4.od.nih.gov/oba/sacghs/sacghsdocuments.html. Accessed on December 28, 2006.
3. Burgess, M. Starting on the right foot: public consultation to inform issue definition in genome policy. Electronic Working Paper Series. W. Maurice Young Centre for Applied Ethics, University of British Columbia. 2003.
4. Human Genetics Commission, Human Genetics Commission Fifth Report from April 2005 to March 2006. www.hgc.gov.uk/UploadDocs/DocPub/Document/Final%20PDF.pdf. Accessed on December 19, 2006.
5. Dominick, L., Frosch, P.M., and Caryn, L. Behavioral consequences of testing for obesity risk. *Cancer Epidemiol Biomarkers Prev.* 2005; 14(6): 1485–1489.
6. Debusk, R., Fogarty, C.P., Ordovas, J.M., and Kornman, K.S. Nutritional genomics in practice: where do we begin? *J Am Diet Assoc.* 2005; 105: 589–598.
7. Bowen, D.J., Battuello, K.M., and Raats, M. Marketing genetic tests. *Health Educ Behav.* 2005; 32(5): 676–685.
8. Kaput, J. and Rodriquez, R. Nutrients and norms: ethical issues in nutritional genomics in *Nutrition Genomics Discovering the Path to Personalized Nutrition.* Wiley, 2006, pp. 419–434.
9. International Food Information Council Foundation, Institute of Food Technologists. Guidelines for communicating the emerging science of dietary components for health. 2005. www.ific.org/nutrition/functional/guidelines/guidelinesfulldoc.cfm. Accessed on December 19, 2006.

# 16 Ethics of Personalized Nutrition

*Michiel Korthals*

## CONTENTS



## 16.1 INTRODUCTION

Personalized nutrition focuses on the value of health in choosing food, and prejudges an individualizing policy instead of a public health nutrition policy; it is faced with many uncertainties and is difficult to reconcile with research outcomes. Personalized nutrition raises many issues of ethical concern. The three main issues are mostly approached from a utilitarianist or rights-based perspective of individual autonomy (informed consent or informed choice) that aims at protecting individuals against harmful interventions. However, it is also fruitful to develop a more collective and proactive ethical perspective, because of the collective consequences of individual choices. The first ethical issue is that of the relationship between food and health (drugs), which is at present subject to rather strict regulation. Owing to the rise of nutrigenomics, new gray zones emerge, for instance, when food becomes a preventive drug or when drugs are used by nonpatients, as in the case of enhancement medicine. There are no compelling arguments against new developments, but we are in need of debate about coping with the ethical impacts. The second issue is that of the relations between personalized and public health nutrition, which requires new responsibilities of both consumers and producers in incorporating health concerns into pluralist food styles. The third one covers ethical issues of making use of personalized nutrition and requires consultations between consumers and professionals. Moreover, independent gatekeepers are necessary to safeguard the independence of testing, marketing, communicating, and providing the services.

In the 1980s, nutrigenomics started with the idea of improving general diets of inhabitants of Western countries. By enhancing the quality of food such as common crops and meat products, the goal was to raise the quality of public health. It was the time of "vitamin-enriched food" and sugar beets without sweets, or, as the article in *Time* of June 1999 said, guilt-free, nondigestible sugar: "Sweet Taste of Success." Genetic engineers in Holland claim they have finally come up with the holy grail of the food industry: a plant that provides sugar and can be used to make nonfattening and guilt-free cakes. Unlike normal sugar beet, whose content is easily digested, a new form has been created that can make fructans, sugars that come in long molecule chains that are more difficult for the body to absorb [1]. Even 8 years later, this guilt-free sugar beet still does not exist, so the promise of the engineers was made a bit too early.

Nevertheless, very soon after the promising start on the level of public health (compare Reference 2), nutrigenomics made a more individualizing turn toward personalized nutrition, with the idea that genetic profiles differ very much, and that the genetic profile of individual consumers should determine what they eat. Personalized nutrition has, in a certain sense, already a long history as part of public health nutrition policies, particularly during industrialization because of the health condition of the urban labor force. General practitioners made "food charts" that signaled food deficiencies [3]. Food diseases were proved to be connected with bad food and undernourishment, and good food could cure these diseases.

However, nowadays personalized nutrition nutrigenomics is driven by *individual prevention*, not the cure, of food-related risks such as vitamin deficiencies, alcoholism, obesity, allergies, and food-related diseases such as diabetes mellitus type 2, hypertension, gallstones, osteoporosis, problems of lipid metabolism, and cancer. Overweight is, in particular, a case in point that is said to be preventable by individualized nutrition. The World Health Organization (WHO) wrote a report in 2004 in which it was stated that in 2020, 50% of the world population is expected to become overweight. For instance, in the U.S., in general, 15 to 20% of the adults in some states are obese, and in some even more than 25% of the inhabitants (BMI > 30) are obese. The personal factors that determine overweight and obesity are the imbalance between energy intake and expenditure because of high intake of saturated fat and sugar; but inactivity (computer and television), social economic factors such as urbanization, educational level of parents, and the lifestyle of parents do play a role as well [4,5,6].

In this chapter I will first analyze the main structure of personalized nutrition, which covers fours aspects: laying bare general relationships between genetic profiles, organisms, and environment such as food intake and lifestyle; testing and screening of individuals to understand their vulnerabilities; giving personal nutrition advice to individuals and, lastly, producing innovative food products. I will next describe two ethical perspectives that in literature on food and health are mostly mentioned, i.e., the utilitarianist perspective of individual autonomy (informed consent or informed choice) and the rights-based (Kantian) and communicative perspective that develops a more collective ethical outlook emphasizing the collective consequences of individual choices. I will subsequently show that personalized nutrition focuses on the value of health in food choice, and seems to prejudge an individualizing policy instead of a public health nutrition policy; this focus results in three main areas of ethical concern. The first is the relationship between food and health (or food and drugs), the second is the relations between personalized and public health nutrition, and the third issue covers items that emerge in making use of personalized nutrition. I will finish with future prospects of personalized nutrition and its ethics.

## 16.2 OPENING THE BLACK BOX OF PERSONALIZED NUTRITION

The first assumption of personalized nutrition is that food is predominantly not seen as positive, having pleasurable features or even as neutral, but as having impacts on human health in the long run in preventing or even accelerating risks for diseases such as cardiovascular diseases, cancer, and allergies. The second main idea is that people should choose their diet on the basis of their genetic profile and that diet-induced diseases should be detected as early as possible and should be prevented by a change in diet.

Personalized nutrition covers four aspects (see also Reference 7). The first aspect is the complex relationship between the genetic makeup of individuals and their food intake. Second, the screening and testing of an individual to find out in how far he or she runs any risk. To this aspect belong questions such as, how to interpret the chances and how to share this information with your relatives, who are possibly affected as well. Another question is the privacy of the screening and test results. Third, there is the personalized advice to eat in a certain way, or more broadly, to follow a healthy life style that this same person gets from some professional. The fourth aspect covers the products (foods or drugs) that are the innovative fruits of nutrigenomics research. These products again can have multiple effects, and it is often unclear in how far these are taken into account. Long-term health effects of products are mostly not tested, and therefore not known.

## 16.3 TWO ETHICAL PERSPECTIVES

Everyone wants to be healthy, but many of us differ in what role health should play in life, what the meaning of health is, and also refuse to act in healthy ways. What bearing, if any, should our food, health, and life choices have on the ethics and policy of food production, food regulation, clinical practice, and health policy? What do personal freedom, responsibility, and solidarity mean here? Should risk-takers have the same claim on scarce resources, such as organs for transplant, as those whose plight is owing to no choices of their own?

With respect to the issues at hand, we can discern at least two ethical perspectives that are rather common now in medical ethics and can shed some light on nutrigenomics oriented toward personalized nutrition. The first one emphasizes the protection of consumer/citizens by viewing all ethical issues from the point of view of informed consent or informed choice, i.e., from the point of view of individual freedom and autonomy, which seeks to limit social powers that threaten to transgress the boundaries of privacy and of private freedom. Although issues of justice, i.e., the socially fair distribution of resources plays a role here, the idea is primarily that social powers should not be allowed to dominate individual consumers. Patients and consumers should be enabled to protect themselves against powers that invade their personal responsibility, by giving them rights [8]. In the alternative model, the emphasis is on coordination and interaction between consumers, producers, and other stakeholders, which means that individual consent and choice can play a role, but in the social context of interaction and social learning, and of distributing responsibilities according to issues and needs. Consultations and deliberations with stakeholders (as a matter of fact, including consumers) to pinpoint agreement and disagreement play an important role here. The aim is not to protect patients and consumers against professional powers; patients and consumers are invited and encouraged to take part in consultations and are given the opportunity to tell their narratives, interests, and anxieties.

In both models, the concept of autonomy plays a pivotal role; however, in the first as individual autonomy and, in the second, as social or collective autonomy.

The first concept of individual autonomy (and protection) is more connected to utilitarianism, which emphasizes individual utility and happiness as the most important criterion for the outcome of ethical decisions. The concept of personal autonomy lies at the heart of the utilitarian doctrine of, for example, John Stuart Mill (1806–1873)[9]:

> The only freedom which deserves the name is that of pursuing our own good in our own way, so long as we do not attempt to deprive others of theirs, or impede their efforts to obtain it. Each is the proper guardian of his own health, whether bodily, or mental or spiritual [10].

As long as one can do what one thinks is in favor of one's own health and as long as one does not harm others, then actions are ethically seen allowed. Harm toward others is the category that marks the distinction between personal autonomy and social life, and harm is the indicator that something is ethically wrong. This means that individuals first and foremost should be protected from the harmful actions of others or should be enabled to protect themselves from those harmful actions.

Of the two alternative models, the second one, of social autonomy, is directly linked to the German philosopher Immanuel Kant (1724–1804) [11], the foremost thinker of autonomy. Kant thinks more positively than Mills about the relation between individual and society, in terms of enrichment and humanization and not in terms of harm. Kant argues:

> Laziness and cowardice are the reasons why such a large part of humanity, even long after nature has liberated it from foreign control (*naturaliter maiorennes*), is still happy to remain infantile during its entire life, making it so easy for others to act as its keeper. It is so easy to be infantile. If I have a book that is wisdom for me, a therapist or preacher who serves as my conscience, *a doctor who prescribes my diet*, then I do not

> need to worry about these myself. I do not need to think, as long as I am willing to pay [11] (my italics).

As food choices are a component of one's autonomy, consumers should determine their own food (diet); as a consequence, the food markets and food professionals should follow suit, and they should act as our keeper. Only paying for your food, without acting according to your autonomy, is a sign of infantility, or of having no control over your mouth. Autonomy not only encompasses what goes out of the mouth but also what goes into the mouth.

Kant gives some more interesting clues on what "autonomous food choice" means elsewhere [12]. In general, he considers humans to be subject to both Nature and Reason. Man has neither only capacities from nature nor capacities from reason but from both, where nature stands for passions and sensual experience and reason for transcending nature by using the reasoning faculty in knowing, willing, and appreciating (judging). For instance, enjoying art and food socially means transcending nature by assessing something that is given and subsequently structured according to the judgmental structure that you share with other rational beings. This type of (communicative) assessing is what autonomy means, so autonomy has nothing to do with informed consent or choosing or doing what you want. Human beings are involved in a development toward standing on their own feet, although hesitating and stumbling. Taste has, according to Kant, the extraordinary feature that it stimulates solidarity in enjoying. Enjoying food is related to culture and society. But there is more. A good meal enjoyed over a long period with congenial people is an occasion where experience and reason are united and which can be repeated again and again. Through having common meals, reason acts upon the experiences, because they stimulate solidarity and humanity. Meals are a stimulus to come together and share your thoughts with other rational beings. Kant takes into account that we do not have the same taste for food: some like this and others like that. However, he introduces the concept of comparative universality to make clear that on closer inspection, by experiencing and talking, many of our tastes overlap. *Comparative universality* is a term that refers to the narrative overlapping of our food preferences. It recognizes both that taste is personal, which you have to personally recognize in food, and that tastes have some commonality, proved by the fact that we enjoy the meal together [12, p. 567].

## 16.4 THREE MAIN AREAS OF ETHICAL CONCERN

On the basis of these ethical perspectives one can discern at least three main areas of ethical issues connected with nutrigenomics-based personalized nutrition. With these two perspectives in mind, we can tackle the three main areas of ethical concern connected with nutrigenomics.

### 16.4.1 The Relationship between Food and Health (Drugs)

The first area of ethical concern covers the relationship between food and health or between food and drugs, and addresses all the aspects of personalized nutrition mentioned earlier. Although there has always been in the past some overlap between food and health (see the case of food in curing diseases), in general, the distinction between the two up to now has been rather strict. The most important distinctions between food and health (drugs) are located in the dimensions of personal lives, culture, politics, organizations, and market forces. First, food is for everyone, drugs only for the ill; food should not have too severe negative effects, because of its lifelong intake, and drugs sometimes have (acceptable) negative effects because of their temporary intake; food choices involve multiple reasons, whereas drugs are chosen for only one reason (to be cured); foods are freely available for all, and drugs only on prescription; and finally, food is not tested for efficacy, but only for safety, whereas drugs are tested for both efficacy and safety. When food is indeed becoming a drug in a preventive way, it is possible for persons to get side effects caused by their food choice; they are expected to choose their food only for health reasons; they should consult their physicians before eating and have to learn new types of behavior that redistribute responsibilities, duties, and rights in a fundamental way. People will have to deal with the blurring of these important cultural, political, personal, social, and scientific distinctions and their ethical implications [14,15] (Table 16.1).

People have a complex set of considerations governing their food choice, which are different from the considerations that determine their use of drugs. At least four factors determine our food preferences, in general: genetic factors, social and cultural factors, bodily history, and personal historical factors [17]. The genetic factors, depending on genetic makeup, are generally not changeable; they determine taste in general (like bitter and sweet) and, partially, taste development. The social and cultural factors consist of determining organizational structures and values, such as family relationships and health or nationalistic values. The bodily history influences tongue and mouth, but also nose and ear, which are part and parcel of food choices. When one is tasting food, one is also tasting one's own body. Finally, there are

**TABLE 16.1**
**Some Differences between Food and Drugs**

| | Food | Drugs |
|---|---|---|
| 1. Side effects | Not accepted | Accepted |
| 2. For whom? | All | Groups of patients |
| 3. Choice | Multiple reasons (lifestyle) | Health reasons |
| 4. Time taken | Over lifetime | During illnesses |
| 5. Delivery | Freely available | Over-the-counter/prescription |
| 6. Activities | Shopping, talking, preparing, sharing | Pill taking |
| 7. Testing | Safety, not efficacy | Safety and efficacy |
| 8. Production | Food companies, farmers (open production systems) | Drug companies: closed lab |
| 9. Responsibility | Governments and food sector | Physicians, drug companies, governments |
| 10. Trust [16] | Low trust in sector | Sector trusted |

personal historical factors, such as the family history and how it is internalized. Moreover, when actually having a meal, additional factors do play a role as well, such as the present conditions of the meal, the present condition of the body, and the actual pleasure and displeasure in tasting. Gustatory taste and food choice are strongly intentional and cognitive: it matters what one eats and to know what one eats. They comprise the visual, the smell (olfactory), tongue senses (gustatory), and the auditory (e.g., crunchy or not). The fact that taste is cognitive implies that taste can be learned, and can develop in a certain direction. A yellowish substance with a rotting smell turns suddenly into a delicious cheese upon tasting it, preferable with nice and knowledgeable people.

More generally, in the domains of food and health culture, politics, science, and society, the most important distinctions between food and drugs are that food is for everyone, drugs only for the diseased; that food should not have negative effects, because of its lifelong intake, and drugs sometimes have (acceptable) negative effects because of their temporary intake; that food choices are motivated by multiple reasons (see earlier text) and drugs by only one (to be cured or protected); that food is freely available and drugs only on prescription available, and that food is not tested for efficacy, but only for safety.

However, from an ethical point of view, objections against the identification of food and health (drugs) can be heard; for example, food should not be seen as a drug and society is not a hospital, meaning that health should not be the all-determining value in food choices. For instance, Crawford [18] warns of the medicalization of daily life, which leads to a narrowing of perspective. As an observer notices: "For some decades the doctor–patient relationship has been the central concern of medical ethics. This focus has marginalized public health issues by concentrating on individual patients and individual practitioners, and thereby on one aspect of medical structures in the richer parts of the world" [19]. The British Food Ethics Council views the exclusive orientation on health in food choices as a transformation of society into a hospital [20], which is in the case of prevention of obesity not desirable and not necessary as well, because physical activity is a good recommendation as well [21]. Petrini [22], the founder of Slowfood, and a fierce defender of the social and cultural aspects of enjoying food, quotes Madame Sevigny approvingly, "Health is enjoying the other enjoyments. When the other enjoyments are taken away, we live longer, but we lose our health. "

However, because of the development of the food sciences, traditional truths regarding healthy food collapse: the health value of wine, chocolate, vegetable oils, and milk are reevaluated. Food intake should correspond with changes in lifestyles: What to eat in the new situation of sedentary work and other changing social contexts?

The exact boundaries between food and health (drugs) are unclear, and there have always some blurred boundaries (the ancient Greek thinker Hippocrates said: "Let food be your medicine!"[23]. Moreover, we are facing now two new gray areas: food as drugs and drugs as enhancements, and we cannot eliminate them. This means that the relationship between food and drugs needs to be reconsidered: the refusal to reconsider the traditional distinction between food and drugs looks like sheer dogmatism. Even with Kant [11] in hand, one could argue thus: There is a difference

**TABLE 16.2**
**New Gray Zones between Food and Drugs**

| | Food | Drugs | Gray Zone: Food as Drugs and Drugs for Nonpatients (modafinil, Ritalin, enhancement drugs) |
|---|---|---|---|
| 1. Side effects | Not accepted | Accepted | ?? |
| 2. For whom? | Everybody | Groups of patients | Quasi patients |
| 3. Choice | Multiple reasons | Health reasons | Health prevention, enhancement |
| 4. Time taken | Over lifetime | During illnesses | Preventive against susceptibilities; over lifetime |
| 5. Delivery | Freely available | Over the counter | Both |
| 6. Testing | Only safety, not efficacy | Safety and efficacy | ? |
| 7. Activities | Shopping, talking, preparing, sharing | Taking pills | Testing, getting advice, shopping |
| 8. Production | Food companies, farmers (open production systems) | Drug companies: Closed lab | Mixed drugs in greenhouses/ pharmadrugs |
| 9. Responsibility | Governments and food sector | Physicians, drug companies, governments | ?? |
| 10. Trust | Sector not highly trusted | Sector trusted | ? |

between obeying a physician and taking into account the advice of experts on food. Moreover, the Eurobarometer [16] shows that the association of food with health is in the EU only made by one person in five; the idea that society should transform into a hospital is not very realistic. As long as health remains one of the considerations in food choice and supply, and the multiple functions of food stay in place, there is some reason to reconsider the intricate relationship between the two [14]. When personal nutrition on a modest scale is implemented, then the first area of ethical concern can be overcome, is our final assessment. This allows for reflection on the new gray zones between food and health when personalized nutrition on a modest scale is implemented in certain fields. This reflection can begin by analyzing the second and third main areas of ethical concern (Table 16.2).

### 16.4.2 The Second Main Area of Ethical Concern: The Relationship between Personalized and Public Health Food Policies

The second main area of ethical concern is the relationship between personalized or individualized nutrition and social or public nutrition (and health). Many argue on the basis of ethical and empirical arguments that a population or public health nutrition and public health policy should have precedence over an individualist health approach for reasons of efficacy [24] or for ethical reasons [25]. Moreover, they argue that personal nutrition and health care have collective effects. When most rich people in the Western world only want personal nutrition and care, the danger emerges that the public nutrition and health system will seriously be damaged as a result of a kind of personal/collective dilemma [18]. We will run the risk that the food and medical problems of the poor in the West and the South will be neglected because the richer people all will choose according to their own personal nutrition and health projects. Because of these enormous collective effects, personalized nutrition is not only a personal decision up to the individual, but affects the whole population. Social responsibility seems to require that the whole population be considered. For instance, it is a well-known fact that socioeconomic status (SES) and health expectancy are strongly linked. The rich always have more opportunities to look after their health than the poor and have therefore a longer life expectancy. International public health (for example, World Health Organization [4]) aims at improving health on a populational level. How far should personal responsibility for health be taken into account in setting the agenda for national and global public health nutrition policies, and what role has collective responsibility to play?

The answer of many food scientists and food industrialists to this question is that personalized nutrition and its concomitants, such as a gene passport, comprising the results of screening and testing, are means of individual empowerment and should replace public health nutrition policies [26,27]. Moreover, insurance companies and many governments are of the opinion that consumers should take more responsibility for their health and not rely too much on governmental health regulations. They are arguing: "You're responsible to do what is healthy" and call this self-control and autonomy (see the Blair government paper [28]).

However, some food companies are rather hesitant to enter the market of personalized nutrition. In an adjacent field, that of personalized medicine, which is already more developed, it is very often the case that personalized medicines are not commercially viable. Personalized medicine means that companies will have to be content with only a (small) share of the market and cannot cover all the (potential) patients. As a result, few new pharmagenomic drugs are filed for license in the U.S. According to the FDA [29], the number of new drugs and biological applications submitted to it has declined significantly. Moreover, the U.K.-based Public Health Association [25] argues in its reaction to the Blair government's policies [28] that public health should be the main target of governmental policies. This association argues that in the long run the poorer parts of the population, and health itself, will lose in a health and food system in which individual responsibility is the main organizing principle [31]. In the same vein, Lang [24] also makes a strong case for the primacy of public vs. individualized health nutrition politics. "Targeting whole populations provide governments with better chances of public health success, whereas targeting 'at risk' individuals could be socially divisive" [24, p. 110]. But in the end he concedes that "individual tendencies" [24, p. 120] do have to play a role in a public health system.

Moreover, from an ethical point of view, one could argue with Kant [11] that personalized nutrition in the sense of a gene passport or chart means disempowerment and not enrichment of social autonomy, because one makes oneself dependent on a physician. Only as a socially autonomous member of a rational community can personalized nutrition be given a try, and the issues boil down to the balanced relationship between autonomy and solidarity, not an either/or relationship [14].

Concluding, there are some arguments in favor of personalized nutrition, as long as it does not displace public health nutrition [30]. Also, from a utilitarian standpoint, there is place for personalized nutrition as long as individual responsibility can defray the costs.

### 16.4.3 Third Main Area of Ethical Concern: Personalized Nutrition for the Consumer

Granted that there is indeed a role for personalized nutrition in health, we are faced with ethical issues concerning the development of personalized nutrition, such as the protection of privacy (input, use, and sharing of databases) and misuse of information (as in the example on the DNA pill hype; this concerns the second and third aspect of personalized nutrition); the regulation of health claims (regarding the fourth aspect of personalized nutrition, i.e., the development of foods); and the balance of personal and social responsibility (regarding the second, third, and fourth aspects). Also, issues related to communication on personalized services and products such as claims, right to know and not to know, and informed consent need to be discussed. Preparation for optimal consumer protection brings up issues related to intellectual property and equal access. On the level of food choice, expression of identity with food and the functions of food other than for staying healthy will with personalized nutrition undergo dramatic changes that will challenge established ethical routines [31]. The notion of personal responsibility for health is vulnerable to intentional manipulation by self-interested (commercially interested) parties [36,37].

The scientific peculiarities of personalized nutrition and nutrigenomics, in particular, the huge complexities of the interactions between genome, genetic profiles, and environments, such as diets and lifestyles, reduce severely the possibility of reproducing experiments in other locations, because food and lifestyles differ so much and are difficult to exclude [32,33]. It means that validation and falsification of scientific relationships are confronted with extremely difficult and expensive research designs. Nutrigenomics is not about a single relationship between a single gene and its expression, but about the reactive genome, contextualizing at all levels. Genes influence the expression of other genes in proteins and the organism and *vice versa*, so the genome is not one, stable, all-determining commando post. Food has multiple effects on the genetic profile, and is dependent on the food choices, which in turn are influenced by lifestyle factors. It is not only that risks abound, such as the now established connection between smoking and increased chance of lung cancer, but also that ambiguities are quite normal; for example, two glasses of wine give a higher risk of breast cancer but a lower risk of cardiovascular disease. However, so far this evidence, which has led to some widely promoted dietary recommendations, has come from mainly observational epidemiologic studies. The complexity of multifactorial diseases and other interwoven complex causal relations between genetic factors, omics factors, and the environment (lifestyle, social context) confronts ethics with the necessity of transforming itself from a "taken for granted" discipline to a "searching and experimenting discipline." Ethics will need to incorporate these uncertainties and ambiguities into the use of nutrigenomics services and products in the daily life of consumers, in adequate policy measures and in ethical acceptable research agendas for research institutes.

An ethics for consumers can draw inspiration from Kant's adage, "don't obey your doctor" [11], which in a certain sense is right, but does not assist in establishing the new necessary connections between food and health (drugs). The traditional ethical concepts such as "informed choice" and "individual responsibility" are not adequate for this new task [10]. When the collective implications of the individual choice for personalized nutrition are so huge, more collective ways of opinion and decision making should be tried in which all stakeholders have to readjust their opinions and interests according to the ongoing discussion. This implies that the ethics of protection of the individual against the apparently mighty powers of state and professionals is not appropriate; more desirable is an ethics of participation in continuous discussion on the intricacies of nutrigenomics.

Moreover, consumers need an ethics of dealing with uncertainties in the sense of identifying and selecting between important, major, minor, and unimportant choices. There are no general tools or guidelines to deal with that process of selection, but there are general procedures such as consultations, deliberations, and exchange of war stories and anecdotes. The main purpose of these procedures is to discern commonalities and particularities in your own life and that of other affected individuals (Kant's comparative universality! [12]). Some ethical support can be given by Putnam's distinction between commonsense doubt, meaning the selecting of more and less certain cases, and philosophical doubt, i.e., the radical denial of all certainties, which is most of the time not meaningful [34]:

> We have to remind ourselves of the distinction between common sense doubt and philosophical doubt. Finishing in believing in something is not really a human possibility. Criticism cannot be a reason for universal skepticism. The fact that sometimes we are wrong is not a reason to really doubt every particular conviction.

The reason that informed choice is not a good ethical concept in this context has to do with the fact that it does not say anything about selecting the more certain and less certain recommendations and the incorporation of well-established health considerations into one's diet and personal health. The needed ethics of cooperation between consumers and professionals and of sharing life experiences implies that consumer groups should try to bridge the gap between production and consumption of food and new technologies and to incorporate the new health considerations into their food style together with the main stakeholders such as governments and food industry [35].

With respect to the ethics for governments and their food policy, the uncertainties in the gray zone between food and health are best tackled not by prohibiting the gray zone but by regulating these on a social and technological level (coevolution) [14]. Governments should organize the research agenda of nutrigenomics in a democratic way, not exclusively oriented toward personalized nutrition, but oriented toward the prevention of common illnesses, common conditions, and chronic diseases. There is a role to play for public health nutrigenomics, directed at general risk profiles. Governments should regulate the three sectors, food, drugs and the newly emerging gray zone, improve research ethics and medical testing of health foods, and allow only affordable health foods. Its main aim in nutrition policy should be the encouragement of the formal and informal ties between pleasurable eating and fundamental health. Health should be a secondary goal in eating, and consumers and their associations should be empowered as stakeholders (most trusted according to Reference 16: 33%) and be given a voice not only downstream of nutrigenomics (with respect to the end products) but also upstream of the nutrigenomics research agenda. To tackle the issue of easy expectations and hype, it is necessary to establish independent gatekeepers to safeguard the independency of testing, marketing, communicating, and providing the services of nutrigenomics. Trust of citizen-consumers in the food and health sector can be best maintained by the establishment and maintenance of independent bodies fixing and monitoring rules with respect to claims.

With respect to ethics for scientists, scientists are in need of codes of practice governing forward ethically acceptable research agendas and validating nutrigenomics scientific claims. Research focusing on common illnesses should not be disrupted, as also research on affordable and common drugs and food. Making healthy food accessible for everyone remains an important challenge for nutrigenomics.

Of course, these three areas overlap with each other; how far food should be connected with health considerations, or even identified with it, is both an issue for collective consideration as well as a personal affair. The issue of responsibility is also to be considered in these three main areas. But some issues (such as those of the last area) demand more individualistic concepts, such as informed consent and autonomy and protection, and others more collective ethical concerns such as trust and justice.

## 16.5 FUTURE PERSPECTIVES

Nutrigenomics has still an uncertain future, and a lot depends on the interaction of research developments and priorities, prospects for profits, and ethical concerns. An important first issue to be settled for the future of nutrigenomics is the relationship between food and health (drugs). Although there are good reasons to be careful and to make this distinction, there is room for taking into account new connections between food and health; this gray zone is in need of regulation and requires additional attention on the part of consumers and producers. Attention is in particular needed so that health does not socially and personally function as the only motive behind food choices, and health policies should not move in that direction. Second, the issue of the relation of public health vs. personalized nutrition requires a balance between solidarity and individual autonomy. In many societies, one is motivated to look for such a balance, and only processes of continuous consultation and deliberation can find out what this implies. It is unmistakably the case that a more personal appeal to customers of food and medicine to incorporate recent health standards into their food styles can have some effect. From this perspective, it seems ethically desirable that consumers learn to cope with the hype [36,37], the uncertainties, and relative certainties of this new approach to identifying and selecting their chief vulnerabilities and be able to incorporate these in their narrative life plans. This implies not only room for informed choice, but also for consultations and deliberations on these uncertainties. The ethics of these issues is still in its infancy, because until now the ethics of food (and of health) has had a strong defensive, and not proactive outlook. However, from a public health point of view, the potentialities of nutrigenomics in improving the health of the population, in particular of the least well off, should be developed as well. Governmental policies and research institutes should allow their research agendas to be shaped not only by personalized nutrition but by common nutritional issues as well.

## KEY READINGS

Castle, D., Cheryl Cline, Abdallah S. Daar, Peter A. Singer, and Charoula Tsamis, 2006, *Science, Society and the Supermarket : The Opportunities and Challenges of Nutrigenomics*, Wiley.

Food Ethics Council, 2005, *Getting Personal: Shifting Responsibilities for Health*, Brighton.

Korthals, M., 2004, *Before Dinner: Philosophy and Ethics of Food*, Springer, Berlin.

Korthals, M. (Ed.), *Genomics and Obesity*, Dordrecht, Springer, forthcoming.

Müller, M. and Kersten, S., 2003, Nutrigenomics: goals and strategies, *Nature Reviews Genetics*, 4, 4, 315–322.

## REFERENCES

1. *TIMES*, Sweet Taste of Success, June 24, 1999.
2. Della Penna, D., Nutritional genomics: manipulating plant micronutrients to improve human health, *Science* 285: 375–379, 1999.
3. Porter, R., *The Greatest Benefit of Mankind*, Norton, New York, 1999.
4. WHO (2004): Global strategy on diet, physical activity and health. Fifty-seventh World Health Assembly. WHA57.17. May 22, 2004; WHO (2005): The Bangkok Charter for health Promotion in a Globalized World. WHO, August 2005. Available on www.who.int.
5. Friedman, J.F., Modern science versus the stigma of obesity. *Nature Medicine*, 10(6): 563–569, 2004.
6. Roth, J., Qiang, X. et al., The obesity pandemic: where have we been and where are we going? *Obesity Research* 12(Suppl.): 88S–100S, 2004.
7. Kaput, J. and Rodriguez, R.L., Nutritional genomics: the next frontier in the postgenomic era. *Physiological Genomics*. 16, 166–177. PMID: 14726599, 2004.
8. Chadwick, R., Nutrigenomics, individualism and public health. *Proceedings of the Nutrition Society*, 63(1): 161–6, 2004.
9. For a general discussion on utilitarianism and other ethical perspectives. Singer, P., *Practical Ethics*, Cambridge University Press, Cambridge, 1979; 2nd ed., 1993.
10. Mill, J.S., *On Liberty*, Oxford, Oxford University Press, 1859, 1978.
11. Kant, I., What is enlightenment?, Guyer, P. Ed. *The Cambridge Companion to Kant*. Cambridge University Press, 1992. Translation from 'Was ist Aufklärung?' 1785.
12. Kant, I., Anthropologie in pragmatischer Hinsicht (Anthropology from Pragmatic Point of View) (1798/1790), idem, Kants Werke, Darmstadt, 1975.
13. ibidem, p. 567.
14. Korthals, M., *Before Dinner*, Dordrecht: Springer, 2004.

15. Castle, D., Cline, C., Daar, A.S., Singer, P.A., and Tsamis C., *Science, Society and the Supermarket : The Opportunities and Challenges of Nutrigenomics*, Wiley, 2006.
16. Eurobarometer, 2005, Risk issues, http://ec.europa.eu/public_opinion/archives/ebs/ebs_238_en.pdf.
17. Korsmeyer, C., Making Sense of Taste, Cornell University Press,1999; Korsmeyer doesn't take into account the personal history of tasting in listing factors that determine food preferences, p. 82, 98.
18. Crawford, R., Healthism and the medicalization of every day. *International Journal of Health Services*, Vol. 10, No. 3, 1980.
19. O'Neill, Onora, Public health or clinical ethics: thinking beyond borders, *Ethics and International Affairs*, 16, 2002.
20. Food Ethics Council, Getting personal: shifting responsibilities for health, Brighton, 2005.
21. Hillsdon, M., Foster, C., Naidoo, B., and Crombie, H., The effectiveness of public health interventions for increasing physical activity among adults: a review of reviews. Evidence briefing of the NHS Health Development Agency. www.hda.nhs.uk/evidence. 2004.
22. Petrini, *The Pleasures of Slow Food: Celebrating Authentic Traditions, Flavors and Recipes*, Chronicle Books, 2002.
23. Foucault, M., *History of Sexuality*, Vintage, Part 2, 1990.
24. Lang, T. and Heasman, M., 2005, *Foodwars*, London: Earthscan.
25. UKPHA, Public Health Association: Choosing Health or Losing Health? 2003.
26. German, J.B. and H.J. Watzke, Personalizing foods for health and delight. *Comprehensive Reviews in Food Science and Food Safety* 3: 145–151, 2004.
27. Koelen, M.A. and Lindström, B., Making healthy choices the easy choices: the role of empowerment. EJCN. 59, Suppl. 1, S10–S16, 2005.
28. U.K. Department of Health, Choosing Health, London, 2004.
29. Darnton-Hill, I., Margetts, B., and Deckelbaum, R., Public health nutrition and genetics: implications for nutrition policy and promotion, *Proceedings of the Nutrition Society*, Vol. 63, No. 1, February 2004, pp. 173–185(13).
30. Khoury, M.J. and Mensah, G.A., Genomics and the prevention and control of common chronic diseases: emerging priorities for public health action. *Prevention of Chronic Diseases* (serial online) April 2005. Available from http://www.cdc.gov/ pcd/issues/2005/apr/05_0011.htm.
31. Cain, M. and Schmid G., From nutrigenomics science to personalized nutrition: The market in 2010. The Institute for the Future, CAL.; Castle (2003). Clinical challenges posed by new biotechnology: the case of nutrigenomics. *Post-Graduate Medical Journal*, 79: 65–66, 2003.
32. Sinha, G., the diet that fits — analyzing metabolism for personalized nutrition, *Scientific American* 292(3): 22 March 2005; DeCamp, M. and Sugarman, J. (2004). Ethics and research assessing the relative roles of genes and the environment. *Accountability in Research: Policies and Quality Assurance* 11: 161–182.
33. Tate, T.K. and Goldstein, D.B., Will tomorrow 's medicines work for everyone? *Nature Genetics* 36(11): S34–S42, 2004.
34. Putnam, H., *Pragmatism: An Open Question*, Oxford: Blackwell, pp. 57–81, 1995.
35. Liakopoulos, M. and Schroeder, D., Trust and functional foods. New products, old issues, Poiesis & Praxis: *International Journal of Technology Assessment and Ethics of Science*, Vol. 2, No. 1, 41–52, 2003.
36. Meek, J., Public 'misled by gene test hype'. In *The Guardian*, March 12, 2002.
37. *BBC-News*. (July 17, 2005). DNA test for diabetes and obesity. Health. Retrieved November 7, 2005.

# Section III

## The Future of Personalized Nutrition

# 17 International Efforts on Nutrigenomic Health for Individuals in the Global Community

*Jim Kaput*

## CONTENTS

## 17.1 INTRODUCTION

Nutrigenomics is the study of how constituents of the diet interact with genes, and their products, to alter phenotype and, conversely, how genes and their products metabolize these constituents into nutrients, antinutrients, and bioactive compounds. The data and results from nutrigenomics research are predicted to provide individuals with knowledge for optimizing nutrient intakes with the goal of preventing or delaying the onset of diseases. The research and application path to personalized nutrition faces the challenges of the chemical complexity of food, genetic heterogeneity of human populations, intricacies of biological processes, and the need for new methods of analyzing high-dimensional data sets generated by omics technologies. With the success of the Human Genome and HapMap projects, many scientific disciplines are beginning to develop best practices and share data sets for understanding biological processes. A number of large-scale collaborative programs focusing on nutrient–gene interactions have been initiated within the past 3 years. Nutrigenomic researchers individually, in centers, and in multi-institutional programs have recognized the need for developing best practices, fostering international collaborations, and sharing data sets. The scientific and humanitarian need for forming a network of networks and the initial steps on that pathway are reviewed in this chapter.

The excitement caused by the unparalleled international collaborations to analyze the human genome (1,2) and its variability (3) created lofty expectations in the medical and pharmaceutical sectors, food industries, media, and informed public. Information obtained with genetic and emerging omic tests are predicted to personalize medical treatments (4), drug selection (5), and nutritional advice (6–9), and perhaps lead to the development of healthier processed foods targeted to individuals (10,11). Although many believe these goals will be realized, expectations have given way to the sobering recognition of the challenges of understanding genetic causes of complex traits such as chronic diseases and the role of environment in regulating expression of genetic makeup.

Results from genetic studies attempting to associate a gene or its variants to a disease or specific metabolic phenotype illustrate the challenges: many published gene–disease associations could not be replicated in subsequent studies [e.g., (12,13)]. This led one accomplished epidemiologist to publish a report entitled "Why Most Published Research Findings Are False" (14), identifying experimental designs where sample sizes lacked appropriate statistical power, control groups were not appropriately matched to cases, study participants had differing genetic admixtures (populations stratification), and data that were overinterpreted (among others, see References 15 to 18). Researchers working at the intersection of nutrition and genetics added that diet–gene interactions are major contributors to the control of gene expression and could influence associations among genes–phenotype and dietary intake (7,19–21). Reaching the goal of personalized nutrition will require an understanding of the scientific challenges of identifying nutrient–gene interactions involved in health or disease development and realistic solutions to surmount those challenges.

## 17.2 THE SCIENTIFIC DIVERSITY CHALLENGES

### 17.2.1 Chemicals in Foods

Humans have adapted to almost every nutritional environment on earth, including northern tundra, equatorial, and high-altitude ecosystems. Based on this adaptability, one could conclude that as long as minimum amounts of energy and micronutrients were consumed, the most significant contribution to health and disease susceptibility would be one's genetic makeup, However, environment, and specifically nutrients, alters the expression of genetic makeup leading to promotion of health or the development of chronic diseases (7). The most obvious example of the importance of environment on disease is the rise in the incidence of obesity and its complications (http://www.cdc.gov/nccdphp/dnpa/obesity/) over the past 20 years. This time span is not long enough for genetic changes to cause such rapid weight gains in individuals. Rather, changes in diet and physical activity habits have produced the epidemic of obesity, type 2 diabetes (T2DM), and their complications. This conclusion is supported by traditional epidemiologic and immigration studies (e.g., Reference 22) that associate environment with chronic diseases. However, the underlying molecular mechanisms cannot be ascertained by these statistical associations.

Numerous *in vitro*, animal, and human studies have demonstrated that chemicals classified as macronutrients, such as certain fatty acids, and micronutrients such as genistein, sterols, and vitamins regulate gene expression directly (reviewed in Reference 23) or through changes in signal transduction pathways (7,24). Hence, for the specific chronic disease of obesity, overconsumption of calories (25) and subsets or specific bioactive chemicals (e.g., Reference 26) alter the regulation of genes that cause increased weight deposition in genetically susceptible individuals.

In addition to chemicals present in unprocessed foods, our diets are now greatly influenced by modern food production methods. Humans have been able to extract and recombine food chemicals for mass markets only since the onset of the industrial revolution. Designing new foods was done primarily for taste and economic purposes. Hence, it is not surprising that our current national and international food systems have not produced the most healthful foods. Nevertheless, modern food production provides enough calories and most macro- and micronutrients, at least for a large proportion of the world's population.

Regardless of the type of food, identifying the specific pathways and the effect of different amounts of these bioactive chemicals is a critical part of understanding of how diet maintains health or leads to disease in each individual. For more complete analyses of gene–disease (or phenotype) associations, studies must assess food intake as well as genetic differences. Quantifying nutrient intake in epidemiologic studies is challenging because free-living humans do not regard daily life as a science experiment where the amount and type of food is accurately and precisely recorded. It is generally accepted in the nutrition community that food frequency questionnaires (FFQs) for assessing intakes are less than ideal (27). Nevertheless, FFQs are likely to be the most convenient assessment for large-scale studies. Quantitative biological measurement tools for nutrient intakes need to be developed for more accurately assessing nutrient intake. (28,29).

Converting food intake to nutrients is done using food composition databases. The most complete is the USDA Food Composition Database (http://www.nal.usda.gov/fnic/foodcomp/Data/SR18/sr18.html). However, plant species, similar to other organisms, respond to their environments, which may result in different nutrient contents depending on the genotype of the plant and its growth conditions (30). Because a full nutrient profile costs about $2000 (per sample in 2002, from Reference 31) and it is typical to average six samples, a ranking scheme (31) will be needed to prioritize analyses of foods. Progress in developing national and international food composition databases is being made, as noted by the International Life Sciences Institute (ILSI) Crop Composition Database (http://www.cropcomposition.org/), the International Network of Food Data Systems (http://www.fao.org/infoods/directory_ en.stm), and the European Food Information Resource Network (EuroFIR—http://www. eurofir.net/).

An added layer of complexity occurs when comparing across populations. Cultural differences in food manufacturing, preparation, and eating customs differ not only among nations and ethnic groups, but also among different religions (e.g., Reference 32). Personal choices such as various vegetarian practices will also confound assessments of nutrient intakes. Other aspects of culture and personal habits [e.g., sleep time and continuity (33,34), activity levels (35–38), and other factors (reviewed in Reference 39)] are all known to alter expression of genetic information. Individual studies have successfully included one or more of these variables, but to date, no study has been published with complete environmental analyses. The development of admixture mapping (40), a genetic method that uses differences among ancestral groups to identify chromosomal regions involved in disease, provides an example of using comparative methods to identify causal factors in complex systems. Similar comparative analyses might be developed for nutrient components involved in health and disease.

### 17.2.2 Genetic Diversity

Genetic analyses showed that Africans have the most DNA sequence variations compared to other populations, a result consistent with the hypothesis that modern humans evolved on that continent (41,42). During the stepwise migrations from east Africa and subsequent population centers, migrating groups carried subsets of the genetic diversity to each new location. Rapid growth of these isolated populations produced populations that share 99.9% of genomic sequences. Examination of the remaining 0.1% indicated that there is a 12 to 14% difference between geographically distinct populations (42) — for example, between Asia and Europe, whereas the majority of human variation (estimated range of 86 to 88%) occurs within a geographic population (Europe, for example).

Food availability and other factors contributed pressures for selecting and maintaining specific gene variants in new environments. Lactase persistence is a prime example of this natural selection process. In many adult humans, severe gastrointestinal discomfort and diarrhea result when milk is ingested because adults cannot metabolize lactose. Certain populations, such as Europeans and many of their descendents, have the ability to drink milk because the gene encoding lactase is expressed in adults. A polymorphism in the promoter [C-13910T (43)] of the lactase phlorizin hydrolase gene (*LCH*) that arose as a mutation around 9000 years ago is responsible for the altered expression pattern of the gene. Individuals not descended from the founding European population retain the normal metabolism of being unable to metabolize lactose as adults: less than 5% of the individuals in southeast Asia can safely drink milk (7). Certain populations in Africa also exhibit lactase persistence even though the African and European populations have been separated for at least ~35,000 years. DNA sequence analyses showed that a large percentage of Africans in certain populations have a G-14010C polymorphism 5′ to the *LCH* gene. This polymorphism arose about ~7000 years ago (44). The maintenance of these *LCH* promoter variants may confer selective advantages that include improved nutrition, prevention of dehydration, and improved calcium absorption in environments that are nutrient poor. The independent selection and maintenance of separate mutations in African and European populations are a prime example of convergent natural selection (44). Different alleles conferring the same phenotype (lactase persistence) have practical consequences for both pharmacogenomics and nutritional genomics: gene variant–phenotype associations may be population specific because members of different ancestral groups may have different polymorphisms affecting the same gene.

The implications of this genetic similarity and diversity are also significant for nutrigenomic researchers because the frequency of gene variants differs among populations. Perhaps as importantly, gene variants and their products (either RNA or DNA) interact with other genes and their products in pathways and networks. Such gene–gene interactions [or epistasis (45–47)] work at the protein and enzyme [and probably iRNA (48)] levels to "buffer" biochemical reactions (49,50). The concept of buffering is important because the presence or absence of a particular gene variant (i.e., SNP) is not an all or none phenomenon. For example, the activity of a gene A variant may be affected by a second gene B (through its protein product) that is inherited separately (i.e., that is, on an unlinked chromosomal region). The result of epistasis is that a single SNP is not deterministic but expresses itself within the background of the individual's genome (that is, the total set of all variations in their DNA). Hence, SNP analyses of individual genes must be accompanied by analyses of genomic variations, an analytical approach that has yet to be developed.

A specific example is illustrative: a specific group of SNPs (called a haplotype, and in this case, HapK) in leukotriene A4 hydrolase (*LTA4H*) was associated with increased risk of myocardial infarction (MI). However, the risk of MI was significantly greater in African Americans who carried the HapK haplotype derived from Europe (51) compared to the presence of the HapK in a European genetic background. The genetic explanation is that SNPs in *LTA4H* affect the activity of that enzyme product and its interaction with other genes whose variants are found more frequently in Africans. These results demonstrate the concept that a SNP or haplotype is "context specific" (52); that is, a SNP or haplotype may contribute different amounts to disease risk depending on ancestral background because of epistatic (gene–gene) interactions. Because some of the genes that cause disease are influenced by diet, the same nutrients may differentially affect individuals with different ancestral backgrounds. Researchers have used self-described ethnicities as proxies for genetic architecture, but skin color is a poor substitute for genetic analyses (53,54).

### 17.2.3 Complexity of Health and Disease Processes

Chronic disease is often thought of as an all or none phenomenon — one is either healthy or has the symptoms of some disease. This dichotomous view of health and disease does not accurately describe biological processes. Complex traits, such as the chronic diseases obesity, diabetes, cardio- or cerebrovascular diseases, Alzheimer's, and certain cancers are caused by the contribution of many genes interacting with multiple environmental factors (reviewed in references 20 and 55). Many of these diseases manifest with complications. For example, T2DM is often caused by, or associated with obesity, a proinflammatory condition that will introduce additional variation in physiology and responsiveness to diet and drugs. Symptoms associated with the metabolic syndrome — dyslipidemia, hypertension, insulin resistance and hyperinsulinemia (56–59) — further complicate even sophisticated classification schemes for diabetes (60). Many of the primary causes of T2DM, such as glycemic control and insulin regulation, change gradually over many years in genetically susceptible individuals exposed to improper diets and lack of physical activity. The resulting physiologies and responses to increased glucose in turn create conditions for the development of complications. These physiological abnormalities may have overlapping molecular and genetic causes to further confuse diagnosis and the development of targeted treatment options (4).

As an example of the genetic and molecular complexities of chronic diseases, genetic analyses suggest that at least 24 chromosomal regions are linked to T2DM. Seven are statistically significant (log of the odds = $LOD > 3.6$), and 17 others suggestive [$2.0 < LOD < 3.6$; (61)]. One or more genes at each of these loci contribute to the development of the T2DM but to different amounts in different individuals depending on function, gene–gene interactions, and gene–environment interactions. Association studies have linked 51 genes to T2DM or metabolic conditions associated with this disease, some but not all of which map to the T2DM loci (reviewed in Reference 4). It is not surprising, then, that chronic diseases and their complications are difficult to study accurately, diagnose precisely, and treat effectively. Similarly, there may be multiple "healthy states," each produced by different combinations of genes at different chromosomal loci. Developing optimal diets to maintain health in different healthy individuals is the flip side of nutrigenomic efforts to understand disease processes caused by imbalanced nutrient intakes in genetically susceptible individuals.

### 17.2.4 Complexity of Data Sets

Although these challenges seem intractable, high-throughput technologies of genomics, transcriptomics, proteomics, and metabolomics, will produce large data sets (also called high-dimensional) of nutrients, gene variants, genetic ancestry data, physiological measurements of proteins and metabolites, as well as physical activity levels and other personal habits. Results will than have to be extracted from these interacting data sets to produce knowledge of gene–environment interactions for each individual. The existing paradigm of analyzing biological data often assumes linear relationships, such as dose-dependent effects. However, genes, nutrients, and their interactions may not necessarily be related linearly.

Analyzing complex data sets is not limited to biological data, and other disciplines have developed algorithms that can discover nonlinear patterns in high-dimensional data. Dimensionality reduction is a mathematical method of mapping multidimensional data into a space of fewer dimensions (62,63), generating a deeper understanding of complex biological processes (e.g., Reference 64 and review in Reference 65). Among these methods are isomap (46,62,63), factor analysis (http://www2.chass.ncsu.edu/garson/pa765/factor.htm), and classification tree analysis (http://www.statsoft.com/textbook/stclatre.html), all of which can be used to analyze complex patterns of gene variants and their influence on subphenotypes (insulin levels or fasting glucose levels, etc.) in response to different dietary intakes. The behavior of interacting genetic and environmental systems cannot yet be predicted accurately and, hence, multiple approaches may be needed to extract knowledge from experimental data. Nevertheless, data generated from different high throughput technologies may be analyzed with more confidence when other paradigms (nonlinearity) are considered possible.

## 17.3 THE CHANGING SHAPE OF BIOMEDICAL RESEARCH

The cultural and scientific view that science is conducted by a lone researcher developed during the early part of the scientific revolution. The practice of conducting science began to change in the early 20th century with the development of teams consisting of a senior mentor, technicians, graduate students, and postdoctoral fellows, usually at one academic institution or company. Although there are lab-to-lab collaborations within a nation and internationally, these typically result from friendships and contacts and are *ad hoc*. The U.S. government–sponsored Manhattan project and subsequent development of national laboratories focusing on high-energy physics and its applications accelerated an era of collaboration consisting of specialized teams within a country and sometimes across national boundaries.

Biological research has been slower to adopt this large-scale collaboration model. However, the complexities of understanding health and disease processes in light of the nutritional, genetic, and cultural variation are changing the structure of science teams. Many current scientific experimental designs and projects are reductionist in nature, which still allows single-investigator-led teams. Focusing on one pathway of a complex process is unlikely to determine the full spectrum of gene–nutrient interactions that produce health or lead to disease (14). A systems biology approach (66) using technologies that analyze DNA variation, transcription regulation, protein amounts or activities, or metabolite concentrations (67–69) will be required for progress to be made. No single research team has the expertise or resources for completely analyzing how the many environmental factors, including thousands of food chemicals, alter the expression of genetic information in an individual.

Hence, the new paradigm emerging in the 21st century for biological research is based on the model of the large-scale genome projects (1–3). Spurred by these successes, scientists in many disciplines are organizing national and international efforts for their individual fields of research for providing resources and best practices (examples in Table 17.1).

**TABLE 17.1**
**Examples of Investigator and Center Networks**

| Topic or Field | Title | Goal | Reference |
|---|---|---|---|
| Mouse genetics | Collaborative Cross Project | Develop inbred and congenic strains as a community resource for complex trait analyses | 108 |
| Pharmacogenetics | Pharmacogenetics Research Network | Database for pharmacogenomics results | http://www.nigms.nih.gov/pharmacogenetics/goals.html |
| Heart, lung, blood, and sleep disorders study | PROGENI Program for Genetic Interaction | Administrative and data coordinating center | http://www.biostat.wustl.edu/progeni/ |
| Human epidemiology | HuGENet | Analyses of human genome variation on population health | 109,110 |
| Human epidemiology | P3G the Public Population Project in Genomics | International network promoting transparency and collaboration for human epidemiology studies | http://www.p3gconsortium.org |
| Inflammatory bowel disease | IBD Network | Consortium for understanding the genetic contributions to this disease | 111 |

Nutrigenomics researchers have also been successful in developing collaborative centers supported by national governments (Table 17.2). Centers and multi-institutional programs supplement the extensive national and international collaborations that several individual laboratories have developed (reviewed in Reference 70).

The new model emerging from these collaborative projects is one in which individually funded laboratories in separate institutions contribute expertise to a large study that analyzes multiple biological parameters. For example, an epidemiologic study of nutrient–gene interactions affecting some phenotype may require biostatisticians for designing the experiments with science specialists and ethicists (and perhaps nonscience community members), clinicians who see patients, geneticists for analyzing SNPs and chromosomal inheritance, nutritionists monitoring and assessing dietary intakes, metabolomics researchers determining serum and urine metabolite concentrations, proteomic specialists studying multiple enzymatic pathways in various tissues, neuroscientists examining NMR brain spectra, physiologists interpreting hormone levels, bioinformaticists capturing and managing the data sets, and biocomputationists using high-dimensionality reduction and other algorithms for analyzing the data. A type of specialist — currently in short supply in our scientific communities — is the individual who can organize the team and interpret the data and results from multiple disciplines. Funding such an enterprise would add to the development of this integrative science and, more importantly, to the type of data and results that could be applied to complex

**TABLE 17.2**
**Examples of Multi-Institutional Centers for Studying Gene–Nutrient Interactions**

| Partners/Host Institution[a] | Agency | Focus |
|---|---|---|
| **AFMNet — Advanced Foods and Materials Network** **http://www.afmnet.ca/** | | |
| Fourteen universities across Canada | Networks of Centres of Excellence<br>Canadian National Government | Structure dynamics function of foods and biomaterials<br>Functional foods and nutraceuticals<br>Genetics, ethics, economics, environment, law, and society (GE3LS) |
| **ARS Children's Nutrition Research Center** **http://www.ars.usda.gov/main/site_main.htm?modecode=62-50-00-00** | | |
| Baylor College of Medicine<br>Texas Children's Hospital<br>United States Department of Agriculture — Agricultural Research Service (USDA — ARS) | USDA | Natural products and nuclear receptors |
| **DIoGenes — Diet, Obesity, and Genes** **http://www.diogenes-eu.org/** | | |
| Thirty research partners<br>Four major industries | European Union<br>Sixth Framework projects:<br>Food Quality and Safety Priority | Obesity and<br>Macronutrient composition of diet<br>Gene–nutrient interactions<br>Genes and diet at the population level<br>Consumer attitudes and behavior<br>Food technology<br>Ensure that science yields applications<br>Data hub |
| **EARNEST — Early Nutrition Programming Project** **http://www.earlynutrition.org** | | |
| Thirty-eight research partners<br>Sixteen European countries | European Union<br>Sixth Framework projects:<br>Food Quality and Safety Priority | Effects of early programming on later chronic diseases<br>Definition of critical periods in fetal and early life on later disease |

*(continued)*

**TABLE 17.2 (CONTINUED)**
**Examples of Multi-Institutional Centers for Studying Gene–Nutrient Interactions**

| Partners/Host Institution[a] | Agency | Focus |
|---|---|---|
| | | Genetic determinants on early programming effects and on subsequent outcome |
| | | Role of specific nutrients and their interactions in the maternal and infant diet on programming |
| | | Mechanisms for early programming of later disease and their risk factors |
| | | Development strategies for treating and preventing adverse programming effects of early nutrition |
| | | How knowledge about early programming affects consumer behavior |
| | | Impact of early nutrition on the economic burden of adult ill-health<br>New technologies for potential economic advantage. |
| **EuroFIR — European Food Information Resource Network** **http://www.eurofir.net/** | | |
| Forty academic and small- to medium-sized enterprises | European Union<br>Sixth Framework projects: | Authoritative source of food composition data in Europe |
| Twenty-one European countries | Food Quality and Safety Priority | |
| **HealthGrain — Exploiting Bioactivity of European Cereal Grains for Improved Nutrition and Health Benefits** **http://www.healthgrain.org/pub/** | | |
| Forty-three organizations | European Union | Consumer research |
| Fifteen European Countries | Sixth Framework projects:<br>Food Quality and Safety Priority | Plant breeding and biotechnology |
| | | Technology and processing |
| | | Nutrition |
| | | Dissemination and training |

**TABLE 17.2 (CONTINUED)**
**Examples of Multi-Institutional Centers for Studying Gene–Nutrient Interactions**

| Partners/Host Institution[a] | Agency | Focus |
|---|---|---|
| **HEPADIP — Hepatic and Adipose Tissue in the Metabolic Syndrome http://www.hepadip.org/** | | |
| Twenty-seven partner institutions<br>Thirteen countries | European Union Sixth Framework projects: Food Quality and Safety Priority | Biology of adipose and liver tissue<br>Integrative studies of adipose and liver in rats<br>Integrative studies of adipose and liver in humans<br>Clinical and genetic epidemiology studies<br>Development and integration of omics and bioinformatics<br>Target validation and development |
| **LipGene Diet, genomics, and the metabolic syndrome: an integrated nutrition, agrofood, social, and economic analysis http://www.lipgene.org** | | |
| Twenty-five partners<br>Ten European countries | European Union Sixth Framework projects: Food Quality and Safety Priority | Role of dietary fats and genetic variation<br>Create agrofoods of LC n-3 PUFA<br>Alter milk fat from cows and fats in poultry<br>Consumer attitudes: MS and agrofood technologies<br>Economic barriers to new agrofood technologies<br>Diet vs. drug costs in management of the MS<br>Dissemination and education program |
| **NCMHD Center of Excellence in Nutritional Genomics http://nutrigenomics.ucdavis.edu** | | |
| University of California–Davis<br>Children's Hospital of Oakland Research Institute<br>USDA Western Human Nutrition Research Center<br>Ethnic Health Institute<br>University of Illinois Chicago Laboratory of Nutrigenomic | NIH — National Center for Minority Health and Health Disparities | Biological basis of health disparities<br>Education and outreach |

*(continued)*

**TABLE 17.2 (CONTINUED)**
**Examples of Multi-Institutional Centers for Studying Gene–Nutrient Interactions**

| Partners/Host Institution[a] | Agency | Focus |
|---|---|---|
| **NuGO — European Nutrigenomics Organization http://www.nugo.org** | | |
| Twenty-three partner institutions in ten European countries | European Union Sixth Framework projects: Food Quality and Safety Priority | Develop and integrate genomic technologies for European nutritional sciences |
| One collaborative center | | Facilitate the application of technologies in nutritional research worldwide |
| | | Create the leading international virtual center of excellence in nutrigenomics |
| | | Train a new generation of European scientists to use postgenomic technologies |
| **Nutrigenomics New Zealand http://www.nutrigenomics.org.nz/** | | |
| University of Auckland | New Zealand Foundation for Research and Science Technology (FRST) | Inflammatory bowel diseases |
| Crown Research Institutes: | | |
| AgResearch | | |
| HortResearch | | |
| Crop and Food Research | | |
| **The UAB Center for Nutrient Gene Interactions in Cancer Prevention http://207.203.38.82:8888/ssg/cngi2/index.htm** | | |
| University of Alabama Birmingham | NIH — National Cancer Institute Division of Cancer Prevention | Dietary polyphenols and chemoprevention |
| The Northern California Cancer Center | | Soybean |
| The University of Missouri-Rolla | | Statistical analyses of high-dimensional data |

[a] For a full list of partner institutions and countries, see URL for each center.

*Source:* Adapted from Kaput, J. 2007. Nutrigenomics — 2006 Update, *Clinical Chemistry and Laboratory Medicine*, in press.

biological phenotypes such as chronic diseases. A functioning alliance producing evidence-based recommendations to address personal and public health issues must be accomplished first, given the current nation (or region)-based funding mechanisms of the early 21st century.

## 17.4 THE ROAD MAP FOR HARNESSING NUTRIGENOMICS FOR PERSONAL AND PUBLIC HEALTH

The development of regional and national nutrigenomic centers and programs (70), although encouraging and essential, is nonetheless insufficient to address the complexities of nutrient–gene interactions. The reasons were outlined previously in the diversity challenges of nutrient complexity of foods, genetic heterogeneity, intricacies of metabolic processes, and the need for large data sets. This realization led to a call for international strategic alliances to harness nutritional genomics for public and personal health (39), a position statement coauthored by 89 scientists from 22 countries. Table 17.3 provides an outline of key steps in harnessing nutritional genomics data for developing the knowledge for personalized nutrition.

### 17.4.1 The Status of the Nutrigenomics Society — 2006

The shift from small- to large-scale projects will be challenging because of the sociology of modern science, the source of funding, and how they are managed, and how they are executed. These challenges can be met through the creation of a central organizing center focused on promoting, organizing and communicating interest, developing community-based resources, developing best practices, and developing global databases for data sharing.

**TABLE 17.3**
**Road Map for Nutritional Genomics Research**

| Topic | Rationale | Outcome |
|---|---|---|
| Data federation | Scalable databases — share genetic, phenotypic, dietary, nutritional status, and other environmental and cultural information | Allow for greater statistical power across populations |
| Larger study populations | Statistical power limitations | Improve reliability of results |
| Phenotypes | More reliable analyses and consistency | Improve reliability of results |
| Nutrient intakes | Quantitative measurements | Improve reliability of results |
| Genomic controls | Ancestry background analyses | Control for epistasis |
| Study participants | Inclusion of diverse cultures and genotypes | More complete understanding of nutrient–gene interactions |
| Assess other environmental variables | Affects expression of genetic info | Reduce noise in data sets |
| Partnerships among academia, industry, society | Resource building for capturing nontraditional data and interactions among data sets | More complete understanding of nutrient–gene interactions |

*Source:* Adapted from Kaput, J., Ordovas, J.M., Ferguson, L. et al. 2005. *Br J Nutr* 94: 623–32.

#### 17.4.1.1 Promoting, Organizing, and Communicating Interest

The only nutrigenomics organization whose mission is multinational and that is not explicitly linked to a specific research program is The European Nutrigenomics Organisation (NuGO). The mission of NuGO is to develop, integrate, and facilitate genomic technologies, infrastructure, and research for nutritional science, to train a new generation of nutrigenomics scientists, in order to improve the impact of nutrition and genetics in health promotion and disease prevention. NuGO has recently established the Nutrigenomics Society to provide its leadership and resources to all in the international nutrigenomic community.

The first step of this effort was the creation of a central Web site (http://www.nugo.org) that provides information to the researcher in pages called the *Nutrigenomics Information Portal* (*NIP*) (71). Divided into Research, Technology, Outreach, and Partnerships, the *NIP* provides a meeting and resource site for those interested in nutrigenomics topics. A second section of the Web site, labeled *Facts about Nutrigenomics* (*FAN*), is designed for the educated public. *FAN* describes the field, key terms and concepts and information about the collaborative effort. The final section of the public pages are entitled Nutrigenomics Stakeholders (*NS*), which is a section focusing on industry, health professional, regulators, politicians, patient organizations, and government departments. Many who use the Web recognize the need for reliable information from experts, and the content of the Nutrigenomics Society intends to provide balanced and accurate descriptions of nutrigenomics science and its applications. The Web site is an ongoing effort that was initiated in mid-2006 (71). The ultimate goal of the Web site — registration of individuals and projects, resource development, and best practices is — to create data that can be shared across studies.

In addition to the education and outreach efforts of NuGO, the NCMHD Center of Excellence in Nutritional Genomics at the University of California–Davis has a nutrigenomics LISTSERV to alert subscribers to various scientific and public news articles, nutrigenomic activities, and issues facing the field. Started in July of 2002, the LISTSERV currently has over 1600 subscribers (January 2007) in over 50 countries.

#### 17.4.1.2 Best Practices

Many scientists doing research at the turn of the millennium were taught reductionist approaches to science. This philosophy and the associated methods have contributed immensely to scientific progress and will always be needed to understand individual pathways and reactions of complex networks. However, reductionism cannot fully explain complex, interacting systems because expression of genetic information relies on environmental factors that change during life. Developmental and aging processes of biological systems also vary over time, possibly altering gene–environment interactions. Such complexity is rarely accounted for in reductionist experimental designs.

Nutrigenomics projects therefore will require best practices developed by experts in different disciplines. NuGO began this process in early 2004 with ongoing meetings and discussions among European scientists at different institutions. This effort has generated three best practices papers in transcriptomics (72), metabolomics (68), and proteomics (73). These recommendations focus on the technologies of each discipline rather than experimental designs for human, laboratory animal, cell culture experiments, or for pre- and postexperiment biocomputation methods. Because technologies and experience change, these best practices will require ongoing discussions, which will, in the near future, include non-European scientists. Online forums will be created to foster interactions across national and physical divides.

#### 17.4.1.3 Global Biological Databases

The challenges inherent in nutrigenomic studies, specifically genetic variation, population architecture, individual and cultural food preferences, among others, requires large study populations and consistent phenotypes, common data elements, and database interoperability. None of these can be achieved without forethought and planning. Hence, the development of global biological databases focused on data from the omics technologies of genomics, transcriptomics, proteomics, and metabolomics will be necessary. Developing robust nutrient intake databases that account for the many cultural practices associated with food systems throughout the world will be one of the more significant challenges for the nutrigenomic community. The first database to be developed through this effort is the gene–nutrient database, a collaboration between the Genetics and Nutrition Laboratory at Jean Mayer USDA Human Nutrition Research Center on Aging at Tufts University and NuGO. This database will consist of published reports of SNP (gene variant)–nutrient–phenotype associations.

## 17.5 THE EXTRAORDINARY CHALLENGES OF INVOLVING SCIENTISTS AND THE PUBLIC IN DEVELOPING COUNTRIES

Much, if not all of, the research described in this and other review articles about nutrigenomics are derived from studies conducted in developed countries. Caucasians, African Americans (whose ancestors for the most part are West Africans), Asian Americans of various ancestries, and in a few instances, with other ethnicities [e.g., Indians, Malays, and Chinese (74) or Koreans (75)] have been study participants. Representatives from other ancestral and ethnic groups are rare or missing from most nutritional genomic research projects. This is not unique to nutrigenomics, but to nutrition (76), genetics (77) and other scientific disciplines. The rationale for this focus was that funding was obtained from national agencies and also because including other genetic makeups confounded the analyses because ancestral backgrounds could not be quantitatively measured. Based on data from the Human Genome and HapMap projects, no population can serve as the reference group. A full scientific description of nutrient–gene interactions requires inclusion of as many ancestral groups and cultures as possible because epistatic, and perhaps epigenetic interactions (78), may differ in genetic background and may alter statistical gene–nutrient–phenotype associations. The different SNPs responsible for lactase persistence in African and European descendents (see previous text) exemplifies the need to include other genetic makeups in research and application processes.

### 17.5.1 A Humanitarian Need Also Exists

The World Health Organization's (WHO) Child and Adolescent Health Development Web site (http://www.who.int/child-adolescent-health/dev.htm) states, "The future of human societies depends on children being able to achieve their optimal physical growth and psychological development." Data from numerous scientific studies have demonstrated that improper diets block both physical and mental growth and development (reviewed in Reference 59, 79, and 80). Because nutrient intake requirements are usually determined from studies of individuals in developed countries, who represent only a subset of the human genetic diversity (see earlier text), controversy exists as to whether international nutrient intake standards are valid (81,82). Some experimental data pertinent to this controversy exist. Additional dietary folate in individuals with variants of methylene tetrahydrofolate reductase [MTHRF; (83)] individuals with polymorphisms in alcohol-metabolizing genes experience skin flushing (84), and individuals carrying certain variants of angiotensinogen are sensitive to increased salt intakes (85). The likelihood of inheriting these gene variants differs because allele frequencies differ among ethnic populations. If nutrient intakes are to be optimized for health of individuals in developed countries, it follows that this process should also be applied to those in developing countries. One could make a strong argument that nutrigenomics research should first focus on populations in most need of food because delivering the appropriate nutrients would do the most good in terms of personal and public health (86). For example, Neel proposed the thrifty gene hypothesis in 1962 (87), which posited that certain genetic makeups are more susceptible to energy-dense foods because their metabolism utilizes energy from foods more efficiently (88–90). If this is true for calorie intake, it is likely to be true for concentrations of at least some macro- and micronutrients (81,91,92).

Imbalances of nutrient intake may be most devastating during key nutritional developmental windows (59,79,80) Developmental windows are periods during which perturbations of the intrauterine, and probably early postnatal, growth environment have major effects on biological processes. These critical periods may allow for permanent programming of cardiovascular and metabolic functions, and are predicted to determine final health outcomes in adults.

### 17.5.2 Funding Nutrigenomic Research in Developing Countries

Obtaining funds for nutrigenomic research efforts in developing countries will not be easy. The 10/90 gap describes the current biomedical funding scheme in the world: only 10% of the U.S. research budget is spent on conditions and diseases that affect 90% of the world's population (93). This gap is narrowing only because of the rapid increase in obesity and T2DM in developing countries and a significant percentage of the West's research funds are spent on those diseases, although, in populations where the genetic makeups are not reflective of the world's diversity.

Because analyzing gene–nutrient interactions responsible for chronic diseases requires inclusion of many different genetic makeups, the increased funding within developed countries may soon enable inclusion of scientists and citizens of developing countries to participate in the research and its applications. Genetic testing costs are continually falling and economies of scale may allow the analyses of individuals in different populations at only incrementally higher costs. Collaborative efforts will likely allow the transfer of technologies and information which may aid these disadvantaged nations economically (94–96).

Several different groups are exploring the moral issues of doing research in resource-poor countries (97) and in developing ethical statements and procedures for such research. The Nuffield Council on Bioethics (http://www.nuffieldbioethics.org/) has thoroughly reviewed this topic in 1999 (98), with follow-up discussions published in 2005 (99). The Joint Centre for Bioethics of the University of Toronto has provided guidelines for ethics and reasons for using technology and genomics for science and economic development in disadvantaged countries (95,96,100).

The need for addressing the imbalances in nutrient availability, genetic diversity, and economic development in developing countries has been more eloquently expressed by nutritionists (76), geneticists (77), economists (100,101), and ethicists (95–99). Disadvantaged individuals and populations can, and should be, included in new and ongoing studies through appropriate collaborations with scientists, ethicists, public health officials, and institutions in developing countries as can those most vulnerable subpopulations in developed countries. Science and morality justify these efforts.

These efforts are similar to the recent description of the new nutrition project (102–104), an elucidation of the precepts in the Giessen Declaration (105). That declaration calls for the expansion of the definition, concepts, and dimensions of nutritional research and its applications to include biological, social, and environmental principles and methods. The new nutrition would address personal, population, and planetary health through an integrative approach of studying and understanding food systems. The authors of the Giessen Declaration believe that nutrition sciences should be, and are rightfully, involved with addressing global food and nutrition insecurity and inadequacy and the new epidemics of obesity, diabetes, and other chronic diseases whose incidence is rising in developed and developing countries. The sentiments of the Giessen Declaration and its accompanying explanations are similar to those expressed by an informal international network of nutrigenomic and related scientists (39).

### 17.5.3 Issues Facing Collaborative Research in Developing Countries: The Ethiopian Example

Although the case for inclusion and benefit sharing is compelling, the challenges are many. Conditions in Ethiopia may serve as an example of some of these challenges. Ethiopia's Human Development Index (HDI, http://hdr.undp.org/statistics/data/country_fact_sheets/cty_fs_ETH.html) is 0.361 (out of 1), which is a measure of living a long life (life expectancy 47 years in 2003, and falling), being educated (literacy rates are gender specific but average about 45%), and income (GDP US$711). Although these statistics alone would skew statistical analyses of most sociological and biological experiments, the physical and health-care infrastructure issues are even more significant. Approximately 70% of urban dwellers have access to safe drinking water with per-liter consumption of about 7 l. Only 15 to 20% of country or rural inhabitants have access, with some consumption estimates of between 3 and 12 l per day. The recommended amounts for basic needs of drinking, culinary, personal hygiene, and other domestic uses is 20 to 50 l per day for rural and urban residents, respectively (106). Accessibility is defined as the geographic proximity of safe source of drinking water points within *15 minutes walk or a radius of 1 km from users' homes* (106) [Emphasis added]. In Ethiopia, 21% of the rural population, 84% of the urban dwellers, and 30% of the country's inhabitants have access to safe drinking water (called *drinking water coverage*). These numbers translate to significant biological consequences:

- Children under age 5 have 4 to 7 episodes of diarrhea per year (106)
- As many as 92.7% of school-children under the age of 15 in the Lake Awassa area of Southern Ethiopia had at least one helminthic infection. The most prevalent parasites were *A. lumbricoides*, hookworm species, *T. trichura*, and *S. mansoni*.
- Of the estimated 5000 street children (no permanent home or sleeping quarters) in Awassa (Southern Nations, Nationalities, and People Region, Ethiopia), 42.6% had malaria-like febrile illnesses, 33.1% had respiratory illness, and 4.5% had diarrheal illnesses. Almost 50% of the children ate only when meals were available (107); that is, half of the street kids in Awassa did not know where or when their next meal was going to be available.

The federal Ethiopian government promises full health care, but only ~52% of the population has access (Ethiopian Ministry of Health, Annex 1). The number of physicians per 1000 people is 0.029 in Ethiopia, and 2.3 in the U.S. The point of this listing is that examining nutrient–gene interactions, or simply nutrient requirements (76), will require significant planning and adjustments of protocols many researchers take for granted — there are few studies that monitor water intake or energy expenditure of walking to water sources. Nutrigenomics research cannot address all of these issues but can, and should, focus on extending its research and humanitarian efforts to those in developing and transitional countries.

## 17.6 FUTURE PERSPECTIVES

Understanding gene–nutrient interactions and applying that knowledge for personal and public health will require strategic collaborations, resource and data sharing, and joint funding strategies that cross discipline and national boundaries. It is not likely that nutrigenomics will fulfill its promise of personalized nutrition without comparing responses of gene–nutrient interactions across many different genetic makeups. Gene–disease studies have demonstrated the need to study multiple ancestral groups (51). The effort to begin those collaborations and international networking was initiated with the publication of a position statement authored by 89 individuals from 22 countries (39). From this effort, an international Nutrigenomics Society

(71) is emerging that will encourage scientists from any related discipline to join and participate. The organization of this democratic, ground-up approach will be done initially through an international Web site hosted by NuGO (71). The international team is committed to including people of all nations and ethnicities in the research and benefits of that research, in large part to reduce the disparities in health care and living standards across the world. Significant challenges for this research effort must be overcome — in developed economies the effort requires mainly political will. For developing countries facing infectious diseases, lack of access to safe water, food insecurity, poor sanitation and health care, the issues are significantly greater. Genetic variation is likely to produce differences in requirements of micronutrients needed to maintain health and allow for full attainment of physical and mental health. Hence, the perspective for nutrigenomics is not only improved nutrition for individuals in developed countries, but also the potential for evidence-based improvements of public health for citizens of the world.

## ACKNOWLEDGMENTS

The preparation of this manuscript was supported by the National Center for Minority Health and Health Disparities Center of Excellence in Nutritional Genomics, Grant MD 00222 and from the European Union, EU FP6 NoE Grant, Contract No. CT2004-505944.

## KEY READINGS

1. NCMHD Center of Excellence in Nutritional Genomics Web site: http://nutrigenomics.ucdavis.edu.
2. NuGO Web site: http://www.nugo.org.
3. The Case for Strategic International Alliances to HarnessNutritional Genomics for Public and Personal Health (39).
4. A variant of the gene encoding leukotriene A4 hydrolase confers ethnicity-specific risk of myocardial infarction (51).
5. Developmental origins of the metabolic syndrome: prediction, plasticity, and programming (59).

## REFERENCES

1. Lander, ES, Linton, LM, Birren, B et al. 2001. Initial sequencing and analysis of the human genome. *Nature* 409: 860–921.
2. Venter, JC, Adams, MD, Myers, EW et al. 2001. The sequence of the human genome. *Science* 291: 1304–51.
3. The International HapMap, C. 2005. A haplotype map of the human genome. *Nature* 437: 1299–1320.
4. Kaput, J, Noble, J, Hatipoglu, B, Kohrs, K, Dawson, K, and Bartholomew, A. 2007. Application of Nutrigenomic Concepts to Type 2 Diabetes Mellitus. *Nutrition, Metabolism, and Cardiovascular Disease*, 17: 89–103.
5. Kaput, J, Perlina, A, Hatipoglu, B, Bartholomew, A, and Nikolsky, Y. 2007. Nutrigenomics: Concepts and Applications to Clinical Medicine. *Pharmacogenomics*, 8: 369–390.

6. Willett, W, *The Pursuit of Optimal Diets: A Progress Report*, in *Nutritional Genomics. Discovering the Path to Personalized Nutrition*, J Kaput, Rodriguez, RL, Eds., 2006, John Wiley and Sons: Hoboken, NJ, pp. 37–56.
7. Kaput, J and Rodriguez, RL. 2004. Nutritional genomics: the next frontier in the postgenomic era. *Physiol Genomics* 16: 166–77.
8. Ordovas, JM. 2004. The quest for cardiovascular health in the genomic era: nutrigenetics and plasma lipoproteins. *Proc Nutr Soc* 63: 145–52.
9. DeBusk, RM, Fogarty, CP, Ordovas, JM et al. 2005. Nutritional genomics in practice: where do we begin? *J Am Diet Assoc* 105: 589–98.
10. Fogg-Johnson, N and Kaput, J. 2003. Nutrigenomics: An Emerging Scientific Discipline. *Food Technology* 57: 61–67.
11. Ferguson, LR and Kaput, J. 2004. Nutrigenomics and the New Zealand Food Industry. *Food New Zealand (the journal of the New Zealand Institute of Food Science and Technology)*: 29–36.
12. Hirschhorn, JN, Lohmueller, K, Byrne, E et al. 2002. A comprehensive review of genetic association studies. *Genet Med* 4: 45–61.
13. Newton-Cheh, C and Hirschhorn, JN. 2005. Genetic association studies of complex traits: design and analysis issues. *Mutat Res* 573: 54–69.
14. Ioannidis, JP. 2005. Why most published research findings are false. *PLoS Med* 2: e124.
15. Cardon, LR and Bell, JI. 2001. Association study designs for complex diseases. *Nat Rev Genet* 2: 91–9.
16. Lander, E and Kruglyak, L. 1995. Genetic dissection of complex traits: guidelines for interpreting and reporting linkage results [see comments]. *Nat Genet* 11: 241–7.
17. Tabor, HK, Risch, NJ, and Myers, RM. 2002. OPINION: Candidate-gene approaches for studying complex genetic traits: practical considerations. *Nat Rev Genet* 3: 391–7.
18. Risch, N. 1997. Evolving methods in genetic epidemiology. II. Genetic linkage from an epidemiologic perspective. *Epidemiol Rev* 19: 24–32.
19. Ordovas, JM and Corella, D. 2004. Nutritional genomics. *Annu Rev Genomics Hum Genet* 5: 71–118.
20. Kaput, J. 2004. Diet-disease gene interactions. *Nutrition* 20: 26–31.
21. Ordovas, JMaC, D., Gene-Environment Interactions: Defining the Playfield, in *Nutritional Genomics. Discovering the Path to Personalized Nutrition*, J Kaput, Rodriguez, RL, Eds. 2006, John Wiley and Sons: Hoboken, NJ. pp. 57–76.
22. Kolonel, LN, Altshuler, D, and Henderson, BE. 2004. The multiethnic cohort study: exploring genes, lifestyle and cancer risk. *Nat Rev Cancer* 4: 519–27.
23. Schuster, GU, *Nutrients and Gene Expression*, in *Nutritional Genomics. Discovering the Path to Personalized Nutrition*, J Kaput, Rodriguez, RL, Eds. 2006, John Wiley and Sons: Hoboken, NJ. pp. 153–176.
24. Guo, SaS, G., *Green Tea Polyphenols and Cancer Prevention*, in *Nutritional Genomics. Discovering the Path to Personalized Nutrition*, J Kaput, Rodriguez, RL, Eds. 2006, John Wiley and Sons: Hoboken, NJ. pp. 177–206.
25. Goldberg, JP, Belury, MA, Elam, P et al. 2004. The obesity crisis: don't blame it on the pyramid. *J Am Diet Assoc* 104: 1141–7.
26. Jequier, E. 2002. Pathways to obesity. *Int J Obes Relat Metab Disord* 26(Suppl. 2): S12–7.
27. Rutishauser, IH. 2005. Dietary intake measurements. *Public Health Nutr* 8: 1100–7.
28. Corella, D and Ordovas, JM. 2005. Single nucleotide polymorphisms that Influence lipid metabolism: interaction with dietary factors. *Annu Rev Nutr* 25: 341–390.
29. Corella, D and Ordovas, JM. 2004. The metabolic syndrome: a crossroad for genotype-phenotype associations in atherosclerosis. *Curr Atheroscler Rep* 6: 186–96.

30. Reynolds, TL, Nemeth, MA, Glenn, KC et al. 2005. Natural variability of metabolites in maize grain: differences due to genetic background. *J Agric Food Chem* 53: 10061–7.
31. Haytowitz, D, Pehrsson, PR, and Holden, JM. 2002. The Identification of Key Foods for Food Composition Research. *J Good Composition Anal* 15: 183–194.
32. Kim, KH and Sobal, J. 2004. Religion, social support, fat intake and physical activity. *Public Health Nutr* 7: 773–81.
33. Irwin, M. 2002. Effects of sleep and sleep loss on immunity and cytokines. *Brain Behav Immun* 16: 503–12.
34. Redwine, L, Hauger, RL, Gillin, JC et al. 2000. Effects of sleep and sleep deprivation on interleukin-6, growth hormone, cortisol, and melatonin levels in humans. *J Clin Endocrinol Metab* 85: 3597–603.
35. Gleeson, M, Nieman, DC, and Pedersen, BK. 2004. Exercise, nutrition and immune function. *J Sports Sci* 22: 115–25.
36. Nieman, DC, Davis, JM, Henson, DA et al. 2003. Carbohydrate ingestion influences skeletal muscle cytokine mRNA and plasma cytokine levels after a 3-h run. *J Appl Physiol* 94: 1917–25.
37. Nieman, DC, Dumke, CI, Henson, DA et al. 2003. Immune and oxidative changes during and following the Western States Endurance Run. *Int J Sports Med* 24: 541–7.
38. Nieman, DC, Davis, JM, Brown, VA et al. 2004. Influence of carbohydrate ingestion on immune changes after 2 h of intensive resistance training. *J Appl Physiol* 96: 1292–8.
39. Kaput, J, Ordovas, JM, Ferguson, L et al. 2005. The case for strategic international alliances to harness nutritional genomics for public and personal health. *Br J Nutr* 94: 623–32.
40. Patterson, N, Hattangadi, N, Lane, B et al. 2004. Methods for high-density admixture mapping of disease genes. *Am J Hum Genet* 74: 979–1000.
41. Tishkoff, SA and Verrelli, BC. 2003. Patterns of human genetic diversity: implications for human evolutionary history and disease. *Annu Rev Genomics Hum Genet* 4: 293–340.
42. Jorde, LB and Wooding, SP. 2004. Genetic variation, classification and 'race'. *Nat Genet* 36(Suppl. 1): S28–33.
43. Enattah, NS, Sahi, T, Savilahti, E et al. 2002. Identification of a variant associated with adult-type hypolactasia. *Nat Genet* 30: 233–7.
44. Tishkoff, SA, Reed, FA, Ranciaro, A et al. 2007. Convergent adaptation of human lactase persistence in Africa and Europe. *Nat Genet* 39: 31–40.
45. Chiu, S, Diament, A.L., Fisler, J.S., and Warden, C.H., Gene-Gene Epistasis and Gene Environment Interactions Influence Diabetes and Obesity, in *Nutritional Genomics. Discovering the Path to Personalized Nutrition*, J Kaput, Rodriguez, RL, Eds. 2006, John Wiley and Sons: Hoboken, NJ. pp. 135–152.
46. Moore, JH. 2004. Computational analysis of gene-gene interactions using multifactor dimensionality reduction. *Expert Rev Mol Diagn* 4: 795–803.
47. Carlborg, O and Haley, CS. 2004. Epistasis: too often neglected in complex trait studies? *Nat Rev Genet* 5: 618–25.
48. Nakahara, K and Carthew, RW. 2004. Expanding roles for miRNAs and siRNAs in cell regulation. *Curr Opin Cell Biol* 16: 127–33.
49. Hartman, JL, Garvik, B, and Hartwell, L. 2001. Principles for the buffering of genetic variation. *Science* 291: 1001–4.
50. Hartman, JL, IV, Genetic and Molecular Buffering of Phenotypes, in *Nutritional Genomics. Discovering the Path to Personalized Nutrition*, J Kaput, Rodriguez, RL, Eds. 2006, John Wiley and Sons: Hoboken, NJ. pp. 105–134.

51. Helgadottir, A, Manolescu, A, Helgason, A et al. 2006. A variant of the gene encoding leukotriene A4 hydrolase confers ethnicity-specific risk of myocardial infarction. *Nat Genet* 38: 68–74.
52. Klos, KLE, Kardia, SLR, Hixson, JE et al., *Linkage Analysis of Plasma ApoE in Three Ethnic Groups: Multiple Genes with Context-Dependent Effects*. 2005. p. 157–167.
53. Kittles, RA and Weiss, KM. 2003. Race, ancestry, and genes: implications for defining disease risk. *Annu Rev Genomics Hum Genet* 4: 33–67.
54. Shriver, MD, Mei, R, Parra, EJ et al. 2005. Large-scale SNP analysis reveals clustered and continuous patterns of human genetic variation. *Hum Genomics* 2: 81–89.
55. Kaput, J. An Introduction and Overview of Nutritional Genomics: Application to Type 2 Diabetes and International Nutrigenomics, in *Nutritional Genomics. Discovering the Path to Personalized Nutrition*, J Kaput, Rodriguez, RL, Eds. 2006, John Wiley and Sons: Hoboken, NJ. pp. 1–36.
56. Steinmetz, A. 2003. Treatment of diabetic dyslipoproteinemia. *Exp Clin Endocrinol Diabetes* 111: 239–45.
57. Cordain, L, Eades, MR, and Eades, MD. 2003. Hyperinsulinemic diseases of civilization: more than just Syndrome X. *Comp Biochem Physiol A Mol Integr Physiol* 136: 95–112.
58. Curtis, J and Wilson, C. 2005. Preventing type 2 diabetes mellitus. *J Am Board Fam Pract* 18: 37–43.
59. McMillen, IC and Robinson, JS. 2005. Developmental origins of the metabolic syndrome: prediction, plasticity, and programming. *Physiol Rev* 85: 571–633.
60. Rosenzweig, JL, Weinger, K, Poirier-Solomon, L et al. 2002. Use of a disease severity index for evaluation of healthcare costs and management of comorbidities of patients with diabetes mellitus. *Am J Manage Care* 8: 950–8.
61. Florez, JC, Hirschhorn, J, and Altshuler, D. 2003. The inherited basis of diabetes mellitus: implications for the genetic analysis of complex traits. *Annu Rev Genomics Hum Genet* 4: 257–91.
62. Roweis, ST and Saul, LK. 2000. Nonlinear dimensionality reduction by locally linear embedding. *Science* 290: 2323–6.
63. Tenenbaum, JB, de Silva, V, and Langford, JC. 2000. A global geometric framework for nonlinear dimensionality reduction. *Science* 290: 2319–23.
64. Dawson, K, Rodriguez, RL, and Malyj, W. 2005. Sample phenotype clusters in high-density oligonucleotide microarray data sets are revealed using Isomap, a nonlinear algorithm. *BMC Bioinformatics* 6: 195.
65. Kaput, J and Dawson, K. 2007. Complexity of type 2 diabetes mellitus data sets emerging from nutrigenomic research: a case for dimensionality reduction? *Mutation Research.* In press.
66. Hood, L, Heath, JR, Phelps, ME et al. 2004. Systems biology and new technologies enable predictive and preventative medicine. *Science* 306: 640–3.
67. Bijlsma, S, Bobeldijk, I, Verheij, ER et al. 2006. Large-scale human metabolomics studies: a strategy for data (pre-) processing and validation. *Anal Chem* 78: 567–74.
68. Gibney, MJ, Walsh, M, Brennan, L et al. 2005. Metabolomics in human nutrition: opportunities and challenges. *Am J Clin Nutr* 82: 497–503.
69. van Ommen, B. 2004. Nutrigenomics: exploiting systems biology in the nutrition and health arenas. *Nutrition* 20: 4–8.
70. Kaput, J. 2007. Nutrigenomics — 2006 Update. *Clinical Chemistry and Laboratory Medicine*, 45: 279–287.
71. Kaput, J, Astley, S, Renkema, M, Ordovas, J, and van Ommen, B. 2006. Harnessing nutrigenomics: development of web-based communication, databases, resources, and tools. *Genes Nutr.* 1: 5–12.

72. Garosi, P, De Filippo, C, van Erk, M et al. 2005. Defining best practice for microarray analyses in nutrigenomic studies. *Br J Nutr* 93: 425–32.
73. Fuchs, D, Winkelmann, I, Johnson, IT et al. 2005. Proteomics in nutrition research: principles, technologies and applications. *Br J Nutr* 94: 302–14.
74. Qi, L, Tai, ES, Tan, CE et al. 2005. Intragenic linkage disequilibrium structure of the human perilipin gene (PLIN) and haplotype association with increased obesity risk in a multiethnic Asian population. *J Mol Med.*
75. Shin, HD, Kim, KS, Cha, MH et al. 2005. The effects of UCP-1 polymorphisms on obesity phenotypes among Korean female subjects. *Biochem Biophys Res Commun* 335: 624–30.
76. Uauy, R. 2005. Defining and addressing the nutritional needs of populations. *Public Health Nutr* 8: 773–80.
77. Consortium, IH. 2004. Integrating ethics and science in the International HapMap Project. *Nat Rev Genet* 5: 467–75.
78. Jiang, YH, Bressler, J, and Beaudet, AL. 2004. Epigenetics and human disease. *Annu Rev Genomics Hum Genet* 5: 479–510.
79. Lucas, A. 1998. Programming by early nutrition: an experimental approach. *J Nutr* 128: 401S–406S.
80. Gallou-Kabani, C and Junien, C. 2005. Nutritional epigenomics of metabolic syndrome: new perspective against the epidemic. *Diabetes* 54: 1899–906.
81. Victora, CG, Morris, SS, Barros, FC et al. 1998. The NCHS reference and the growth of breast- and bottle-fed infants. *J Nutr* 128: 1134–8.
82. Hughes, RG and Lawrence, MA. 2005. Globalization, food and health in Pacific Island countries. *Asia Pac J Clin Nutr* 14: 298–306.
83. Wilcken, B, Bamforth, F, Li, Z et al. 2003. Geographical and ethnic variation of the 677C>T allele of 5,10 methylenetetrahydrofolate reductase (MTHFR): findings from over 7000 newborns from 16 areas world wide. *J Med Genet* 40: 619–25.
84. Chen, WJ, Chen, CC, Yu, JM et al. 1998. Self-reported flushing and genotypes of ALDH2, ADH2, and ADH3 among Taiwanese Han. *Alcohol Clin Exp Res* 22: 1048–52.
85. Nakajima, T, Wooding, S, Sakagami, T et al. 2004. Natural selection and population history in the human angiotensinogen gene (AGT): 736 complete AGT sequences in chromosomes from around the world. *Am J Hum Genet* 74: 898–916.
86. Darnton-Hill, I, Margetts, B, and Deckelbaum, R. 2004. Public health nutrition and genetics: implications for nutrition policy and promotion. *Proc Nutr Soc* 63: 173–85.
87. Neel, JV. 1962. Diabetes mellitus: a "thrifty" genotype rendered detrimental by "progress"? *Am J Hum Genet* 14: 353–62.
88. Lieberman, LS. 2003. Dietary, Evolutionary, and Modernizing Influences on the Prevalence of Type 2 Diabetes. *Annu Rev Nutr*:
89. Epping-Jordan, JE, Galea, G, Tukuitonga, C et al. 2005. Preventing chronic diseases: taking stepwise action. *Lancet* 366: 1667–71.
90. James, PT, Leach, R, Kalamara, E et al. 2001. The worldwide obesity epidemic. *Obes Res* 9(Suppl. 4): 228S–233S.
91. Iannotti, LL, Tielsch, JM, Black, MM et al. 2006. Iron supplementation in early childhood: health benefits and risks. *Am J Clin Nutr* 84: 1261–76.
92. McCann, JC and Ames, BN, Is docosahexaenoic acid, an n-3 long-chain polyunsaturated fatty acid, required for development of normal brain function? *An overview of evidence from cognitive and behavioral tests in humans and animals.* 2005. pp. 281–295.
93. Research, GFfH, *The 10/90 Report on Health Research 2001 — 2002.* 2002, Global Forum for Health Research, World Health Organization: Geneva, Switzerland.

94. Acharya, T, Daar, AS, Thorsteinsdottir, H et al. 2004. Strengthening the role of genomics in global health. *PLoS Med* 1: e40.
95. Daar, AS, Thorsteinsdottir, H, Martin, DK et al. 2002. Top ten biotechnologies for improving health in developing countries. *Nat Genet* 32: 229–32.
96. Singer, PA and Daar, AS. 2001. Harnessing genomics and biotechnology to improve global health equity. *Science* 294: 87–9.
97. Marshall, PA. 2005. Human rights, cultural pluralism, and international health research. *Theor Med Bioeth* 26: 529–57.
98. Bioethics, NCo. 2002. The ethics of research related to healthcare in developing countries: 190.
99. Bioethics, NCo. 2005. The ethics of research related to healthcare in developing countries: a follow-up Discussion Paper:
100. Sachs, JD and Reid, WV. 2006. Environment. Investments toward sustainable development. *Science* 312: 1002.
101. Sachs, JD, *The End of Poverty. Economic Possibilities for Our Time*. 2005, New York: The Penguin Press.
102. Leitzmann, C and Cannon, G. 2005. Dimensions, domains and principles of the new nutrition science. *Public Health Nutr* 8: 787–94.
103. Beauman, C, Cannon, G, Elmadfa, I et al. 2005. The principles, definition and dimensions of the new nutrition science. *Public Health Nutr* 8: 695–8.
104. Cannon, G and Leitzmann, C. 2005. The new nutrition science project. *Public Health Nutr* 8: 673–94.
105. 2005. The Giessen Declaration. *Public Health Nutr* 8: 783–6.
106. Kunie, A and Ahmed, A. 2005. An overview of environmental health status in Ethiopia with particular emphasis to its organization, drinking water and sanitation: a literature survey. *Ethiop J Health Dev* 19: 89–103.
107. Sorsa, S, Kidanemariam, T, and Erosie, L. 2002. Health Problems of street children and women in Awassa, Southern Ethiopia. *Ethiop J Health Dev* 16: 129–137.
108. Churchill, GA, Airey, DC, Allayee, H et al. 2004. The Collaborative Cross, a community resource for the genetic analysis of complex traits. *Nat Genet* 36: 1133–7.
109. Khoury, MJ. 2004. The case for a global human genome epidemiology initiative. *Nat Genet* 36: 1027–1028.
110. Ioannidis, JPA, Gwinn, M, Little, J et al. 2006. A road map for efficient and reliable human genome epidemiology. *Nat Genet* 38: 3–5.
111. Cavanaugh, JA. 2003. IBD International Genetics Consortium: international cooperation making sense of complex disease. *Inflamm Bowel Dis* 9: 190–3.

# 18 The Future of Foods

*Heribert J. Watzke and J. Bruce German*

## CONTENTS



## 18.1 INTRODUCTION

Although not typically appreciated, processed foods are perhaps the most critical elements to the success of modern civilization. In fact, it is a tribute to the success of the processed food industry that urbanized societies are largely blissfully unaware of the multiple values inherent in their foods that make life as we know it possible. The core values of processing of foods are primarily to convert unstable, unsafe, and sparingly nutritious agricultural commodities into safe, stable, and completely nourishing foods. Industrialized societies continue to add and combine more values within the foods that they consume. This chapter will first examine the core values of industrialized foods and then suggest where the most obvious opportunities lie to increase or add value in the future. Finally, the chapter will examine the advances in science and technologies that are emerging, or would be necessary, to enable such a future.

## 18.2 THE VALUES OF INDUSTRIAL FOODS

Over the past century, as income levels have risen and societies have been able to invest in the science and technologies of food production, additional values have been added to processed foods. Foods are increasingly more convenient, freeing a larger and larger segment of the population from the need to prepare foods for immediate consumption. Foods are becoming progressively more delicious. Eating is a physiologically pleasurable experience, and safe, nourishing foods also enhance the quality of daily life through enhanced taste, flavor, texture, and even color. With greater income, society is able to afford increasingly more diverse foods in which the various elements of food delight (flavor, texture, color, etc.) are simultaneously enhanced. Foods are becoming more and more nutritious. In the latter half of the 20th century, a growing awareness of the ability of different food components to alter physiology, metabolism, and immunologic functions has led to the development of "functional foods" in which these health values are explicitly added to foods targeted at subsets of consumers (e.g., athletes, the infirm, the elderly) (Clydesdale, 1997).

The processed food industry of today is based on a remarkable depth and breadth of scientific research and development. Modern processed foods are possible only because of the detailed knowledge that this scientific activity has produced. This is certainly in part a detailed compositional description of the agricultural commodities that underpin foods as well as the compositions of the assembled final products. Information detailing the compositions of commodities include the amount and types of different proteins (from plant, animal, and microbial sources), carbohydrates (glucose, simple sugars, complex polymers of different sugar backbones, and polysaccharides), lipids (triacylglycerides as fats and oils from plants and animals, complex membrane lipids, and sterols), nucleic and organic acids, alcohols, and a wide array of plant secondary metabolites (carotenoids, flavonoids, anthocyanins, etc.). These are the basic ingredients of foods.

The knowledge of food components also extends to their macroscopic structures. The processing of basic commodities and their formulation into food products can alter both the relative composition of the basic molecules and also their cellular and biological structures. Food processing is designed to reformulate the compositions of foods, mixing ingredients from diverse commodity resources, and to remodel and synthesize new structures. Gels, fibers, emulsions, and foams are highly desirable food structures that are explicitly formed during food processing and preparation. These structures contribute to the stability, shape, texture, and organoleptic quality of the final foods. Considerable research has been directed toward understanding these basic structures, their formation, stability, and organoleptic properties (Tolstogustov, 1987).

The basic compositional and descriptive knowledge of commodities now also extends to detailed genomic sequences of an increasingly complete subset of agricultural commodities (European Plant Science Organization, 2005; Womack, 2005; McCarthy et al., 2006) and the molecular composition of these plants, animals, and microorganisms that we convert into the foods that we eat (Catchpole et al., 2005). Equally important, scientific research is building the functional annotation of these components both in terms of their structures, stabilities, and chemical interactions as raw materials and final foods (Sagalowicz et al., 2006; Tolstogustov, 1986) and in terms of their nutritional, safety, and toxicological implications for the humans that finally consume them (German et al., 2006; McCarthy et al., 2006). This remarkably diverse and predictive scientific knowledge is translated into practice by the myriad technologies that are used to process commodities into foods. Technologies that process foods range from careful control of heating and biological fermentations to highly complex engineering systems that simultaneously deliver pressure, temperature, mechanical, and biological inputs to high-throughput, multicomponent, sterile process assembly lines (Bruin and Jongen, 2003).

### 18.2.1 Integrating Food Values

Perhaps the most remarkable requirement of industrialized foods is the need to integrate multiple values within each food. It is not sufficient that a food be just safe or convenient. Foods must be simultaneously safe, nourishing, stable, convenient, affordable, and delightful. Furthermore, this requirement extends to any updation of food products. Any subsequent enhancement in an existing food's value must do so without compromising the other value assets. This places a great deal of pressure on all aspects of the food development process. Improving stability and convenience cannot lead to deterioration of flavor. Nor can improvements in flavor compromise safety. The first generation of functional foods failed because, although they contained added health values, the ingredients and technologies necessary to add these values compromised the perceived values of the foods (taste and convenience). Hence, within the very competitive food marketplace, they simply failed to attract consumers away from their existing choices. The next generation of functional foods recognized this need, and functional health values have been incorporated into foods that also deliver all of the values that consumers have come to expect.

### 18.2.2 Food Values Meeting Consumer Desires

Innovations in processed foods are thus an intersection of (1) desired consumer values, (2) molecular scientific knowledge, and (3) efficient industrial technologies (Figure 18.1). The future will certainly see a continuous series of developments in

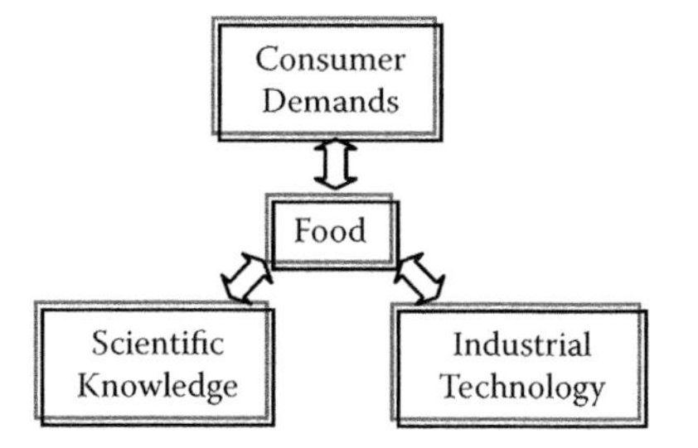


**FIGURE 18.1** Key inputs to food design, formulation, and process innovations.

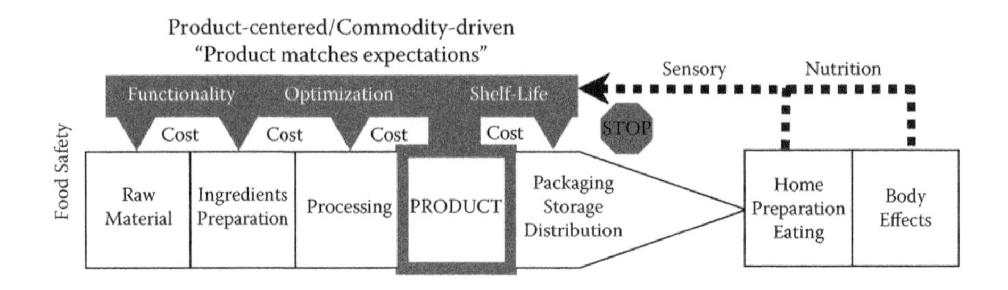


**FIGURE 18.2a** Current approach to food processing, designed to assemble food products according to the consumers' anticipated view of particular products or product categories.

all three of these areas, with progressive enhancements in the values provided by foods. Although many trends will be discernible, one unifying theme is the increasing personalization of foods, and this singular trend toward more personalized food product propositions will transform all of the values of processed foods.

The basic driving forces of the current industrial food sector are illustrated in Figure 18.2a. Food production today is a product-centric, commodity-driven industry. With food safety as the critical, nonnegotiable core, the food product itself is the defining element. Once established in the consumer's mind as a viable product, whether a fast food hamburger or a sweet carbonated beverage, the consumer is buying a familiar product with known organoleptic properties. The profit drivers all lie within the ability of competitors to drive the costs of delivering that same product lower. Nutrition is only considered as an ingredient additive at the end (vitamin-enriched), without compromising the basic product perception. This is a model that, while providing food products at spectacular volumes and low prices, is providing very little net value either to the consumer or to the production chain itself. Agriculture is essentially eating itself alive trying to provide cheaper and cheaper food products, and the consumers are literally eating themselves to death because of the poor nutritional contents. It is now possible to foresee an entirely different model (Figure 18.2b) in which the consumer becomes the defining element. In this model

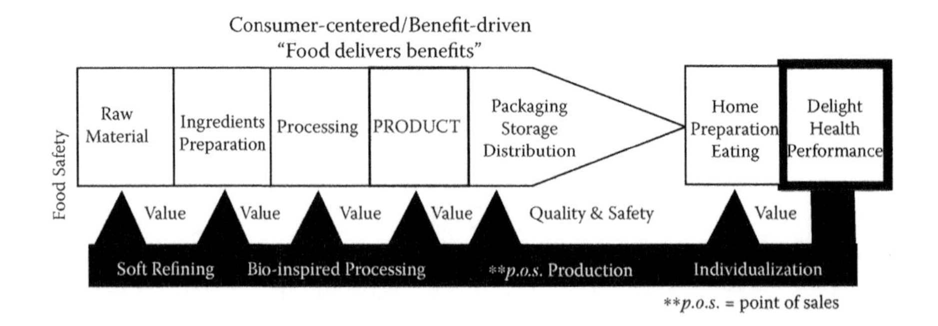


**FIGURE 18.2b** Proposed approach to foods for the future, designed around the consumer and delivering foods that address the specific needs, desires, and aspirations of each consumer for their individual health and well-being.

the goal is to provide values to the consumer. With the consumer as the goal, many values such as health, performance, and even enjoyment and delight become attributes that enhance the overall value proposition to the consumer. In this model, any stage in the agricultural process that is capable of adding, or enhancing, benefits to the consumer creates value at that level, from seed producer through farmer through processor to delivery system. It is critical to such a model that the variation among consumers be recognized, and thus foods must become more personalized.

Consumers themselves will be the major drivers of the trend to personalization. The average consumer is increasingly gaining awareness of his or her wants and needs, and growing scientific knowledge and technological advances will race to meet them. Examples of this ongoing progressive trend are numerous, yet the diversity of foods and consumers makes it difficult to predict the future. Nonetheless, it is possible to categorize innovations within each of the previously stated areas (desired consumer values, molecular scientific knowledge, and efficient industrial technologies) to gain a sense of predictability. From the consumer perspective, the major trend is toward individualization of health. The last decade has seen an explosion in the personalization of consumer products of virtually all kinds from computers to entertainment, from transportation to cosmetics (German et al., 2005b). This trend has been evident in foods, extending to all of the values of foods, but will increasingly include health as a personal value proposition. Consumers know more about their own health issues and the potential of foods to alter them. Although it has been a core value of processed foods to ensure safety, the future safety of foods will take on a more personal dimension. Foods will include means of making consumers themselves safer. Initially this will mean more specific control of food processing and specific labeling (no nuts, gluten-free, etc.). Eventually foods will incorporate various means of ensuring that however consumers choose to assemble their diet, risks to safety will be minimized.

## 18.3 THE TOOLS OF THE FUTURE

### 18.3.1 Life Sciences and Genomics

The major growth dimension in science is the developing biological understanding of virtually all life-forms, because of the genomics revolution and the sequencing of the entire genome of humans, of hundreds of viruses, bacteria, plants, and animals, and even entire ecosystems (Miller et al., 2004; McCarthy et al., 2006; Morris, 2006). This biological knowledge of genomes and the rapidly assembling annotation of their functions are dramatically accelerating the rate at which we are acquiring a truly mechanistic understanding of human health and disease, and how diet impacts both. This knowledge is also much more accessible to other fields of research, and thus this basic genomics knowledge will also empower biotechnologies to interact with our lives in multiple ways. The scientific understanding of microbial, plant, and animal physiology, and metabolism will lead to a greater diversity of agricultural commodities that can serve as input to the food chain (Delmer, 2005). But even greater innovations will come as new biological applications are brought forward to participate in the actual processing of foods, i.e., bioguided processing (Ward et al., 2004).

It is certainly not revolutionary for a wine maker who has used yeast to ferment grape juice into wine to imagine a life-form participating in the processing of an agricultural commodity. Nonetheless, the improvements in molecular dexterity, cost, and control that biological strategies contribute to food processing will lead to a dramatic increase in biologically based innovations in foods. Many of the components of human milk are active catalysts whose benefits to the infant are provided by the catalytic activity itself (e.g., bile-salt-stimulated lipase makes lipids more available for absorption). At present such activities are destroyed during processing, whereas in future they will be retained. Other molecules present in milk are highly dependent on the subtleties of molecular structure lost during processing, for example, the milk fat globule in which surface carbohydrates capable of binding microbial toxins are lost because of homogenization. Again, processes designed to maintain these structures will be valuable but likely only to a subset of consumers; hence, the need to personalize the value chain from processing to product.

### 18.3.2 Computing and Scientific Knowledge Management

Technology continues to be driven by computerization, and the proliferation of all aspects of information technologies is moving rapidly through the food process industry as the cost of acquiring and managing information plummets. Nonetheless, the key to the applications of the massive computing power now available to food-related biotechnologies is to coordinate — if not unify — the terminologies that are used for cross-disciplinary studies in food, agriculture, and nutrition (Lange et al., 2007). Equally important for the successful application of computational mathematics — now bringing remarkable, and genuinely revolutionary, understanding of basic biological processes (Grigorov, 2005) — to improving health through foods is to standardize the database structures of these same fields so that advances in the larger fields of biology and medicine can be readily translated into food and nutrition (Lemay et al., 2007). It is particularly discouraging that health itself remains a poorly defined concept in scientific terms. Computing power is most effective when automated across large and dissimilar data sets. However, if data sets are not comparable, they must be hand-curated, reducing all of the computing power back to the snail's pace of individual comparisons. If we examine fields in which database consolidation has occurred (communication and satellite imaging, for example), it is possible to see that applications can not only be made commercially viable (mobile phone technologies), but astonishing cost-efficiencies are possible (mobile phone technologies have supplanted hard line technologies in the developing world). The example of global financial transactions is not just illustrative of what is possible today in terms of personalized technologies, it is most illuminating by virtue of how little value is necessary to make it commercially viable. The routine use of electronic transactions (credit card purchasing) that has spread throughout the world in order to carry out large financial transactions is now used for on-the-spot payment of a single cup of coffee. If such a trivial value is sufficient to drive globally accessible credit card technology into coffee shops, then it is only the imagination of the scientist that limits what would be possible for foods and health if we could move to a more standardized and computer-friendly information system.

### 18.3.3 Consumer Demands in Future

The last 50 years have seen a continuous trend toward providing products to consumers that maximize their ability to make immediate choices about the foods they wish to eat (Moskowitz et al., 2005). This drive to provide immediate food choices has literally transformed the competitive food marketplace. Not just convenience, but safety, stability, packaging, distribution channels, and now nutrition, all have been driven relentlessly forward by a marketplace catering to individual consumers wishing to customize their personal eating opportunities. The emerging demand for nutritious foods is now moving not simply away from foods that are perceived as unhealthy but the trends are instead toward foods that can improve the personal health of consumers (Sloane, 2006). This desire is in part being driven by the reality of the worsening health of the average consumer.

The aging, sedentary population in the Western world is increasingly becoming overweight, hypertensive, and diabetic, and all of these conditions are accelerated by poor diets (Alberti, 2001). Importantly, these poor diets are not deficient in essential nutrients (vitamins, minerals) but are instead unbalanced in terms of calories and macronutrients (Popkin, 2006). These macronutrient imbalances lead to chronic dysregulation of normal metabolism within susceptible individuals. Although such metabolic disorders are eventually devastating to health and lead to diseases different from deficiencies of essential nutrients, they develop gradually as endogenous, noncommunicable diseases (Quam et al., 2006). Furthermore, whereas the first wave of metabolic disease — atherosclerosis — was caused by an invisible, progressive accumulation of lipoproteins in artery walls, and thus was not evident to consumers, obesity, hypertension, and diabetes are readily sensed or measured, and consumers are vividly aware of their own deteriorating health although they do not know how to change their health trajectories (Petrovici and Ritson, 2006). This crisis in health-care problems owing to chronic degenerative diseases is becoming rapidly evident as the population ages. Even if the formal policies and infrastructures of public health are unable to mount an effective change that resolves these health issues, consumers are increasingly demanding that their food provide health protection. It has not escaped the attention of the food industry that the only significant growth in food marketing value is occurring in the health-promoting food sector (Clydesdale, 2004). Consumers are increasingly recognizing the importance of diets to their health, and will be demanding products and services to meet their desires.

### 18.3.4 The Technologies for the Future

The genomics revolution has enhanced not only the knowledge of biology, but has dramatically altered the way research in the life sciences is conducted. Various aspects of biology are being discovered at unprecedented rates — from the development of diseases in humans to the production of biofuels by plants and microorganisms (Collins et al., 2003; Pharkya et al., 2004). Although the initial stages of the biological revolution in agriculture has been to narrow genetic diversity of crops due largely to the agronomic success of genetically modified core commodities such as soy and corn, this is not sustainable in the long term. What our rapidly growing knowledge of plant and animal genomics portends for the future is the increased domestication of a much larger and more diverse agriculture. Human agriculture is based on a very limited subset of all living organisms. The reason for this is that most organisms evolved under the constant Darwinian selective pressure to avoid being eaten. As a result of this pressure, most plants elaborated secondary metabolism leading to the production of compounds to discourage animal predation. Antinutritive, and overtly toxic alkaloids, flavonoids, protease inhibitors, phytates, etc., render most existing wild plants inedible. However, as we gain mastery of the genomics of plants and the history of their evolution becomes clear, it will be possible to selectively eliminate the antinutritional and toxic elements. With such tools, plant geneticists will be able to dramatically expand the available genetic stocks for agriculture and increase the diversity of inputs to the food supply. What the organic food movement of today is struggling to provide as value propositions, with increased sustainability, environmental protection, and species diversity will be dramatically enhanced by the ability to understand the genetics of all of the agricultural players from plants to animals, and even microorganisms.

In addition to making plant diversity an asset to food production, genomics will increase our biotechnology dexterity with a wide array of microorganisms. Bacteria, yeasts, and molds represent a very successful traditional means of food processing providing increased safety, stability, and nutritional quality while modifying many of the taste, flavor, and textural properties of biomaterials from cultured vegetables, meats, cheeses, and cereals. The combination of knowledge and biological tools that microbial genomics is providing will revolutionize the bioprocessing of foods. Not only bacteria, yeasts, and molds but viruses too will be recruited to the task of improving food values.

Although agricultural species diversity will increase dramatically, one of the interesting outcomes of this knowledge explosion involves understanding the diversity within species. Research is revealing all of the ways that humans differ from each other, one of them certainly being the way different humans respond to diet. The fields of nutrigenomics and nutrigenetics are rapidly compiling examples of genetic variation in the normal population that predicts variation in health outcome. From dietary fat and lipoprotein atherogenicity (Krauss, 2001; Ordovas, 2003) to dietary carbohydrate and weight loss (Martinez et al., 2003), to dietary vitamins and risk of birth defects (Whetstine et al., 2002), genetic variation is being demonstrated to be a key component of the variation in human health that is ascribable to diet. The most widely used index of metabolic health is the level of circulating lipids in blood, primarily cholesterol and triglycerides. Just by looking at the mechanisms by which lipids are cleared from blood, we see a vivid story of the genetic variation within the human population. Clearance of triglyceride-rich lipoproteins is affected by polymorphisms at several gene loci, including apoB (Rantala et al., 2000), apoAV (Lai et al., 2003), apo E (Ostos et al., 1998), and lipoprotein lipase (Mero et al., 1999). The consequences of these genotypic differences are that individuals can be assigned to varying responses to, for example, high- and low-fat diets. The size and atherogenicity of cholesterol-rich, low-density lipoproteins, and their response to diet are mitigated by heritable genes that can be demonstrated to persist in the offspring of phenotypic carriers (Krauss, 2001). Again, as a result of defining these genotypes, individuals who vary in response to diet will eventually be assigned/guided to lower or higher saturated fat-containing diets.

The success of these emerging studies implies that parts of our health will be predictable from simple genotypic analyses. However, this is not the only basis on which individuals in the population differ with respect to responses to diet. We are all exposed to different environments, (exercise, diets, etc.), and these are now recognized as increasingly important to the net effects of dietary choices on our health (Bateson et al., 2004). If multiple variables relate to the response of health to diet beyond genotype of individuals, then health itself will have to be explicitly measured using technologies akin to disease diagnostics. However, these assessors will need to be more accurate and capture the fluctuations in metabolism and physiology that correspond to variations in aspects of health, not simply the diagnostics of disease (German et al., 2005a).

### 18.3.5 Analytic Technologies for Health Assessment

Currently, diagnostic tests use the measurement of surrogate endpoints, or biomarkers of a disease process, to assess the progress of an individual toward a disease state or to monitor the effectiveness of a treatment. This approach is successful and becoming increasingly automated for diagnosing many of the diseases of humans — including infection and overt toxicities — where a specific molecule or group of molecules present in blood or tissues are uniquely characteristic of the disease state, and are otherwise foreign to the matrix being sampled in healthy individuals (Sajda, 2006). Diseases that are caused by an imbalance in endogenous metabolism are more difficult to diagnose and predict because they lack unambiguous markers and are, instead, characterized by changes only in the absolute concentration of metabolites that are otherwise always present in the tissue or fluid (Schoenhagen and Nissen, 2006). In these cases, the absolute, measured concentration of the metabolites must be compared to a database of metabolite concentrations for the entire population. Even when these databases are assembled and the utility of a single biomarker for monitoring disease risk is well established (e.g., plasma cholesterol in atherosclerosis and plasma glucose in diabetes), these single measurements cannot by themselves identify the biochemical pathway responsible for the problem (e.g., in this individual, why is glucose high?). Ideal assessment technologies are more comprehensive and reflect the spectrum of metabolic states that dictate overall immediate health as well as predict future health risk. Assessment should be capable of identifying both the presence of a dysregulation and the responsible molecular mechanism, and ideally predict a logical strategy for intervening in the process in each individual (German et al., 2005a). For example, cholesterol levels are now routinely measured in a substantial fraction of the population as a means of identifying those at risk for developing heart disease. However, the basic technologies that measure cholesterol, even when ascribing the cholesterol to specific lipoprotein classes, are unable to distinguish the underlying mechanisms in each individual that are responsible for the elevated cholesterol. They simply note that the individual is potentially at risk because of this reading. If the measures of cholesterol were broadened to include a relatively few additional metabolites, much more information could be gained as to the underlying cause. For example, it has been well established that the basic causes of elevated cholesterol in humans are not all the same.

Some individuals have high levels of circulating cholesterol because their hepatic and peripheral biosynthesis rates are high (Schmitz and Langmann, 2006). Some have high cholesterol because they absorb inordinately high levels from the intestine, and still others have high cholesterol because they secrete less sterol both as cholesterol and bile acids from the liver as bile (Plosch et al., 2005). By measuring sterol biosynthesis intermediates quantitatively in plasma, relative sterol synthesis rates can be estimated, thus identifying those who synthesize high levels of cholesterol; by measuring the immediate products of bile acid synthesis in plasma, those who produce and excrete less bile can be identified, and by measuring phytosterols in plasma, those individuals who hyperabsorb sterols can be identified (reviewed in German et al., 2005a). Now, with each of the different causes of high cholesterol identified within individuals, appropriate strategies for effective intervention can also be designed. Cholesterol synthesis drugs are highly effective in those who oversynthesize cholesterol, but are relatively ineffective in those who hyperabsorb. Similarly, sterol absorption inhibitors are highly effective in those who hyperabsorb sterols.

The new sciences of omics — genomics, transcriptomics, proteomics and metabolomics — have emerged as a result of the developments of complete databases of genomes and their products, and the technologies to simultaneously analyze all, or significant subsets of all members of a biological class of molecules (genes, mRNAs, proteins, and metabolites) (Raamsdonk et al., 2001). These tools have dramatic implications for the routine assessment of health because of their potential to literally measure a complete picture of functional biology in a tissue or fluid compartment at once (Nicholson and Wilson, 2003). Omic assessment technologies, and in particular metabolomics, thus offer a unique opportunity for clinical chemistry not only to monitor the progress of disease states but also to characterize and define how to maintain health. With such information on health status, individuals will be able to gain knowledge of their unique metabolic needs, and most importantly, will be able to act on these needs with diet as the major intervention. Assessment conducted routinely (e.g., monthly, yearly) will also provide feedback regarding the success of all food, drug, and lifestyle changes within a time frame that reinforces them or redirects them as appropriate. Again, this type of assessment will bring a much more empowered consumer population to the marketplace for agriculture and its products — foods. Even more importantly, with assessed health status of individuals in place as a consumer asset, it will be possible for diets to be much more effective in preventing diseases long before they occur, at which points foods become a competitive alternative to drugs in maintaining health and preventing disease.

There is an important economic argument for disease prevention that undermines most attempts to bring preventive medicine into practice. How much will a consumer pay for a drug/therapeutic/bioactive substance to prevent a disease that they will never have? The answer is discouragingly simple, very little. Drugs are perceived to be a valuable product category precisely because they are designed to cure existing disease. In prevention, you are currently healthy and by following a particular regimen of food consumption, behavior, or lifestyle, you are unlikely to develop a future disease. Hence, the value of any single therapeutic preventive is very low. In order to be successful, preventive strategies have to be very cost-effective. In fact, it is precisely because foods are already routinely consumed, carry an existing value proposition, and can easily deliver multiple biological activities that they are so appropriate as the "engines of prevention."

### 18.3.6 Technologies for Food Production

The technological advances of the first half of the 20th century saw the burgeoning science of chemistry yielding a wide range of applications, for example, the petroleum chemistry revolutionizing fuel and transportation, and the fertilizer chemistry driving the green revolution. This was also true for the food processing industry. From the separation and use of chemicals as ingredients and processing aids that improved the safety, quality, and stability of agricultural commodities and food products (acids, gases, emulsifiers, colors flavors, etc.), to the synthesis and enrichment of vitamins for nutrient adequacy, the food processing industry was able to apply the breakthroughs of chemistry to the improvement of food process operations and the routine manufacturing of foods. Today's research in food engineering is actively pursuing various means of expanding the ways in which foods are processed within the existing unit operations, and with the same goals in mind. There are many examples of novel technologies that could potentially enhance the cost and effectiveness of existing unit operations in food processing. For example, it is possible to render pathogenic bacteria inactive by high pressure, and the use of high-pressure sterilization of processed foods is being studied intensively (Gould, 2000). Nonetheless, these cannot be considered to be the major focus of today's technological innovation in foods. The true technological innovation that is emerging is information itself. The technological developments of computing in the latter half of the 20th century are driving incredible progress in the acquisition, storage, and mathematical manipulation of information. Such information is providing levels of control of food production, processing, distribution, and marketing not previously possible. Interestingly, information management of health is the largest growth industry of the world's largest information highway, the Internet. It is certainly inevitable that the future will move toward information transfer so effectively that personal health knowledge becomes part of each individual's daily decision making, of which diet will be a part. The only questions are how fast and how the food industry will accelerate this trend.

### 18.3.7 Self-Assembly Processes in Food Biomaterials

The gradual migration of food processing from large centralized factories producing large numbers of identical products to processing that is capable of assembling more customized formulations appropriate for a more individualized health proposition will require that foods be assembled in smaller unit operations. Although it is currently assumed that this will require factory-like operations, this is not necessarily true. The goals of current processing of ensuring microbial safety while maintaining basic nutrient composition will broaden to include the added value of retaining many of the inherent biological properties of the commodities from which the biomaterials originally derive (Ward et al., 2004). Furthermore, although considerable external energy is input during processing to manipulate food materials in order to produce multiple phases (foams, emulsions, etc.) as the means to formulate, stabilize, and texturize food products, many of these desired goals could be achieved without the macroscopic, high-energy unit operations currently used today. In fact, to the extent possible, food processing will take advantage of the properties of the molecules within biomaterials to spontaneously self-assemble into desired forms (Leser et al., 2006). Self-assembly of biomolecules is not a new concept invented for the food sciences — life itself is based upon it. The most remarkable property of life is that every organism, from the smallest to the largest, is ostensibly self-assembled from simple biopolymers. As the sciences of genomics begin to understand the more structure-specific properties of molecules as gene products, the self-assembly properties of biomolecules even complex colloidal properties will similarly be understood with sufficient accuracy to control them (de Campo et al., 2004). There are already many examples of adapting the natural properties of biopolymers for the net benefit of food products. Cheese is an obvious illustration of this principle: the properties of casein micelles are captured for aggregation into three-dimensional gel networks.

## 18.4 APPLYING CONSUMER HEALTH, BIOLOGICAL KNOWLEDGE, AND ADVANCED TECHNOLOGIES PRACTICE TO PERSONALIZED FOODS

### 18.4.1 Individual Health

The personalization of health will require three elements: assessment technologies, health trajectory prediction, and intervention strategies. Assessment was discussed earlier, and it is clear from the rapid rise of personalized medicine that the technologies to assess health are emerging for therapeutic medicine and will be immediately translated into other aspects of health care. However, managing an existing disease is not the same as projecting the health trajectory of healthy individuals according to an assessment even of a large number of metabolites. Decades of research were needed to recognize that high levels of cholesterol in blood were predictive of future heart disease, that altered hepatic cholesterol metabolism was responsible for high cholesterol levels in blood, and that intervening in this metabolism through diet or drugs led to a lower risk of heart disease. Nonetheless, this success provides confidence that it is possible to act on systemic health without having a full mathematical, systems biology solution for the entire organism's physiology. In essence, health solutions can be pursued empirically to a large extent, both in populations and in individuals. This will be possible if (1) assessment technologies are developed and put in place at high throughput to measure large numbers of individuals, (2) databases chronicling the outcomes of assessment with health outcomes are constructed and annotated appropriately, and (3) individual assessment results are able to be compared with outcomes from the larger databases, and assessment converted to projections and interventions as appropriate. The advantages of a combined empirical–mechanistic approach to health assessment and improvement are that we can start now; the discovery process will "find" the most common health issues first, thus providing value to the largest number of individuals immediately, and value can be gained as both health improvement and commercial development proceed and as results emerge.

### 18.4.2 Personalizing Foods and Diets

The food processing industry today has achieved unprecedented success in providing safe and affordable foods based on manufacturing large quantities of relatively standardized products in factory operations engineered to deliver well-defined and validated unit operations. The advantages of the economies of scale that are possible with this process model have led to not only cost of production efficiencies — extending from agricultural commodity production to food product assembly to market distribution — but to dramatic improvements in other aspects of manufacturing, including waste management, environmental protection, and worker safety. This very visible success would seem to be incompatible with a personalized approach to food production. In fact, an important unanswered question is whether personalization of diets according to individual needs for health is even possible both technologically and within the economic framework of modern society. Although we cannot be certain how the development of personalizing foods will proceed, it is appropriate to examine models of existing successes in personalizing consumer products based on science, technology, and consumer values. Perhaps the most extreme example of employing very sophisticated technology to deliver a frankly minor consumer value is global positioning satellite (GPS) localization of golf course distances. At various golf courses throughout the U.S. today, the carts that conduct individual golfers around the course are equipped with a GPS-locating system whose only consumer value is to indicate the distance from the cart (or the device when held in the golfer's hand) to the hole. The technology necessary to this product is truly astonishing. An orbiting satellite network, using Einsteinian mathematics to triangulate distance coordinates accurately against the massive database of the earth's geographical surface that both the individual (personal) device on the fairway and the hole in the green can be measured to within a meter's distance. With this "personalized golf location" system already in place as an example, it is difficult to argue that a more personalized approach to dietary guidance for health is either scientifically or technologically impossible. The question is simply, how will it be done?

## 18.5 PERSONALIZING FOOD: FUTURE PERSPECTIVES

There are unquestionably important hurdles to the widespread conversion of industrial food processing into a more personalized food delivery system. Traditional food preparation within families was obviously very personal as each individual within the family unit ate according to the expertise of the family representative (typically, the mother) who acted as the diet designer for each family member and processed raw commodities into foods within family meals. Anecdote and cultural history combined with close individual inspection were the basis of diet decisions. The question is thus not whether diets and foods themselves can be personalized, but how can the modern, highly efficient industrial processing of food, which gained its value largely by centralizing food processing and achieving economies of scale, be converted to an industrial system of personal food production. The values — safety, affordability, convenience, and delight — that brought industrialized foods such success will continue to operate. To succeed, food production will invariably need to maintain all of these values and yet become more personal with respect to health.

First and foremost for any personalization is flexibility in product composition. No matter what the differences in individual human health problems and requirements are, they will be resolved in large part by consuming diets of different molecular compositions. How then can one imagine that different compositions of foods, decided now at the stage of factory formulation, can be delivered to different consumers at the point of their purchase, or even the point of consumption?

One model would be to increase the number and diversity of food products that are produced by the existing factory manufacturing processes. In such a model, the customization would be performed at the point of distribution using a system of guided choices. A customer would employ a personal knowledge device (the handheld computer is often cited), and a computer would indicate from the wide range of specific food choices those that are appropriate for each individual to select. Although such a model seems attractive in that it would create minimal disruption in existing manufacturing and distribution, it fails in many respects to deliver on the potential values that personalized foods could, and should, provide. It is also unlikely that the added inventory control, dilution of market space, and factory flexibility necessary to such a system would maintain cost-effectiveness.

An alternative model would be to alter the processes of food formulation such that much of the final compositions would be dictated at the point of purchase, preparation, or consumption. Such a model would require that intelligent systems assemble foods much nearer the point at which they are consumed. Although sounding somewhat outrageous for application to existing food products, there are examples where such a conceptual change has already occurred. Nespresso™ is a product category in which a substantial part of the processing of espresso coffee (highly controlled temperature and pressure extraction of ground beans) is accomplished within the kitchen or even at the table of the consumer. Different flavor options are available to "personalize" the coffee-drinking experience, and the processing is in large part performed immediately before consumption. In fact, moving from a one-size-fits-all model to a more plastic and dynamic system of food formulation would not be limited to compositions for health. All of the consumer food values that could be discerned as being desirable for each consumer could also be potentially available. For example, if the composition of a meal/food were being customized for a single individual, its composition for health (macronutrients, micronutrients, and bioactive molecules) would be obvious, but so too would its composition for a more personal preference for flavor, texture, and even convenience. So too would safety be a customized value, assuring individuals with allergies or intolerances to particular food components that these have been eliminated.

## 18.6 CONCLUSIONS

The growing emphasis in the food industry in the 21st century is, and will continue to be, to deliver safe, convenient, affordable, and delicious food products that provide the means to assemble diets that maintain and improve the health of consumers. The power of nutrition research and food processing to solve health problems is illustrated by the success of identifying the essential nutrients, recognizing their absolute requirements, and retaining, enriching, and fortifying the food supply to ensure that deficiency diseases could be prevented. The success is vividly illustrated by the observation that the population is now unaware of, i.e., has never seen the phenotypes of diseases caused by classic deficiency diseases: iodine–goiter, vitamin C–scurvy, and vitamin A–blindness. Through the past three decades, diseases caused by unbalanced diets have become literally epidemic across the developed world (Alberti, 2001). These diseases, attributed at least in part to poorly balanced diets, include atherosclerosis, obesity, diabetes, atherosclerosis, hypertension, and osteoporosis. Food and nutrition research must now adapt to this new challenge and consider strategies that can reverse this trend. A combination of research knowledge and food applications must provide consumers with diets that maintain the value systems of safety, quality, stability, convenience, and cost. These values are not sufficient; diets must also ensure that each consumer as an individual maintains optimal health within the lifestyle that he or she chooses to pursue. The growing scientific knowledge of the diversity of human genetics, lifestyles, and environments is leading to the conclusion that humans are sufficiently different that the same diet will not be optimal for all, and that some form of personal diet is necessary. This realization would appear to be devastating to the current system of industrial food production based on large factories producing homogeneous products with high tolerances of safety, quality, and cost. Indeed, the components associated with personalizing diet and health are substantial. First and foremost, personal human health assessment is necessary. The obvious first step, measuring cholesterol, proved to be the key to identifying individuals with high cholesterol and at risk of future heart disease. Now it will be necessary to assess various other aspects of health and identify those individuals who are at risk of metabolic disorders (obesity, diabetes, hypertension, and osteoporosis) and other health implications, including, for example, immunological issues such as immune senescence, allergy, and inflammation. Second, once an individual is assessed and the scientific knowledge of what the assessment results imply in terms of dietary composition is in place, it will be necessary to provide that individual with foods customized to that composition. Such a customization of industrial food processing seems at first impractical. Nevertheless, the food industry is already highly plastic in many aspects. Dispensing technologies are already in place to apportion sweetener and whiteners to coffees, and hence the expansion of such capabilities into a first-generation personal dispensing system could be done immediately. What will drive the rate of arrival and acceptance of these technologies will be the ingenuity and creativity of scientists, technologists, and engineers throughout the food industry, and the values that they provide to consumers.

## KEY READINGS

Collins FS, Green ED, Guttmacher AE, Guyer MS; U.S. National Human Genome Research Institute. 2003 A vision for the future of genomics research. *Nature*. 24; 422(6934): 835–47.

Morris CE, Sands DC. The breeder's dilemma — yield or nutrition? *Nat Biotechnol*. September 2006; 24(9): 1078–80.

Sturino JM, Klaenhammer TR. Engineered bacteriophage-defence systems in bioprocessing. *Nat Rev Microbiol*. May 2006; 4(5): 395–404.

## REFERENCES


Alberti G., 2001, Noncommunicable diseases: tomorrow's pandemics, *Bull. WHO* 79, 907.

Bateson P., D. Barker, T. Clutton-Brock, D. Deb, B. D'Udine, R. A, Foley, P. Gluckman, K. Godfrey, T. Kirkwood. M. M. Lahr, J. McNamara, N. B. Metcalfe, P. Monaghan, H. G. Spencer and S. E. Sultan, 2004, Developmental plasticity and human health, *Nature* 430(6998), 419–421.

Bruin S. and ThRG Jongen, 2003, Food process engineering: the last 25 years and the challenges ahead, *Crit. Rev. Food Sci. Food Safety* 2, 42–81.

Catchpole G. S., M. Beckmann, D. P. Enot, M. Mondhe, B. Zywicki, J. Taylor, N. Hardy, A. Smith, R. D. King, D. B. Kell D.B., O. Fiehn and J. Draper, 2005, Hierarchical metabolomics demonstrates substantial compositional similarity between genetically modified and conventional potato crops, *Proc. Natl. Acad. Sci. USA* 102, 14458–14462.

Clydesdale F. M., 1997, A proposal for the establishment of scientific criteria for health claims for functional foods, *Nutr. Rev.* 55, 413–422.

Clydesdale F., 2004, IFT Expert Panel Report on Functional Foods: Opportunities and Challenges, *Food Technol.* 58, 35–40.

Collins F.S., E.D. Green, A.E. Guttmacher and M.S. Guyer; US National Human Genome Research Institute. 2003 A vision for the future of genomics research. *Nature*. 24; 422(6934): 835–47.

de Campo L., A.Yaghmur, L. Sagalowicz, M.E. Leser, H. Watzke and O. Glatter, Reversible phase transitions in emulsified nanostructured lipid systems. *Langmuir*. June 22, 2004; 20(13): 5254–61.

Delmer D. P., 2005, Agriculture in the developing world: Connecting innovations in plant research to downstream applications, *Proc. Natl. Acad. Sci. USA* 102, 15739–15746.

European Plant Science Organization, 2005, European plant science: a field of opportunities, *J. Exp. Bot.* 56, 1699–709.

German J. B, F. L. Schanbacher, B. Lönnerdal, J. Medrano, M. a. McGuire, J. L. McManaman, D. M. Rocke, T. P. Smith, M. C. Neville, P. Donnelly, M. C. Lange and R. E. Ward, 2006, International milk genomics consortium, *Trends Food Sci.Technol.* 17, 656–661.

German J. B., B. D. Hammock and S. M. Watkins, 2005a, Metabolomics: building on a century of biochemistry to guide human health, *Metabolomics* 1, 3–8.

German J. B., C. Yeretzian and H. J. Watzke, 2005b, Personalizing foods for health and preference, *Food Technol.* 58, 26–31.

Gould G. W., 2000, Preservation: past, present and future, *Br. Med. Bull.* 56, 84–96.

Grigorov M. G., 2005, Global properties of biological networks, *Drug Discov. Today* 10, 365–372.

Krauss R. M., 2001, Dietary and genetic effects on low-density lipoprotein heterogeneity, *Annu. Rev. Nutr.* 21, 283–295.

Lai C. Q., E. S. Tai, C. E. Tan, J. Cutter, S. K. Chew, Y. P. Zhu, X. Adiconis and J. M. Ordovas, 2003, The apolipoprotein A5 locus is a strong determinant of plasma triglyceride concentrations across ethnic groups in Singapore, *J. Lipid Res.* 44, 2365–2373.

Lange M. C., D. G. Lemay and J. B. German, 2007, A multi-ontology framework to guide agriculture and food towards diet and health, *J. Sci. Food Agric.* (in press).

Lemay D. G., A. M. Zivkovic and J. B. German, 2007, Building the bridges to bioinformatics in nutrition research, *Am. J. Clin. Nutr.* 13 Apr 2007, online, 10.1002/jsfa. 2832.

Leser M. E., L. Sagalowicz, M. Michel, and H. J. Watzke, Self-assembly of polar food lipids. *Adv. Colloid Interface Sci.* 2006 Nov 16; 123–126: 125–36.

Martinez J. A., M. S. Corbalan, A. Sanchez-Villegas, L. Forga, A. Marti and M. A. Martinez-Gonzalez, 2003, Obesity risk is associated with carbohydrate intake in women carrying the Gln27Glu beta2-adrenoceptor polymorphism, *J. Nutr.* 133, 2549–2554.

McCarthy F. M., N. Wang, G. B. Magee, B. Nanduri, M. L. Lawrence, E. B. Camon, D. G. Barrell, D. P. Hill, M. E. Dolan, W. P. Williams, D. S. Luthe, S. M. Bridges and S. C. Burgess, 2006, AgBase: a functional genomics resource for agriculture, *BMC Genomics* 7, 229.

Mero N., L. Suurinkeroinen, M. Syvanne, P. Knudsen, H. Yki-Jarvinen and M. R. Taskinen, 1999, Delayed clearance of postprandial large TG-rich particles in normolipidemic carriers of LPL Asn291Ser gene variant, *J. Lipid Res.* 40, 1663–1670.

Miller W., K. D. Makova, A. Nekrutenko and R. C. Hardison, 2004, Comparative genomics, *Annu. Rev. Genomics Hum. Genet.* 5, 15–56.

Morris R. M., 2006, Environmental genomics: exploring ecological sequence space, *Curr. Biol.* 6, R499–501.

Moskowitz, H. R., J. B. German and I. S. Saguy, 2005, Unveiling health attitudes and creating good-for-you foods: the genomics metaphor, consumer innovative web-based technologies, *Crit. Rev. Food Sci. Nutr.* 45,165–191.

Nicholson J. K. and I. D. Wilson, 2003, Opinion: understanding 'global' systems biology: metabonomics and the continuum of metabolism, *Nat. Rev. Drug Discov.* 2, 668–676.

Ordovas J. M., 2003, Cardiovascular disease genetics: a long and winding road, *Curr. Opin. Lipidol.* 14, 47–54.

Ostos M. A., J. Lopez-Miranda, J. M. Ordovas, C. Marin, A. Blanco, P. Castro, F. Lopez-Segura, J. Jimenez-Pereperez and F. J, Perez-Jimenez, 1998, Dietary fat clearance is modulated by genetic variation in apolipoprotein A-IV gene locus, *J. Lipid Res.* 39, 2493–2500.

Petrovici D. A. and C. Ritson, 2006, Factors influencing consumer dietary health preventative behaviours, *BMC Public Health* 6, 222.

Pharkya P., A.P. Burgard, and C.D. Maranas 2004 OptStrain: a computational framework for redesign of microbial production systems. *Genome Res.* 14(11): 2367–76.

Plosch T., A. Kosters, A. K. Groen and F. Kuipers, 2005, The ABC of hepatic and intestinal cholesterol transport, *Handb. Exp. Pharmacol.* 170, 465–482.

Popkin B. M., 2006, Global nutrition dynamics: the world is shifting rapidly toward a diet linked with noncommunicable diseases, *Am. J. Clin. Nutr.* 84, 289–298.

Quam L., R. Smith and D. Yach, 2006, Rising to the global challenge of the chronic disease epidemic, *Lancet*, 368, 1221–1223.

Raamsdonk L. M., B.Teusink, D. Broadhurst, N. Zhang, A. Hayes, M. C. Walsh, J. A. Berden, K. M. Brindle, D. B. Kell, J. J. Rowland, H. V. Westerhoff, K. van Dam and S. G. Oliver, 2001, A functional genomics strategy that uses metabolome data to reveal the phenotype of silent mutations, *Nat. Biotechnol.* 19, 45–50.

Rantala M., T. T. Rantala, M. J. Savolainen, Y. Friedlander and Y. A. Kesaniemi, 2000, Apolipoprotein B gene polymorphisms and serum lipids: meta-analysis of the role of genetic variation in responsiveness to diet, *Am. J. Clin. Nutr.* 71, 713–724.

Sagalowicz L., M. E. Leser, H. J. Watzke and M. Michel, 2006, Monoglyceride self-assembly structures as delivery vehicles, *Trends Food Sci. Technol.* 17, 204–214.

Sajda P., 2006, Machine learning for detection and diagnosis of disease, *Annu. Rev. Biomed. Eng.* 8, 537–565.

Schmitz G. and T. Langmann, 2006, Pharmacogenomics of cholesterol-lowering therapy, *Vascul. Pharmacol.* 44, 75–89.

Schoenhagen P. and S. E. Nissen, 2006, Identification of the metabolic syndrome and imaging of subclinical coronary artery disease: early markers of cardiovascular risk, *J. Cardiovasc. Nurs.* 21, 291–297.

Sloane E. A., 2006, Top ten functional food trends, *Food Technol.* 60, 33.

Tolstoguzov V., 1986, Functional properties of protein-polysaccharide mixtures, *in Functional Properties of Food Marcomolecules*, Eds. J. R. Mitchell and D. A. Ledward, Elsevier Applied Science, London, pp. 385–415.

Ward R. E, H. J. Watzke, R. Jiménez-Flores and J. B. German 2004, Bioguided processing: a paradigm change in food production, *Food Technol.* 58, 44–48.

Whetstine J. R., T. L. Witt and L. H. Matherly, 2002, The human reduced folate carrier gene is regulated by the AP2 and sp1 transcription factor families and a functional 61-base pair polymorphism, *J. Biol. Chem.* 277, 43873–43880.

Womack J. E., 2005, Advances in livestock genomics: opening the barn door. *Genome Res.* 15, 1699–705.

# Index

## D

## E

## N



## O

## Q



## R



## S



## T



## U



## V

## W



## Z